**Oxford Case Histories
in Geriatric Medicine**

Oxford Case Histories in Geriatric Medicine

Dr Sanja Thompson
Consultant geriatrician, Departments of acute general medicine and geratology, Oxford University Hospitals NHS Foundation Trust, John Radcliffe Hospital, Oxford, UK

Dr Nicola Lovett
Specialist registrar in general (internal) medicine and geratology, Oxford University Hospitals NHS Foundation Trust, and Clinical Research Fellow, Stroke Prevention Research Unit, Nuffield Department of Clinical Neurosciences, University of Oxford, UK

Professor John Grimley Evans
Professor Emeritus, Nuffield Department of Clinical Medicine and Clinical Geratology, University of Oxford, Oxford, UK

Professor Sarah Pendlebury
Associate Professor in Medicine and Old Age Neuroscience, Stroke Prevention Research Unit, Nuffield Department of Clinical Neurosciences, University of Oxford and Consultant Physician, Departments of acute general medicine and geratology, Oxford University Hospitals NHS Foundation Trust and the Oxford NIHR Biomedical Research Centre, John Radcliffe Hospital, Oxford, UK

OXFORD
UNIVERSITY PRESS

OXFORD
UNIVERSITY PRESS

Great Clarendon Street, Oxford, OX2 6DP,
United Kingdom

Oxford University Press is a department of the University of Oxford.
It furthers the University's objective of excellence in research, scholarship,
and education by publishing worldwide. Oxford is a registered trade mark of
Oxford University Press in the UK and in certain other countries

© Oxford University Press 2016

The moral rights of the authors have been asserted

First Edition published in 2016

Impression: 1

All rights reserved. No part of this publication may be reproduced, stored in
a retrieval system, or transmitted, in any form or by any means, without the
prior permission in writing of Oxford University Press, or as expressly permitted
by law, by licence or under terms agreed with the appropriate reprographics
rights organization. Enquiries concerning reproduction outside the scope of the
above should be sent to the Rights Department, Oxford University Press, at the
address above

You must not circulate this work in any other form
and you must impose this same condition on any acquirer

Published in the United States of America by Oxford University Press
198 Madison Avenue, New York, NY 10016, United States of America

British Library Cataloguing in Publication Data

Data available

Library of Congress Control Number: 2015938317

ISBN 978-0-19-969926-1

Printed and bound by
CPI Group (UK) Ltd, Croydon, CR0 4YY

Oxford University Press makes no representation, express or implied, that the
drug dosages in this book are correct. Readers must therefore always check
the product information and clinical procedures with the most up-to-date
published product information and data sheets provided by the manufacturers
and the most recent codes of conduct and safety regulations. The authors and
the publishers do not accept responsibility or legal liability for any errors in the
text or for the misuse or misapplication of material in this work. Except where
otherwise stated, drug dosages and recommendations are for the non-pregnant
adult who is not breast-feeding

Links to third party websites are provided by Oxford in good faith and
for information only. Oxford disclaims any responsibility for the materials
contained in any third party website referenced in this work.

To Mark, Noel and George Thompson
–Sanja Thompson

To Lynn Lovett
–Nicola Lovett

To Edward Harry Jarvis
–John Grimley Evans

To [my father] John Michael Pendlebury
–Sarah Pendlebury

A note from the series editors

Case histories have always had an important role in medical education, but most published material has been directed at undergraduates or residents. The *Oxford Case Histories* series aims to provide more complex case-based learning for clinicians in specialist training and consultants, and is now well-established in aiding preparation for entry and exit-level specialty examinations and revalidation. Each case book follows the same format with approximately 50 cases, each comprising a brief clinical history and investigations, followed by questions on differential diagnosis and management, and detailed answers with discussion. At the end of each book, cases are listed by mode of presentation, aetiology, and diagnosis.

We are grateful to our colleagues in the various medical specialties for their enthusiasm and hard work in making the series possible.

Sarah Pendlebury and Peter Rothwell

From reviews of other books in the series:

Neurological Case Histories

"... contains 51 cases that cover the spectrum of acute neurology and the neurology of general medicine—this breadth makes the volume unique and provides a formidable challenge ... it is a heavy-duty diagnostic series of cases, and readers have to work hard, to recognise the diagnosis and answer the questions that are posed for each case ... I recommend this excellent volume highly."
Lancet Neurology

"This short and well-written text is. ... designed to enhance the reader's diagnostic ability and clinical understanding. . . . A well documented and practical book."
European Journal of Neurology

Oxford Case Histories in Gastroenterology and Hepatology

"... a fascinating insight into clinical gastroenterology, an excellent and enjoyable read and an education for all levels of gastroenterologist from ST1 to consultant."
Gut

Oxford Case Histories in Respiratory Medicine

"The *Oxford Case Histories* series presents cases in a most refreshing manner, using the Aristotelian concept of practical knowledge learned through experience and conveyed to those in search of knowledge. We heartily endorse this approach. These cases . . . are real-world cases with good teaching potential. *Oxford Case Histories in Respiratory Medicine* has 44 short cases that cover many interesting topics in pulmonary and sleep medicine. It is not a cookbook or heavily referenced text, but it encompasses a wide breadth of topics. It is neither too superficial nor too deep, and it is both a delight and a challenge to read."
Respiratory Care

Foreword

The authors of this book have compiled a comprehensive set of 48 case studies in Geriatric Medicine. They are to be congratulated in producing a well researched piece of work, which will benefit trainees of all grades, as well as consultants seeking to update their knowledge. Undergraduates will also find the cases a useful addition to their resources during their placements involving older patients.

The material covered matches well to existing postgraduate curricula in Geriatric Medicine and will help prepare candidates for their Specialty Certificate Examinations (Knowledge Based Assessments). The cases also map well to the British Geriatric Society's, European, and other international undergraduate curricula in Geriatric Medicine.

The cases cover not only the common presenting syndromes in older patients (the so-called 'Geriatric Giants') but also the less common yet important presentations where the diagnosis should not be missed. The cases include discussion on possible differential diagnoses, as well as the evidence base that underpins their management.

Professor Tahir Masud
NHS Trust
Professor of Geriatric Medicine, Nottingham University Hospitals
Vice President for Education and Training, British Geriatrics Society
President of the European Union of Medical Specialists (UEMS)—
Geriatric Medicine Section

Preface

The world's population is ageing rapidly with estimates that in the first five decades of the 21st century, the proportion of the world's population over 60 years of age will double from 11% to 22% and the absolute number of older adults will triple from 605 million to 2 billion. Delivery of optimal healthcare services for older people—both in hospital and in the community—is therefore imperative. Recent reports from the Royal College of Physicians highlight the need for staff skill mix and training to reflect the rising numbers of frail older people in the general hospital. The demand for generalists expert in the care of complex older patients is thus likely to continue to rise over the coming decades.

The cases in this volume have been selected to illustrate the wide spectrum of acute medicine in older patients who often present with atypical or non-specific presentations on a background of complex co-morbidity, and the attendant management and ethical dilemmas. The format follows that of other books in the series: case descriptions with questions followed by answers including detailed discussion of the diagnosis, treatment, management, and ethical and holistic aspects of care. This structure was chosen as it is very difficult to illustrate the practical process of clinical management through a conventional textbook format and we believe it is more interesting and educational to consider real cases and one's own management plan than to read a text that does not require the same interactive effort on the part of the reader.

Acknowledgements

We would like to thank the following colleagues for their comments, expert advice and imaging examples for the cases contained in this volume including: Kevin Bradley, Adam Bailey, Lauren Bailey, Sue Burge, Peggy Frith, Matthew Giles, Tess McPherson, Phil Mathieson, Jim Newton, Annabel Nickol, David Okai, Francesco Pezzella, Sanja Popovic-Grle, Najib Rahman, Rustam Rea, John Reynolds, Peter Rothwell, Ku Shah, Sarah Smith, Mark Thompson, Alastair Webb, Chris Winearls, Simon Winner.

Thanks go especially to Raman Uberoi for expert help with the radiology.

Contents

Abbreviations *xii*
Table of normal ranges *xiii*
Cases 1–48 *1*
List of cases by diagnosis *497*
List of cases by presentation/aetiology *499*
Index *501*

Abbreviations

AAFB	Acid and alcohol fast bacilli		IMCA	Independent mental capacity advocate
ABG	Arterial blood gases		K+	Potassium
ACE	Angiotensin converting enzyme		KCO	Carbon-monoxide transfer coefficient
ACTH	Adrenocorticotropic hormone			
AMTS	Abbreviated Mental Test Score		LFTs	Liver function tests
BMI	Body mass index (kgs/metre^2)		MCS	Microscopy, culture and sensitivity
BNP	B-type natriuretic peptide			
CAM	Confusion Assessment Method		MCV	Mean corpuscular volume
COPD	Chronic obstructive pulmonary disease		MMSE	Mini Mental State Examination
			Na+	Sodium
CT	Computerized tomography		NICE	National Institute for Health and Clinical Excellence
CXR	Chest radiograph			
DLB	Dementia with Lewy Bodies		NOF	Neck of femur (fracture)
DSM	Diagnostic and Statistical Manual of Mental Disorders		PA	Pulmonary artery
			PaCO$_2$	Partial pressure of arterial carbon dioxide
DVT	Deep vein thrombosis			
U&Es	Urea and electrolytes		PaO$_2$	Partial pressure of arterial oxygen
FEV1	Forced expiratory volume in one second		PAP	Pulmonary artery pressure
			PET	A positron emission tomography (PET) scan
FRC	Functional residual volume			
FVC	Forced expiratory volume		PTH	Parathyroid hormone
H&E	Haematoxylin and Eosin		SPECT	Single-photon emission computed tomography
Hb	Haemoglobin			
HCO3-	Bicarbonate		T4	Thyroxine
HDU	High Dependency Unit		TB	Tuberculosis
HHS	Hyperosmolar hyperglycaemic state		TIA	Transient ischaemic attack
			TLCO	Carbon-monoxide transfer factor
HLA	Human leukocyte antigen		U&E	Urea and electrolytes
ICU	Intensive Care Unit		UIP	Usual interstitial pneumonia

Table of normal ranges

	Lower limit	Upper limit	Units	Other units	Lower limit	Upper limit
Hb (men)	13	18	g/dL			
Hb (women)	11.5	15	g/dL			
MCV	83	105	fL			
WCC	4	11	×10⁹/L			
Neutrophils	2	7	×10⁹/L			
Lymphocytes	1	4	×10⁹/L			
Eosinophils	0.02	0.5	×10⁹/L			
Platelets	150	400	×10⁹/L			
PTT	10	14	s			
APTT	22	34	s			
ESR	0	about half the age				
Na	135	145	mmol/L			
K	3.5	5	mmol/L			
Urea	2.5	6.7	mmol/L			
Creatinine	70	150	µmol/L			
Bilirubin	3	17	µmol/L			
AST	3	35	IU/L			
ALT	10	45	IU/L			

(continued)

(continued) Table of normal ranges

	Lower limit	Upper limit	Units	Other units	Lower limit	Upper limit
ALP	75	250	IU/L			
Albumin	35	50	g/L			
GGT (men)	11	51	IU/L			
GGT (women)	7	33	IU/L			
Ca (corr)	2.12	2.62	mmol/L			
PO_4	0.8	1.45	mmol/L			
Glucose (fasting)	3.5	5.5	mmol/L			
CRP	0	8	mg/L			
ACE	18	55	IU/L			
α1 antitrypsin	107	209	mg/dl			
PSA	0	4				
PaO_2	12	14	kPa			
$PaCO_2$	4.7	5.9	kPa			
pH	7.36	7.44				
Base excess	-2	2	meq/L			
Bicarbonate	23	27	meq/L			
IgG	6	13	g/L			
IgA	0.8	3	g/L			
IgM	0.4	2.5	g/L			

IgE	5	kU/L
Creatinine Clearance (Cockcroft-Gault Equation)	120	CreatClear = UrineCreat * DaysUrineVolume/SerumCreat/1440
Glomerular Filtration Rate Estimate by the MDRD Equation		GFR = 170 * SerumCreat-0.999 * Age-0.176 * Sex * Race * BUN-0.170 * Albumin 0.318
Amylase	0	IU/L
Brain (B-type) natriuretic peptide (BNP)		<100pg/mL
Carbon dioxide (CO_2), content	23	mmol/L
Creatine kinase	30	IU/L
D-Dimer	<300	mikrogr/L
Ferritin	15	mikrogr/L
Folate	5	nmol/L
Iron	14	mikromol/L women 7	33	mikromol/L
Lactate dehydrogenase 60	60	160	IU/L
Magnesium	0.75	1.05	mmol/L

(continued)

(continued) Table of normal ranges

	Lower limit	Upper limit	Units	Other units	Lower limit	Upper limit
Osmolality (plasma)	275	295	mOsm/kg H_2O			
Parathyroid hormone	<0.8	8.5	pmol/L			
pH blood	7.38	7.44				
Rheumatoid factor	<40		U/mL			
Thyroid-stimulating hormone	0.3	3.8	mU/L			
Free thyroxine	10	26	pmol/L			
Transferrin	212	360	mg/dL			
Triglycerides	<250 mg/dL					
Vitamin B_{12}		>150	ng/L			
Vitamin D, 25-Hydroxycholecalciferol 15		15–80	ng/mL			
International normalized ratio 2 – 3		standard therapy				
International normalized ratio 2 – 3	ratio 3–4.5 higher risk patients, prosthetic cardiac valves					
N-Terminal propeptide of BNP		<125	pg/mL			
Uric acid	0.21	0.48, men	mmol/L	women 0.15	0.39	
RBC (red blood cells)	4.5	6.5 men	10 × 12/L			
RBC (red blood cells)	3.9	5.6 women	10 × 12/L			

LDL cholesterol	1.55	4.4	mmol/L
HDL cholesterol	0.9	1.93	mmol/L
Urine osmolality	350	1000	mosmol/kg
Urine potassium	14	120	mmol/24 h
Urine sodium	100	250	mmol/24 h

Case 1

The medical team was asked to review a 92-year-old man on the orthopaedic ward. He had been admitted four days previously with a fractured hip after being found on the floor at home by his carer. He had undergone a hemiarthroplasty procedure on the day of admission, and his recovery initially went well. However, two days after surgery, he had developed urinary incontinence, become drowsy in the day, aggressive and agitated at night, and had pulled out three intravenous lines. Past history included a myocardial infarction 8 years previously, hypertension, and osteoarthritis. Medications given were aspirin 75mg od, atenolol 50mg od, paracetamol 1g qds, ramipril 2.5mg od, and codeine phosphate 60mg qds had been added during the postoperative period.

The medical team noted that his Abbreviated Mental Test Score (AMTS) had been 8/10 on admission to hospital. He had previously been living alone with a carer coming once a day to help with dressing and washing. The patient was unable to answer questions coherently and appeared to be talking to his wife who had died five years earlier. He was picking at the bedclothes, and appeared restless and agitated. Physical examination was difficult. Observations showed a borderline tachycardia at 94bpm with satisfactory blood pressure, respiratory rate, and oxygen saturations. The chest appeared clear and the abdomen was soft and non-tender. There was no overt focal neurological abnormality and the operation wound appeared to be healing well, with no surrounding erythema, or discharge. The orthopaedic team had commenced oral antibiotics for a presumed urinary tract infection, but there had been no improvement in his mental state.

Investigations showed the following:

- Hb: 13.2g/dL
- WCC: 13.0×10^9/L
- Neut: 9.8×10^9/L
- Na: 126mmol/L
- K: 3.9mmol/L
- Urea: 13mmol/L

- Creat: 132μmol/L
- CRP: 70mg/L
- Urine dipstick: + nitrites, + leucocytes, trace blood.

Questions

1 What syndrome does this man's case illustrate? What are the sub-types of this syndrome?
2 What other conditions may be difficult to differentiate from this syndrome?
3 What further clinical assessments should the medical team undertake?
4 What is the prevalence of this syndrome in acute medicine patients and in patients with hip fracture?
5 What are the main risk factors for the syndrome in this case?
6 How would you manage the patient in this case? Discuss other potential management strategies.
7 What are the prognostic implications?

Answers

1 What syndrome does this man's case illustrate? What are the sub-types of this syndrome?

This patient's case illustrates the characteristic features of delirium. Delirium, sometimes called 'acute confusional state', is a syndrome characterized by an acutely altered mental status that has a characteristic, but variable clinical picture, with no pathognomic features. Attention deficit is prominent, as such the patient appears distracted and inattentive, and is unable to count or recite the days of the week or months backwards. The diagnosis requires information from multiple sources, including family members and carers, to determine the patient's usual cognitive state and the context is usually suggestive, e.g. occurring in an older patient with admission for severe infection. The Diagnostic and Statistical Manual of Mental Disorders (DSM) IV criteria are shown in Box 1.1.

Box 1.1 The DSM IV criteria for delirium

1. **Disturbance of consciousness** (i.e. reduced clarity of awareness of the environment) with reduced ability to focus, sustain, or shift attention
2. **Change in cognition** (e.g. memory deficit, disorientation, language disturbance, and perceptual disturbance) that is not better accounted for by a pre-existing, established, or evolving dementia
3. **Development over a short period of time** (usually hours to days) and disturbance tends to fluctuate during the course of the day
4. **Evidence from the history, physical examination, or laboratory findings that the disturbance:**
    - is caused by the direct physiological consequences of a **general medical condition**
    - developed during **substance intoxication**
    - was aetiologically related to the use of **medication**
    - developed during, or shortly after, **a withdrawal syndrome**
    - was caused by an unknown precipitant (not otherwise specified)

There are three main sub-types of delirium classified according to the change in level of consciousness:
  1. Hyperactive delirium
     - Agitation
     - Disruptive behaviour

2 Hypoactive delirium
- Lethargy
- Sleepiness/drowsiness
- Unawareness

3 Mixed

Hyperactive and hypoactive features fluctuating over time.

Hypoactive delirium is more likely to go unrecognized by medical and nursing staff. Hyperactive delirium often results in challenging behaviour, which may be directly observed by doctors or prompts nursing staff to alert medical staff.

There is less awareness of delirium compared to dementia across medical and nursing staff, the general public, and politicians. The steady and slow decline from normal through mild cognitive impairment to dementia (Fig. 1.1) is the predominant view of non-specialists, whereas in the hospitalized population and/or in patients with multiple co-morbidity, there are often rapid dynamic changes in cognition over time (Fig. 1.2). Furthermore, even in the absence of overt delirium, patients with inter-current illness may show decrements in cognitive function that subsequently recover. This acute cognitive change may identify a subgroup at high risk of later cognitive decline (Fig. 1.3) analogous to the poor cognitive prognosis of patients with delirium.

Fig. 1.1 Graph showing the typical cognitive change over years in a physically fit patient declining from normal through MCI to dementia (Alzheimer's disease).

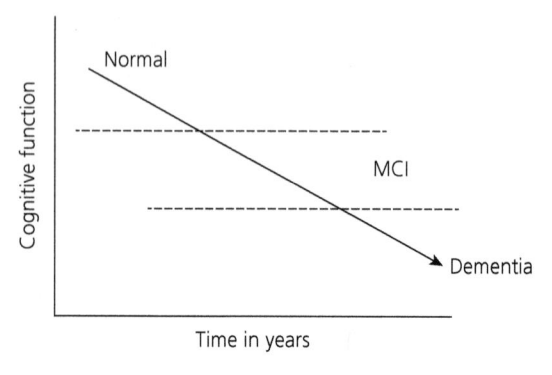

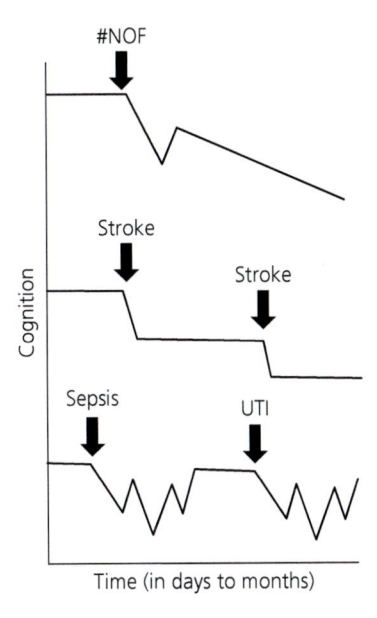

Fig. 1.2 Graph showing examples of cognitive changes over time in patients with co-morbidity including fractured neck of femur (NOF), recurrent stroke, and recurrent infection.

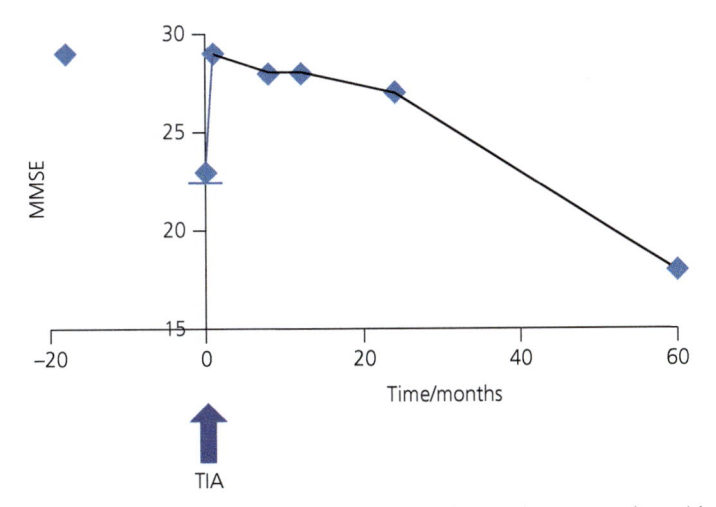

Fig. 1.3 Graph showing cognitive changes over time in a patient presenting with transient ischaemic attack (TIA). The patient had been seen in the geratology clinic with subjective poor memory 20 months prior to the TIA and had had an MMSE, which was 29/30. On repeat testing in the TIA clinic when the focal deficit had resolved, the MMSE was 21/30. One month later it had recovered to the pre-morbid level, but thereafter there was a slow decline to dementia.

2 What other conditions may be difficult to differentiate from this syndrome?

Other conditions which may be difficult to differentiate from delirium include:

Dementia. This most often causes diagnostic uncertainty and commonly co-exists with delirium. Table 1.1 shows the key features that may help differentiate the two syndromes. Dementia with Lewy bodies (see case 25) may be particularly problematic since it is associated with fluctuation and visual hallucinations, and parkinsonism may not be overt in the early stages.

Depression. Hypoactive delirium may appear similar to depression or depression may cause agitation, and mimic hyperactive delirium (see case 18).

Mania. Mania may occasionally be mistaken for hyperactive delirium.

Table 1.1 Differentiating delirium from dementia

Delirium	Dementia
Acute or subacute onset	Insidious onset
Fluctuating course	Progressive
Resolves	Irreversible
Impaired consciousness, which may fluctuate rapidly	Clear consciousness until late in disease
Poor attention span and poor short-term memory	Poor short-term memory with attention less affected
Hallucinations common	Hallucinations rare (except in dementia with Lewy bodies)
Fleeting systematized delusions	Delusions rare (except in dementia with Lewy bodies)
Hyper or hypoactive	May not be psychomotor disturbance

3 What further clinical assessments should the medical team undertake?

The team should:

- Repeat the AMTS to confirm a drop in score from pre-operatively.
- Record that the Confusion Assessment Method (CAM) screen for delirium is positive and that the patient has delirium.
- Obtain a collateral history to determine the patient's usual cognitive state.

The CAM is a useful screen for delirium and is recommended in National and International Guidelines (see Fig. 1.4). It has good sensitivity and specificity for delirium if used in conjunction with a short cognitive test (the Mini Mental State Examination, or MMSE, was the test used in the original publication).The MMSE is now copyright protected and the AMTS (Fig. 1.4) is recommended as an initial pragmatic cognitive screen. Experienced clinicians do not need to go through the CAM in order to make a diagnosis of delirium and it is less sensitive for hypoactive ('sleepy') delirium.

This case illustrates the utility of performing an admission cognitive screen on older people. Pre-admission impairment may not have been recognized in the community (only around half of older in-patients with dementia have had a previous diagnosis) and as seen in Figure 1.2, cognition may change rapidly over time, such that pre-morbid function cannot be assumed to be maintained in the context of acute illness. Further, cognitive impairment may not be overt from the end of the bed. Many patients are able to maintain an effective social façade or may lack insight into their cognitive impairment. The cognitive screen developed at our institution that combines routine AMTS and CAM, along with recording of any known pre-admission diagnosis of dementia or subjective memory complaint, is shown in Figure 1.4.

Medical Admission Proforma

Space for Patient Information Sticker	
	Assessment date/time
	Consultant/team
	Assessing doctor
	GP/ED/other referral

Cognitive screen

MUST be completed on **ALL** patients ≥ 75 years and younger patients with confusion/altered behaviour.

AMTS

Age	Recognise 2 people
Time (nearest hr)	DOB
Recall (42 West Street)	WW2 (start or end year)
Year	Monarch
Location	20 to 1 backwards

CAM (aid to identifying delirium)

1. Acute onset &/or fluctuating confusion/altered behaviour
2. Inattention e.g. unable to do 20 – 1 or distractable
3. Altered conscious level e.g. agitated or sleepy
4. Disordered thinking (e.g. rambling)

AMTS Total = /10.

AMTS not done ☐ Reason:

Delirium = 1+2+(3 or 4) but NOTE that CAM sensitivity is not 100% particularly for hypoactive (SLEEPY) delirium

Does the patient have known dementia? ☐ Y ☐ N ☐ uncertain

Does the patient have delirium (CAM+ve OR clinical diagnosis)? ☐ Y ☐ N ☐ uncertain

If the patient does **NOT** have definite dementia or delirium please ask the following question of the patient or informant: *"Have you/has the patient been more forgetful in the past* 12 *months to the extent that it has significantly affected your/their daily life?"* ☐ Y ☐ N ☐ not assessable

Fig. 1.4 Cognitive screen for routine administration to all older patients admitted as an emergency to our institution combining the AMTS and CAM along with recording of known pre-admission diagnosis of dementia and of delirium, and subjective memory complaint.

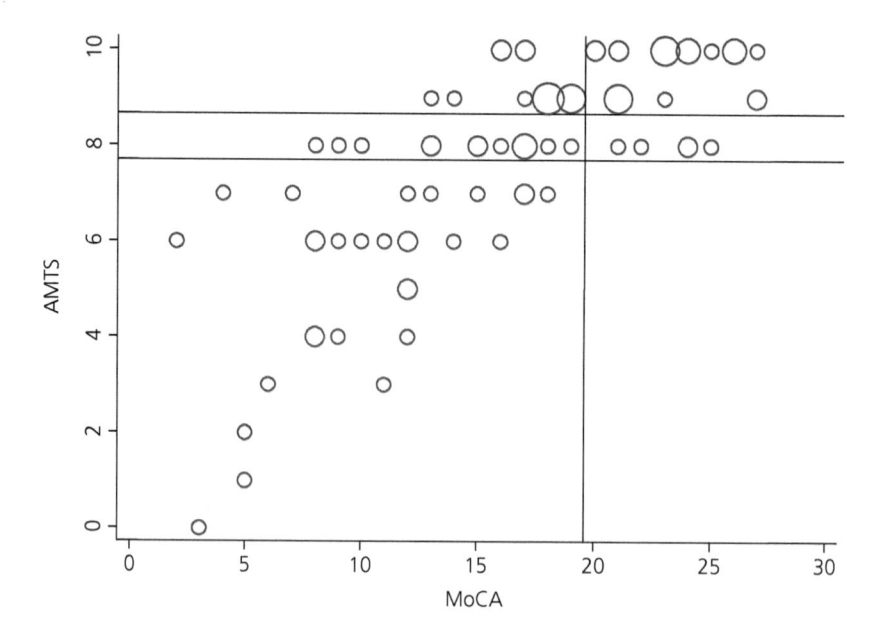

Fig. 1.5 Graph showing the AMTS versus the Montreal Cognitive Assessment (MoCA) in consecutive patients aged >75 years admitted to acute internal medicine. AMTS of </ = 8 indicates a high likelihood of a significant cognitive problem as defined by MoCA<20 (roughly equivalent to MMSE<24). For AMTS = 9 or 10, a cognitive problem is less likely, but cannot be excluded (i.e. the AMTS has a ceiling effect). Reproduced with permission from Pendlebury et al, Age and Ageing ;2015:Oct 13. pii: afv134..

The AMTS was published in 1972 and has been criticized as having culturally specific items and to be out-dated in terms of, e.g. the recognizing two people task: in 1972, the vast majority of doctors were men in white coats, and the nurses were women in obvious uniforms. However, data from our institution suggest it remains a valid test in older in-patients, correlating well with the Montreal Cognitive Assessment (Fig. 1.5) and it has the advantages of being brief, not requiring pencil and paper, motor response, nor good vision in the patient.

4 What is the prevalence of this syndrome in acute medicine patients and in patients with hip fracture?

There are few inclusive studies of the rate of delirium in unselected medical cohorts with reported international prevalence of 18–35% and incidences of 11–14% for cohorts of >100 subjects. Age-specific rates obtained from our institution show rates of ~3% in patients aged <65 years, 16% in 65–75 years and 36% in over 75 years (Fig. 1.6). Therefore, delirium is 10 times more likely in those over 75 years compared to younger people (<65 years).

Rates of delirium are particularly high in older patients with hip fracture with reported rates of up to 50%. Identification of delirium is part of the mandatory screening for dementia for older patients admitted as an emergency in England.

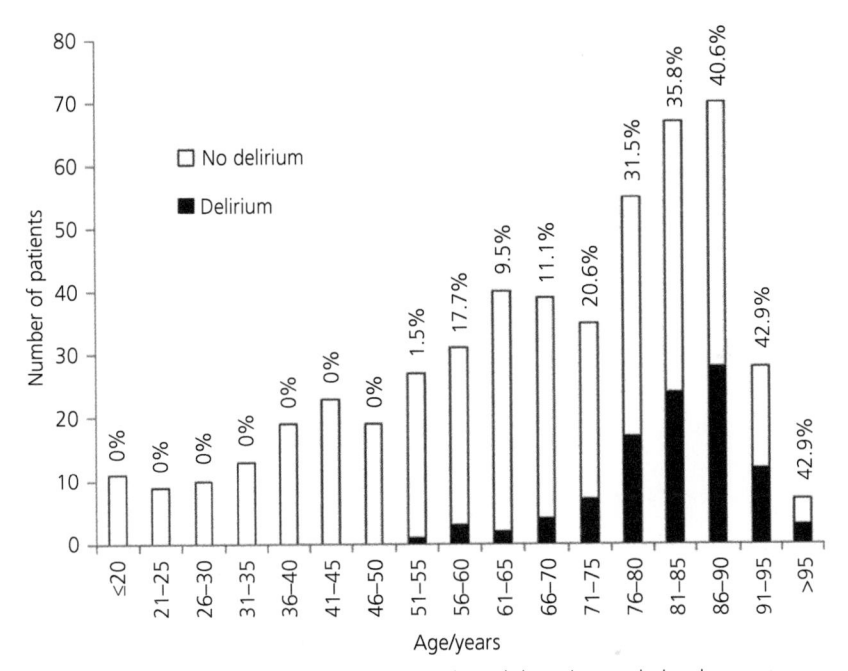

Fig. 1.6 Age-specific delirium rate in consecutive adult patients admitted to acute internal medicine reproduced with permission from the BMJ Publishing Group Ltd from Pendlebury et al, Observational, longitudinal study of delirium in consecutive unselected acute medical admissions: age-specific rates and associated factors, mortality and re-admission, BMJ Open 2015, in press

5 What are the main risk factors for the syndrome in this case?

The risk/precipitating factors for delirium in this case are:
- major trauma and surgery
- urinary tract infection
- hyponatraemia
- codeine phosphate medication
- older age
- pain from the operation site must be excluded.

As illustrated in the current case, delirium is usually multifactorial. Vulnerability (predisposition) to delirium is related to physical and cognitive frailty and delirium may be precipitated by external events (Box 1.2), of which systemic illness (especially infection) is the most important. Delirium may be precipitated by minor events in very vulnerable patients, whereas very severe illness may precipitate delirium in previously robust individuals. Table 1.2 shows factors associated with delirium in consecutive acute medicine patients aged >/=65 years admitted to our institution.

Box 1.2 Factors associated with delirium

Predisposing factors

Age > 65 years

Male

Background cognitive impairment/prior episode of delirium

Visual or hearing impairment

Poor nutritional status

Dehydration

Multiple co-morbidities

Poor functional status

Sleep deprivation

Precipitating factors

Sepsis

Hypoxia

Metabolic disturbance

Electrolyte disturbance

Constipation

Anaemia

Stroke

Surgery

Medication—especially sedatives, narcotics, anticholinergics

Withdrawal from alcohol or barbiturates

Pain

Intravenous access devices, urinary catheters, nasogastric tubes, etc.

Environmental change—moving wards during admission

Table 1.2

Factor	Strength of association
Age ≥75yrs	++
Dementia	++
Falls	+++
TIA/stroke	+
Care package/Care Home	++
Low cognitive test score	+++
Dehydration	++
Severe illness	++
Pressure sore risk	+++
Urinary incontinence	+++
Faecal incontinence	+++
Bedbound	+++
Sleep deprivation	+++
Falls	+++
Urinary catheter insertion	+++
Infection	+++
Stroke	+
Stay >7 days	++
New care home on discharge	+++
Increased care	++
Death	+++

+=OR 1–2,
++=OR 2–3.
+++=OR 4+.

Adapted with permission from Pendlebury et al, Age and Ageing 2015; Oct 13. pii: afv134.

However, many risk factors for delirium will be co-associates and most risk is probably conferred by a few consistent factors. The UK NICE guidelines cite older age, severe illness, hip fracture, infection, visual, and cognitive impairment (cognitive test below cut-off or known dementia/mild cognitive impairment (MCI)) as being key factors. The higher rates of delirium seen in older patients result from greater prevalence of multiple risk factors, and also increased susceptibility. Delirium risk scores have been developed to help predict risk in individual patients in intensive care, internal medicine, and the surgical setting.

6 How would you manage the patient in this case? Discuss other potential management strategies.

The medical team attempted to establish a rapport with the patient and explain the diagnosis to nursing staff and family members, who were encouraged to remain by the patient whenever possible. Appropriate adjustment to the patient's fluid regimen was made to correct the hyponatraemia. A repeat electrolyte screen, including calcium and magnesium, glucose, and thyroid function tests was requested. The patient's requirement for analgesia was assessed with the help of the nursing staff. The codeine phosphate was withdrawn and regular paracetamol substituted without worsening of the pain. Care is needed when making such a change, as the patient may be unable to express the fact that they are in pain and also pain is a potent cause of delirium. The urine culture results were chased, and it was found that the causative organism was resistant to the prescribed antibiotics and the appropriate therapy was instituted. A small dose of haloperidol was prescribed for night-time to treat the patient's distress and prevent injury with a plan to review after 48 hours. Mobilization with the help of the physiotherapists was encouraged.

Regarding treatment of delirium in general, delirium must first be recognized and then the underlying medical disorder(s) identified and treated. In addition, the multi-component intervention programme (Table 1.3) must be applied. In patients with prevalent delirium, transfers within and between wards should be avoided, and continuity of nursing staff is desirable. Pharmacologic treatment should be given if there is distress or risk of injury, despite non-pharmacologic measures being implemented.

Family or friends may be upset by the patient's confusion and it is therefore important to explain the cause to them. The patient may also be distressed after recovery from delirium about their behaviour, for example swearing, or hitting out at nursing staff or by their memory of events while delirious, e.g. misconstruing catheterization as being sexually assaulted.

The evidence for antipsychotic drugs in the treatment or prophylaxis of delirium is conflicting. There is some evidence that delirious patients who receive short-term treatment with low-dose antipsychotics experience positive clinical response across different patient groups and treatment settings. There do not appear to be significant differences in efficacy for haloperidol versus atypical agents. There are few high quality data sources on prophylactic use of antipsychotics, but perioperative use may reduce the overall risk of postoperative delirium. Other interventions meriting further study to prevent delirium in older surgical patients are iliac fascia block, gabapentin, melatonin, and lower levels of intraoperative propofol sedation.

Table 1.3 Multi-component intervention programme to reduce the incidence of delirium in patients at risk

Multi-component interventions	
Clinical factor	Preventative intervention
Cognitive impairment or disorientation	♦ Provide appropriate lighting/clear signage ♦ A clock and calendar should also be easily visible to the person at risk ♦ Reorientate the person by explaining where they are, who they are, and what your role is ♦ Introduce cognitively stimulating activities ♦ Facilitate regular visits from family/friends
Dehydration or constipation	♦ Encourage the person to drink. Offer parenteral fluids if necessary ♦ Seek advice if necessary when managing fluid balance in people with co-morbidities
Hypoxia	♦ Assess for hypoxia and optimize oxygen saturation if necessary
Immobility or limited mobility	♦ Encourage mobilization soon after surgery ♦ Encourage walking (provide aids if needed—these should be accessible at all times) ♦ Encourage all people, including those unable to walk, to carry out active range-of-motion exercises
Infection	♦ Look for and treat infection ♦ Avoid unnecessary catheterization ♦ Implement infection control procedures in line with 'infection control' (NICE CG 2)
Multiple medications	♦ Carry out a medication review for people taking multiple drugs, taking into account both the type and number of medications. Avoid deliriogenic drugs where possible
Pain	♦ Assess for pain and non-verbal signs of pain ♦ Provide appropriate pain management where pain is identified or suspected
Poor nutrition	♦ Follow the advice given on nutrition in 'Nutrition support in adults' (NICE CG 32) ♦ If the person has dentures, ensure they fit
Sensory impairment	♦ Resolve any reversible cause of the impairment (such as impacted ear wax) ♦ Ensure working hearing and visual aids are available, and used by those who need them
Sleep disturbance	♦ Avoid nursing or medical procedures during sleeping hours, if possible ♦ Schedule medication rounds to avoid disturbing sleep ♦ Reduce noise during sleep periods

7 What are the prognostic implications?

Delirium is associated with high mortality after adjustment for age, illness severity, pre-morbid dementia, and dependency. There are also strong associations with morbidity including falls, dehydration, malnutrition, pressure sores and incontinence, sleep deprivation, dependency, and institutionalization. While it is probable that much poor outcome associated with delirium is not preventable, better recognition will facilitate optimal care and also targeting of staffing resources to prevent avoidable deterioration, complications, and deaths in this vulnerable group.

The risk of dementia is significantly elevated on follow-up in patients with delirium (RR ~5). Recent studies suggest that delirium alters the cognitive trajectory in patients with Alzheimer's disease, rather than it simply being a manifestation of ongoing cognitive decline (Fig. 1.7). It is hypothesized that inflammatory mediators released in the periphery cross the blood brain barrier and initiate or accelerate pathologic processes in the brain through interactions with microglia. Rates of delirium are also high in acute stroke, in which inflammation occurs within the brain and this may play a role precipitating post-stroke dementia.

Delirium thus indicates cognitive fragility and denotes a patient at high risk of dementia. In the context of overall under-diagnosis of dementia in the

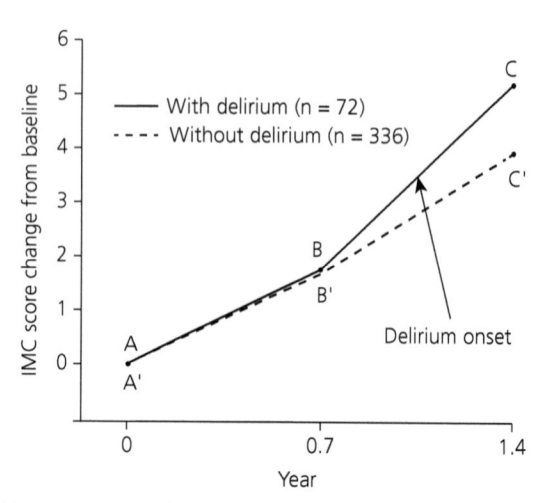

Fig. 1.7 Cognitive trajectories of patients with Alzheimer's disease with and without delirium (Reproduced from Fong, T., et al, Delirium accelerates cognitive decline in Alzheimer disease, Neurology, Vol 72, No 18, Copyright 2009, with permission from Wolters Kluwer Health, Inc.).

community, targeting cognitive assessment at those with a recent episode of delirium would be an effective and low cost route to increasing dementia diagnosis rates. It is therefore important to notify a patient's GP of a delirium diagnosis upon their discharge from care. Since many patients will die or recover to pre-morbid cognitive levels at least in the short term, routine in-patient referral to the memory clinic is not warranted.

Further reading

British Geriatrics Society. Guidelines for the prevention, diagnosis and management of delirium in older people in hospital, 2006. http://www.bgs.org.uk/index.php/clinicalguides/170-clinguidedeliriumtreatment%3Fshowall%3D%26limitstart%3D

Delirium, diagnosis, prevention and management. National Institute for Health and Clinical Excellence (NICE) Guideline CG 103. http://www.nice.org.uk/CG103

Fong TG, Jones RN, Shi P, et al. (2009). Delirium accelerates cognitive decline in Alzheimer disease. *Neurology*; 5;**72**(18): 1570–1575.

Friedman JI, Soleimani L, McGonigle DP, Egol C, Silverstein JH (2014). Pharmacological treatments of non-substance-withdrawal delirium: a systematic review of prospective trials. *Am J Psychiatry*; **171**(2): 151–159.

Hirota T, Kishi T (2013). Prophylactic antipsychotic use for postoperative delirium: a systematic review and meta-analysis. *J Clin Psychiatry*; **74**(12): e1136–e1144.

Hodkinson HM (1972). Evaluation of a mental test score for assessment of mental impairment in the elderly. *Age Ageing*; **1**: 233–238.

Inouye SK, van Dyck CH, Alessi CA, et al. (1990). Clarifying confusion: the confusion assessment method. A new method for detection of delirium. *Ann Intern Med*; **113**: 941–948.

Inouye SK, Westendorp RG, Saczynski JS (2014). Delirium in elderly people. *Lancet*; **383**: 911–922; *see also* http://www.rcplondon.ac.uk/sites/default/files/francis-inquiry-detailed-response.pdf

Kalisvaart KJ, de Jonghe JF, Bogaards MJ, et al. (2005). Haloperidol prophylaxis for elderly hip-surgery patients at risk for delirium: a randomized placebo-controlled study. *J Am Geriatr Soc*; **53**(10): 1658–1666.

Meagher DJ, McLoughlin L, Leonard M, Hannon N, Dunne C, O'Regan N (2013). What do we really know about the treatment of delirium with antipsychotics? Ten key issues for delirium pharmacotherapy. *Am J Geriatr Psychiatry*; **21**(12): 1223–1238.

Pendlebury ST, Lovett N, Smith SC, et al. Observational, longitudinal study of delirium in consecutive unselected acute medical admissions: age-specific rates and associated factors, mortality and re-admission. BMJ Open 2015, in press.

Pendlebury ST, Klaus SP, Mather M, deBrito M, Wharton RM. Routine cognitive screening in older patients admitted to acute medicine: Abbreviated Mental Test Score (AMTS) and subjective memory complaint versus Montreal Cognitive Assessment and IQCODE. Age and Ageing, 2015 Oct 13. pii: afv134. [Epub ahead of print].

Pendlebury ST, Lovett N, Smith SC et al. Delirium risk stratification in consecutive unselected admissions to acute medicine: validation of externally derived risk scores. Age and Ageing, 2015, in press.

Popp J, Arlt S (2012). Prevention and treatment options for postoperative delirium in the elderly. *Curr Opin Psychiatry*; **25**(6): 515–521.

Shakespeare J (2013). An unsafe ward. *BMJ*; 346: f1243; http://www.england.nhs.uk/wp-content/uploads/2013/02/cquin-guidance.pdf;

Teslyar P, Stock VM, Wilk CM, Camsari U, Ehrenreich MJ, Himelhoch S (2013). Prophylaxis with antipsychotic medication reduces the risk of post-operative delirium in elderly patients: a meta-analysis. *Psychosomatics*; **54**(2): 124–131.

van Gool WA, van de Beek D, Eikelenboom P (2010). Systemic infection and delirium: when cytokines and acetylcholine collide. *Lancet*; **375**: 773–775.

Report from the Future Hospital Commission to the Royal College of Physicians, September 2013: https://www.rcplondon.ac.uk/projects/future-hospital-commission

Case 2

An 83-year-old retired receptionist presented to the local community hospital generally unwell and confused. Over the past week, her appetite had decreased, and she had experienced some nausea and vomiting, with increasing shortness of breath on exertion, as well as decreased mobility such that she could now only walk five metres. Her husband reported that she had not been 'quite right' for the past couple of weeks, appearing confused at times. He had also noted increased urinary frequency, but she had not complained of any discomfort when passing urine. A short course of antibiotics for a urinary tract infection (UTI) had been completed 12 days earlier.

There was a history of type 2 diabetes, cataract and transient ischaemic attack, and medications taken were metformin 850mg bd, gliclazide MR 30mg od, pioglitazone 30mg od, aspirin 75mg od, latanoprost eye drops, and beclomethasone nasal spray. She lived with her husband in a three-bedroom house, and mobilized with a stick.

On examination, temperature was 36.4ºC, blood pressure was 105/78mmHg, and heart rate was 112bpm. The mucous membranes were dry with decreased skin turgor and the JVP was not visible. Heart sounds were normal and breath sounds were slightly reduced throughout both lungs. There was neither pedal nor sacral oedema. Examination of the abdomen revealed a distended palpable bladder. There was no focal neurology. Geriatric Depression Scale (GDS) was 14/15 and AMTS 6/10.

Investigations showed the following:

Hb: 17.4g/dL

WCC: 29.56 × 10^9/L, neutrophilia

Platelets: 208 × 10^9/L

Na: 147mmol/L

K: 5.4mmol/L

Urea: 33.1mmol/L

Creat: 338µmol/L (baseline 72µmol/L)

CRP: 96.8mg/L

BM: >27.8mmol/L

Serum ketones: 1.1mmol/L

HbA1c 8 months previously: 69mmol/L (8.5%)

CXR: chest X-ray with normal heart size and clear lungs (see Fig. 2.1)

Urine dipstick: + + + blood (taken post-catheterization).

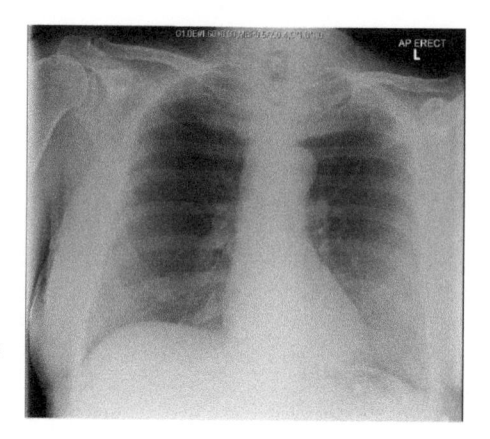

Fig. 2.1 Chest X-ray of the patient showing normal heart size and lungs.

Questions

1 What is the most likely diagnosis and what are the characteristic features?
2 Describe the initial management. What complication should be avoided when correcting the hyperglycaemia?

Answers

1 What is the most likely diagnosis and what are the characteristic features?

The patient has **h**yperosmolar **h**yperglycaemic **s**tate (HHS) with possible partially treated UTI and acute kidney failure.

The patient was given IV co-amoxiclav and IV fluids. Metformin was held and standard gliclazide was given in place of MR (modified release) formulation. Prophylactic low molecular weight heparin was started. A urinary catheter was inserted with 500ml residual, and a renal ultrasound scan (USS) was requested.

HHS is uncommon but life threatening with 15–20% mortality. It may be the mode of initial presentation of type 2 diabetes, but it more commonly affects those with an established diagnosis. HHS was formerly known as hyperglycaemic hyperosmotic non-ketotic coma, the name change reflecting the fact that it exists on a spectrum with diabetic ketoacidosis (DKA), which affects people with type 1 diabetes. Although HHS and DKA are often considered separately, the two conditions can overlap, and a mixed picture is seen in approximately one third of hyperglycaemic emergencies. HHS is more common in older people because of the associated higher incidence of type 2 diabetes, but rates are increasing in younger age groups because of rising obesity and earlier onset of type 2 diabetes. The characteristic features of HHS are:

Hypovolaemia

Hyperglycaemia without significant ketosis or acidosis: glucose > 30mmol/L, ketones <3mmol/L, pH >7.3, bicarbonate >15mmol/L

Hyperosmolar state: osmolality >320mosmol/kg.

The difference between HHS and a transient hyperglycaemic state is the duration of the hyperglycaemia and the presence of severe dehydration. HHS is often precipitated by factors predisposing to dehydration or reduced insulin activity including sepsis, drugs (e.g. glucocorticoids, atypical antipsychotics, thiazide diuretics), and major illness. In this case, the most likely precipitant was a UTI two weeks prior to admission.

2 Describe the initial management. What complication should be avoided when correcting the hyperglycaemia?

The aim of management is to identify and treat the underlying cause, replace the fluid and electrolyte losses, gradually normalizing the osmolality, and blood glucose levels. A urinary catheter should be inserted to allow accurate fluid balance monitoring. Cardiovascular collapse, as well as brain oedema from over-rapid correction of glucose (with insulin) and hyperosmolarity before adequate rehydration must be avoided. No randomized studies have yet been conducted to determine optimal approaches to treatment.

The hyperglycaemia results in an osmotic diuresis with relatively higher losses of water than sodium and potassium. There is usually profound dehydration with reduced intracellular, intravascular, and interstitial volumes, with fluid losses of between 100–220ml/kg (Fig. 2.2, Table 2.1).

Aggressive fluid replacement is required; 1L of 0.9% normal saline should be infused over the first hour and vigorous fluid replacement should continue thereafter, with the aim of replacing 50% of the estimated fluid loss within the first 12 hours. However, care must be taken not to precipitate heart failure in

Fluid balance in HHS:

A. Normal glycaemia and normal hydration

B. Extracellular fluid (ECF) is hyperosmolar causing water to shift from ICF into ECF

C. Continued osmotic diuresis causes dehydration, volume loss and hyperosmolality in both ICF and ECF

D. Insulin therapy without adequate fluid replacement shifts glucose and water from ECF to ICF causing vascular collapse and hypotension

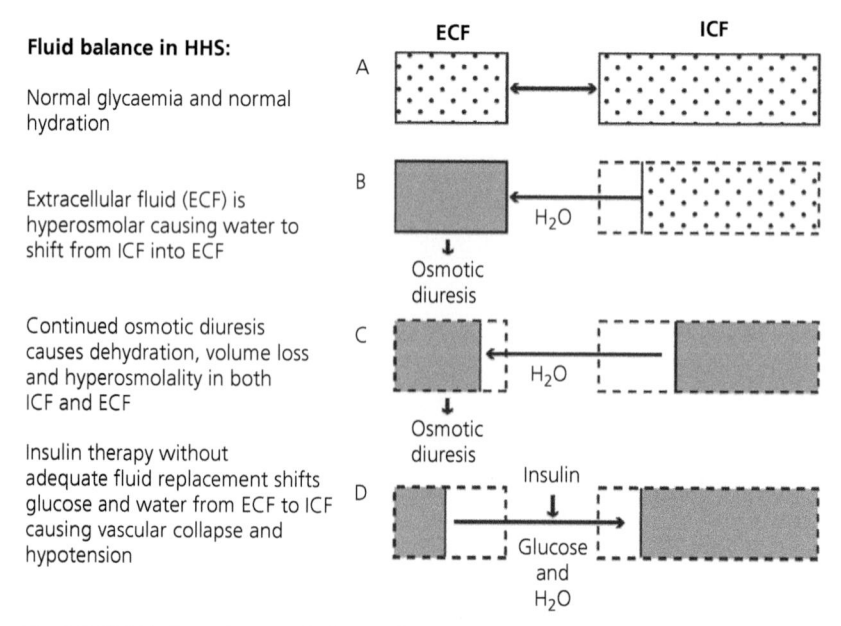

Fig. 2.2 Fluid balance in HHS. (Adapted from: The management of hyperosmolar hyperglycaemic state (HHS) in adults with diabetes. *Joint British Diabetes Societies Inpatient Care Group*, 2012.)
(Reproduced here with kind permission from JBDS)

Table 2.1 The hyperglycaemia results in an osmotic diuresis with relatively higher losses of water than sodium and potassium

Element lost	Estimated losses/kg	For 60 kg patient	For 100 kg patient
Water	100–220ml	6–13L	10–22L
Na +	5–13mmol	300–780mmol	500–1300mmol
Cl-	5–15mmol	300–900mmol	500–1500mmol
K +	4–6mmol	240–360mmol	400–600mmol

(Adapted from: Kitabchi et al. D Care 2009; 32: 1355.)

older patients who may have concomitant heart disease. A urinary catheter allows accurate measurements of fluid balance.

It is important to note that rapid rehydration will correct hyperglycaemia. Therefore, much lower insulin doses are required compared to DKA, or insulin may not be required at all. Over-rapid correction of glucose with high insulin doses before adequate rehydration results in intravascular volume depletion and may precipitate cardiovascular collapse in vulnerable older patients (Fig. 2.2). A target blood glucose of 10–15mmol/L initially is sufficient.

Osmolality should be calculated hourly using the glucose, sodium, potassium, and urea values, aiming for a gradual decline in osmolality of around 3–6mosmol/kg/hr to avoid complications such as cerebral oedema. Potassium replacement may be required.

This patient had few co-morbidities and was previously independent. If adequate monitoring cannot be delivered in a standard ward setting or there is failure to respond to initial therapy, escalation to a high dependency unit (HDU) or intensive care unit (ITU) setting should be considered.

Key points to remember in treating HHS are:

rehydration alone will cause a fall in venous glucose

monitor glucose with serum or VBG samples hourly

aim for a maximum fall in serum/VBG glucose of 5mmol/l/hr

only start insulin if the patient is fully rehydrated and remains hyperglycaemic or develops ketoacidosis.

Case progression

The patient commenced rehydration and was transferred from the local community hospital to the main hospital to the acute medicine team. The blood results from the following days are shown in Table 2.2:

Table 2.2 Blood results

	Day 1	Day 2	Day 3 04:05	Day 3 06:55	Day 3 07:18
Na (mmol/L)	147	163	175	172	166
Glu (mmol/L)		49		7.5	5.6
BM (mmol/L)	>27.4	>27.4		6–13	6–7
Urea (mmol/L)	33	34	31	28	22
Osmolality (mOsm/kg)		409		380	359

Questions continued

3 Why did the BM not fall initially? How has the serum osmolality on day two been calculated?
4 Explain the rise in serum sodium. Would you give hypotonic fluids?
5 Discuss the possible complications of this condition.

Answers continued

3 Why did the BM not fall initially? How has the serum osmolality on day two been calculated?

Conventional point-of-care glucose testing sticks have a ceiling effect, i.e. they measure to a maximum of >27.4. A formal lab glucose is therefore required to accurately measure the glucose level and calculate the osmolality using the following equation:

Serum osmolality = $2Na^+$ + glucose + urea. (Normal extracellular osmolality is between 280–295mOsmol/kg.)

The osmolality on day two is therefore:

$$2(163) + 49 + 34 = 409 mOsm/kg$$

and on day three is:

$$2(172) + 28 + 7.5 = 379.5 mOsm/kg.$$

It is vital to monitor to serum osmolality closely, as rapid changes can be harmful.

4 Explain the rise in serum sodium. Would you give hypotonic fluids?

The serum sodium has increased despite fluid resuscitation. This is not an indication to change from 0.9% normal saline to 0.45% hypotonic saline; the rise in serum sodium is expected. Calculation of the corrected Na level shows that the sodium level in fact falls with treatment:

Corrected Na = Na + 2.4 (glucose/5.5). Therefore the corrected Na is:

Day two: 163 + 2.4(49/5.5) = 184mmol/L

Day three: 172 + 2.4(7.5/5.5) = 175mmol/L

166 + 2.4(5.6/5.5) = 168mmol/L.

As hyperglycaemia develops, the extracellular osmolality rises and is initially greater than the intracellular osmolality owing to slow penetration of glucose across the cell membrane. This causes water to move from the intracellular space to the extracellular space in an attempt to restore homeostasis. Ongoing osmotic diuresis depletes the extracellular compartment and ultimately both intra- and extracellular compartments have reduced volume and increased osmolality (Fig. 2.2).

Restoration of the intravascular volume through rehydration decreases blood glucose and serum osmolality (osmolality = $2Na^+$ + glucose + urea), which causes water to move back into the intracellular space, thus the serum sodium value increases.

A fall of blood glucose level of 5.5mmol/L should equate to a rise in serum sodium of approximately 2.4mmol/L. If the serum sodium is increasing but the osmolality is not decreasing, or is decreasing at a rate of less than 3mosmol/kg/hr, then fluid balance status should be reassessed, and the rate of fluid infusion should be increased.

Therefore, when treating HHS, it should be noted that:

- an initial rise in sodium is expected and not an indication for hypotonic fluids
- absence of a rise in sodium suggests insufficient fluid replacement
- rising sodium is only a concern if the osmolality is not falling
- a fall in osmolality of 3–8mosmol/kg/hr is desirable.

5 Discuss the possible complications of this condition.

Patients with HHS are at high risk of:

- arterial and venous thrombosis
- pressure ulcers (see case 14)
- delirium (illness severity, dehydration, accompanying sepsis—see case 1)
- falls (see cases 24, 27, 47) from hypotension and delirium
- other electrolye deficiencies (see cases 1, 23, 47).

Dehydration, hypernatraemia, and increasing antidiuretic hormone concentrations promote a hypercoagulable state. Prophylactic low molecular weight heparin therapy must be given from admission.

Patients with HHS are often drowsy and are at high risk of pressure ulcers, particularly affecting the heels. These areas should be inspected daily and pressure relieving mattresses or heel protectors should be used as appropriate.

Often patients have hypomagnesaemia and hypophosphataemia. There is currently no evidence to support the routine replacement of these electrolytes. However, many patients are frail with a poor underlying nutritional state and it may be prudent to replace significant deficiency to prevent refeeding syndrome on recovery.

The current patient recovered well with treatment. The AMTS rose to 9/10 and she was able to return home at her pre-admission functional level.

Further reading

Kitabchi AE, Umpierrez GE, Miles JM, Fisher JN (2009). Hyperglycemic crises in adult patients with diabetes. *Diabetes Care*; **32**: 1335.

The management of hyperosmolar hyperglycaemic state (HHS) in adults with diabetes. (2012). Joint British Diabetes Societies Inpatient Care Group.

Pasquel FY, Umpierrez GE (2014). Hyperosmolar hyperglycaemic state: a historic review of the clinical representation, diagnosis and treatment. *Diabetes Care*; **37**: 3124–3131.

Case 3

A 76-year-old retired farmer's wife was brought to the emergency department by paramedics with a two-day history of shortness of breath and a productive cough. A chest infection was diagnosed and she was admitted to the geratology ward for treatment with intravenous antibiotics.

There was a past history of hysterectomy for severe menorrhagia, hypothyroidism, and previous fractures, including of the hip, left clavicle, and radius, occurring on separate occasions over the previous six years. In addition, six months earlier, she had been admitted to the emergency department following a fall at home in which she had sustained a blow to the head resulting in headache, but no loss of consciousness. A computed tomography (CT) scan of the head was reported as normal.

She was teetotal, had never smoked, and was taking paracetamol and thyroxine. She lived alone with her husband on a remote farm, and was independent. There were two children, one daughter who lived abroad, and the other who lived with her severely disabled child in a different part of the country.

During the admission, nursing staff reported that her husband called many times, but she declined to speak to him. He had asked staff about her condition and was very keen for her to return home as soon as possible. He was not able to visit her in hospital as their home was isolated and he was no longer driving. At one point during the admission, she confided to one of the nurses on the ward that her husband had hurt her previously.

On the ward round prior to her planned discharge, she looked well, her temperature was 36.5°C, heart rate was 72bpm (regular), blood pressure 135/70mmHg, without postural drop. The chest examination revealed a few right-sided basal crepitations. The rest of the examination was normal and there were no neurological abnormalities. All the blood tests were normal and the chest X-ray showed improvement. Her MMSE was 30/30 and Geriatric Depression Scale (GDS) was 3/15. When discharge plans were discussed, she expressed reluctance to leave hospital.

Questions

1 Bearing in mind her past medical history, what is the most likely reason for her refusal to talk to her husband and her unwillingness to return home?
2 Define this problem, its prevalence, and associated risk factors.

Answers

1 Bearing in mind her past medical history, what is the most likely reason for her refusal to talk to her husband and her unwillingness to return home?

The most likely reason for her reluctance to go home and refusal to talk to her husband while in hospital was that she was a victim of abuse. There had been many unexplained falls and admissions to the emergency department. On direct questioning, she admitted to having been the subject of physical and psychological abuse by her husband over many years. She had never told anyone about it, owing to fear of the consequences; she had no income or other sources of support, both daughters lived elsewhere, and she was embarrassed to admit the problem to anyone. She felt protected in hospital away from her husband and was able to admit the truth.

Detection of abuse is often dependent on the empathy and intuition of individual members of the multidisciplinary team and their concerns should always be investigated.

2 Define this problem, its prevalence, and associated risk factors.

The World Health Organization defines abuse of older people as: 'A single or repeated act or lack of appropriate action occurring within any relationship where there is an expectation of trust (and) which causes harm or distress to an older person'. It is predicted to increase as the proportion of old and dependent people rises, but the human and financial resources available for looking after them diminish. Around 6% of older people in the general population report suffering abuse in the past month and reported physical violence among couples was found to be 5.6%. The latest estimates of the annual prevalence of abuse among people aged over 65 in the UK is around 3% where perpetrated by a family member, friend, or care worker, rising to 4% if abuse by neighbours and acquaintances is included. However, the true prevalence of abuse in older people is probably higher, as it is often unreported by the victims, unsuspected by doctors and social workers, and also not well researched.

Abuse is two to three times more likely to affect people aged over 80 and those with dementia. It has been estimated by some authors that the mortality of abused older people is three times that of those never reported as abused. A major study of abused older people showed that they had poorer survival than a matched population of people who had no contact with protective services, even though no deaths occurred as a direct consequence of injury. A high level of awareness of the problem is required among clinicians.

Risk factors for abuse in older people are:

- Dementia (particularly in people presenting with behavioural problems such as wandering)
- High dependency, chronic disorders, functional impairment, and carer stress
- Advanced age
- Poor sleeping pattern
- A continuation of long-term domestic violence into old age (e.g. abuse of an older person may be exposed after the new onset of disability of the victim; or sometimes a previous long-term victim may become abuser if a perpetrator becomes disabled and dependent)
- Long-term family conflict (e.g. between the spouses or between child and parent)
- Shared living arrangements with the abuser
- Social isolation and low level of social support
- Financial dependency of the abuser on the victim
- Characteristics of abusers include alcoholism, history of being a victim of child abuse, drug addiction and mental health problems, especially depression.

Given the history of previously undetected abuse of this patient by her husband, answer the following questions:

Questions continued

3. What factors would have made establishing the diagnosis difficult in this patient?
4. List at least five forms of this abuse.
5. Which signs may indicate the existence of abuse?
6. How would you investigate such patients?
7. How would you manage this patient?

Answers continued

3 What factors would have made establishing the diagnosis difficult in this patient?

Abuse was difficult to confirm in this patient because:

- The injuries seemed to have occurred from spontaneous falls with no specific evidence of abuse
- The perpetrator was her spouse, inconspicuous clinically and likely to be protected by her (spouses and adult offspring are the most common perpetrators)
- She felt (as is often the case) ashamed and embarrassed
- She was frightened that if no one believed her, the abuse would become worse
- She did not know what to do, or what her options were
- She was socially isolated with no family members or friends to confide in
- She was financially dependent on her abuser
- In contrast to her response to her other medical conditions, she concealed the abuse, and delayed investigation and management.

Other causes of difficulties in diagnosing abuse include:

- Communication problems or poor cognition
- Fear of being stigmatized
- Fear of institutionalization or being relocated
- Fear of being declared incompetent
- Depression, making resisting or reporting the abuser more difficult
- Tendency of clinical staff and social workers to dismiss complaints as attributed to acute confusion or dementia
- Low levels of awareness among clinicians and lack of knowledge about how to respond
- Lack of a practical screening instrument.

4 List at least five forms of abuse.

Forms of abuse include the following (some of which present breaches of human rights and service standards, criminal offences, or are against professional code of conduct):

1. *Neglect*—failure to care for basic needs including physical (food, money, medicine, personal care, etc.), social (for example leaving an older person for a long time alone) (see Fig 3.1).

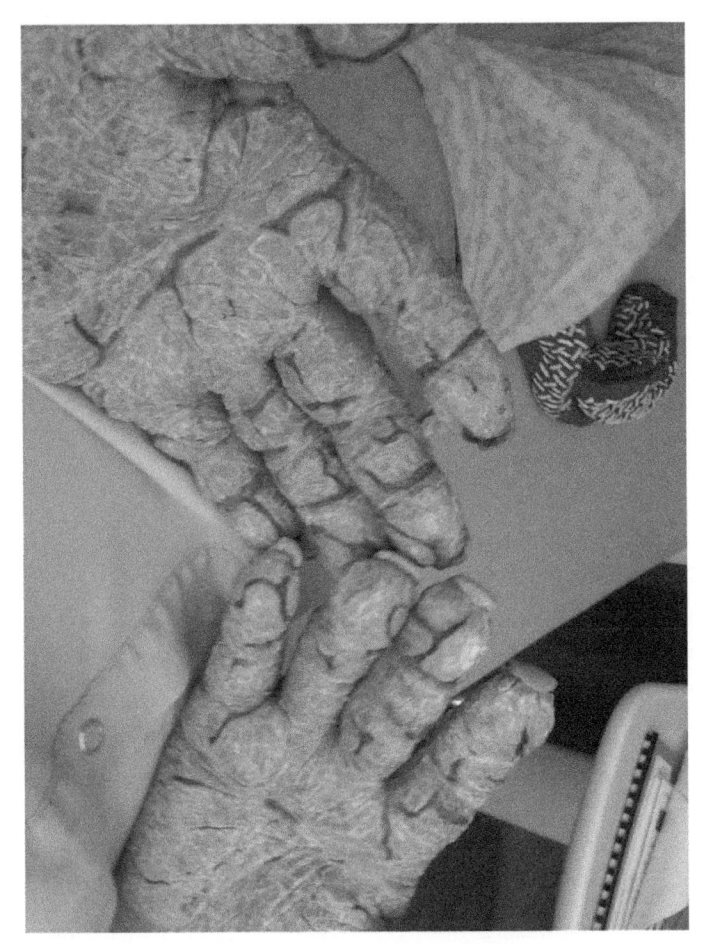

Fig. 3.1 Hands of an older patient with history of schizophrenia and psoriasis, who had been neglected by his family and was not given medications.

2. *Financial*—stealing, extortion, fraud, changing a will, misuse of power of attorney. Recent studies (behavioural and neuroimaging) suggest that vulnerability to financial abuse in older people (when compared to younger people) is most likely biologically determined. Older people display reduced activation of the anterior insula, which is implicated in the assessment of risks and ability to make safe choices, and reduced ability to detect traits of untrustworthiness.
3. *Psychological or emotional*—commonly humiliation, insults, isolation, threats, remaining silent, and ignoring the person. More insidious is infantilization, in which the perpetrator treats an older person as a child, so encouraging the victim to become dependent on the perpetrator.

4 *Physical*—e.g. forceful or improper feeding, kicking, striking, shoving, shaking, beating, restraining, over-medication. Sometimes, only meticulous physical examination, e.g. examining behind ears, under the upper arms, and removal of all clothes will detect injuries.
5 *Sexual*—e.g. touching in a sexual way without consent.
6 *Discrimination*—if treatment is less favourable due to patient age or disability.
7 *Institutional abuse*—various forms of abuse, including poor professional practice, could be suspected if a care home has a higher rate of pressure sores or hospital admissions.
8 *Abandonment*—desertion of an older patient by a person who is providing care.

5 Which signs may indicate the existence of this abuse?

Possible signs of abuse in older patients are:

- Examination findings: unkempt appearance; poor hygiene; inappropriate clothes; traumatic alopecia; bruises in various stages of evolution; pressure sores; dehydration; burns (for example from applied cigarettes, or stocking or glove distribution from scalding); restraint injury on wrists or ankles; skin tears
- Anxiety, agitation, even suicide
- Unexplained pain, fractures, or conflicting accounts of injuries
- Vaginal or rectal bleeding
- Patient withdrawal and/or carer behaviour (such as insistence on providing the history)
- Delay in requesting treatment
- Avoiding or failure to attend appointments
- Carer blaming the patient for difficulties; for example, through resisting or not co-operating with care.

6 How would you investigate such patients?

Where abuse is a possibility, history-taking and examination should be performed with sensitivity, and in the absence of the suspected abuser. Patients should be directly questioned where appropriate e.g. 'Are you frightened of someone?' or 'Has someone harmed you?' or assessed by either a screening form or a self-administered form. However, such forms may be difficult to use in practice, as the majority of existing screening instruments are lengthy to administer, and some require the patient to have an established relationship with the examiner in order to be used. There are several screening scales for abuse (e.g. The Indicators of Abuse—a 22-item tool—to be completed by a health care professional after a home assessment; The Elder Abuse and Neglect Assessment—a 44-item scale), which may aid clinical assessment (see Further reading).

This patient admitted being abused, after being asked a direct question: 'Has someone harmed you?'

Further assessment should include:

- Details of the abuse including type and frequency
- Physical examination should include examination of the inner thighs, soles of the feet, weight loss, new pressure sores, and the inclusion of gynaecological examination in suspected sexual abuse
- Functional assessment including of the current carer's ability to look after the patient
- Carer stress
- Evaluation of the home environment
- Patient's social and financial resources
- Cognitive assessment and mood assessment of the patient (and the carer)
- Laboratory tests (e.g. electrolytes-hydration, albumin-nutritional status, drug levels), X-ray in cases of suspected fracture as appropriate in order to identify and document the abuse.

7 How would you manage this patient?

As soon as the abuse is revealed or suspected, the clinician or other member of the team should alert the hospital social worker or safeguarding adults manager (or adult protection coordinator at the local authority community care or social services department for a patient in the community). The social worker will speak to the patient regarding the abuse (depending on the patient's mental capacity) and will establish whether there has been previous contact with social services. The social worker raises an online 'safeguarding alert'. Access to safeguarding data is available to all social workers in the local area, but not to medical teams. A safeguarding manager is then allocated.

In this case, the patient was offered further support from social services and on their advice, she told her daughters about the abuse. This case was discussed at a further meeting between the social worker, medical team, the patient, and her daughters. The purpose of the meeting was to create a safeguarding plan, which in this case was for the patient to move out of her house and to live near her daughter. She did not want to see her husband ever again, but she did not have any savings or income, and her daughters could not support her financially. Social services therefore provided financial support and accommodation near one of her daughters. The police also investigated the case with a view to possible criminal charges.

The management of abuse in older patients should address each patient's individual circumstances, and may include assessment of mental capacity (see case 13), care input, food provision, use of assistive technology (bed sensors, pendant alarm), supply of clean usable clothes, linen, etc. as well as assessment of the abuser.

Specific management points include:

- Talking openly to patients about the abuse.
- Informing patients about the risks and consequences of different options (e.g. helping them to devise safety plans).
- Meticulous written and photo documentation of all findings (with the clinician's signature and his/her details on each page of the documentation).
- Preserving clothes or other possible evidence if needed for further police investigation, or delaying bathing of a patient until proper examination with samples taking is done by an expert (e.g. DNA sampling in suspected sexual abuse).
- A multidisciplinary team approach involving clinicians, nurses, social workers, and possibly lawyers using a checklist or other framework to facilitate comprehensive assessment.
- Medical or psychiatric assistance as needed.
- Psychological support possibly including formal psychotherapy for victim or abuser.
- Consideration of legal action and involvement of the local domestic violence unit.
- Alternative housing.
- Hospital admission in emergency situations.
- Regular close follow-up, appropriate to the level of risk.
- Clinicians should avoid confrontation with family members or carers in order to keep options open and to avoid increasing the likelihood of further abuse or destruction of evidence by the abuser.
- If the alleged abuser is a member of staff, the individual would usually be suspended from working with patients during the investigation.

Further reading

Castle E, Eisenberger NI, Seeman TE, *et al.* (2012). Neural and behavioral bases of age differences in perception of trust. *Proc Natl Acad Sci USA*; **109**: 20848–20852.

Cooper C, Selwood A. Livingston G (2008). The prevalence of elder abuse and neglect: a systematic review. *Age Ageing*; **37**: 151–160.

Gosney M, Harper A, Conroy S (2012). Oxford Desk Reference: Geriatric Medicine. Oxford, UK: Oxford University Press.

http://www.elderabuse.org.uk

Johannesen MJ, LoGiudice D (2013). Elder abuse: a systematic review of risk factors in community-dwelling elders. *Age Ageing*; **42**: 292–298.

Lachs MS, Williams CS, O'Brien S, Pillemer KA, Charlson ME (1998). The mortality of elder mistreatment. *JAMA*; **280**(5): 428–432.

Manthorpe J (2015). The abuse, neglect and mistreatment of older people with dementia in care homes and hospitals in England: the potential for secondary data analysis: innovative practice. *Dementia (London)*; **14**: 273–279.

Meeks-Sjostrom D (2004). A comparison of three measures of elder abuse. *J Nurs Scholarsh*; **36**(3): 247–250.

O'Keeffe M, Hills A, Doyle M, *et al.* (2007). UK Study of Abuse and Neglect of Older People: Prevalence Survey Report. London: National Centre for Social Research: http://www.natcen.ac.uk/media/308684/p2512-uk-elder-abuse-final-for-circulation.pdf

WHO (2002). The Toronto Declaration on the Global Prevention of Elder Abuse. World Health Organization, Geneva.

Case 4

An 80-year-old woman was admitted to hospital from the emergency department with a two-day history of nausea, loss of appetite, and confusion.

She was previously well and independent in all activities of daily living. Her past medical history included hypertension, osteoarthritis, heart failure, and atrial fibrillation. Medications taken included warfarin, digoxin, furosemide, and paracetamol. Two weeks before admission, her GP had prescribed erythromycin for cellulitis of her left leg and senna for constipation. She was teetotal and had never smoked.

On admission to the ward, she was confused with AMTS 7/10 and CAM was positive consistent with delirium. Blood pressure was 100/60mmHg. The rest of the examination was normal.

Investigations showed the following:

- Urea 8mmol/L; creatinine 160mmol/L; Na 130mmol/L; K 2.8mmol/L; Mg 1.5mg/dL (normal range 1.7 to 2.2mg/dL); INR 2.5
- FBC, liver function tests, calcium, glucose, TFTs, CRP: all normal
- CXR: slightly enlarged heart; clear lungs
- ECG is shown in Figure 4.1:
- CT brain scan performed in the emergency department: unremarkable.

Questions

1 What is the most likely cause of her symptoms?
2 How would you confirm the diagnosis?
3 What factors may contribute to the development of this condition in older patients and what has probably happened in this case?
4 How would you treat this patient?
5 What other condition may cause a similar clinical picture and why is this alternative diagnosis more common in older people?

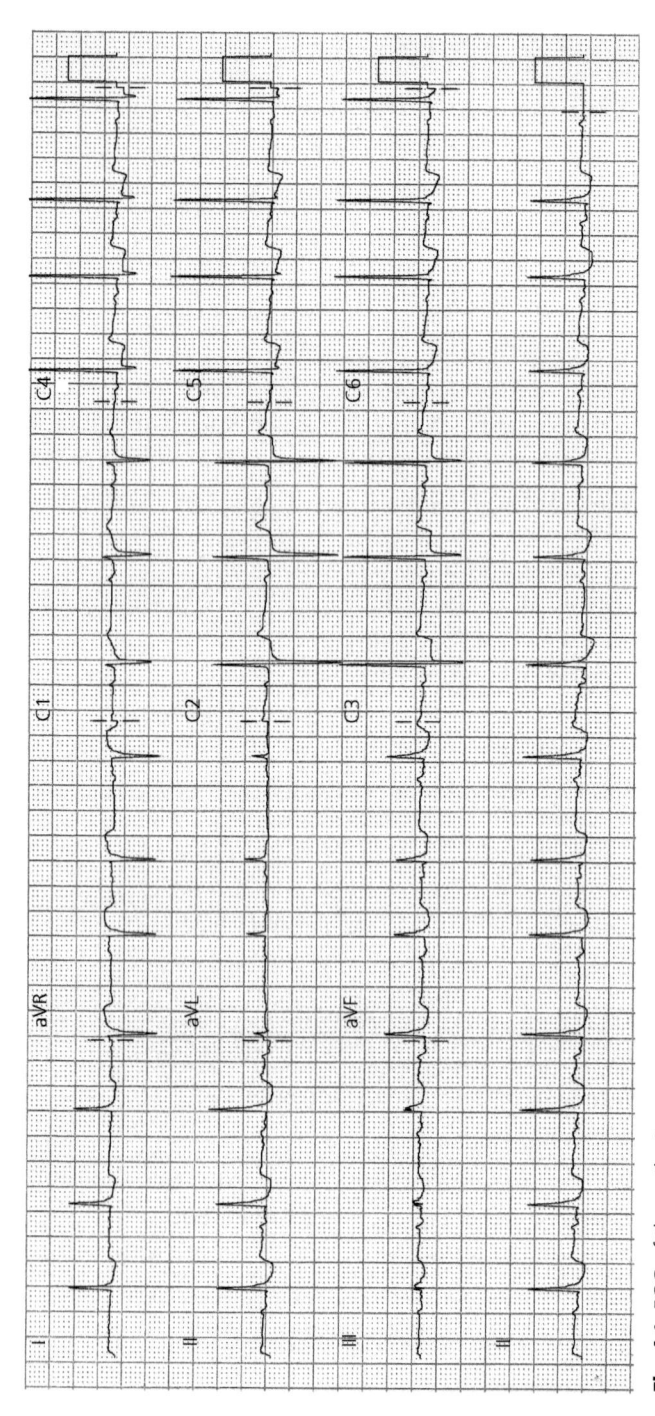

Fig. 4.1 ECG of the patient.

Answers

1 What is the most likely cause of her symptoms?

Digitalis toxicity is the most likely cause as suggested by the clinical symptoms, drug history and ECG changes, and accompanying renal impairment with hypokalaemia and hypomagnesaemia. Digitalis toxicity has various clinical manifestations. Gastrointestinal symptoms are usually first to occur, particularly in acute intoxication, and are usually the most prominent features. In chronic intoxication, malaise and general weakness usually dominate the clinical picture. Abdominal pain, diarrhoea, anorexia, dizziness, headache, seizures, syncope, hallucinations, severe hyperkalaemia, yellow or green visual haloes around objects, and confusion may also occur. Confusion is thought to be caused by cholinergic receptor binding, muscarinic antagonist activity, and inhibition of membrane Na + K + ATPase by digoxin, all of which contribute to disruption of neuronal activity. The symptoms and signs of cardiotoxicity include arrhythmias of virtually any type although bundle branch block is rare. Complete heart block, ventricular ectopics, nodal rhythm, nodal bradycardia, and ventricular tachycardia are most common, but atrial fibrillation with a rapid ventricular response rate or atrial flutter may also occur. The ECG from the patient in Figure 4.1 shows sinus rhythm (with sinus arrhythmia) and widespread down-sloping ST segment depression of a 'reverse tick' pattern while the QT interval remains relatively short and there is borderline PR interval prolongation.

2 How would you confirm the diagnosis?

Digitalis toxicity is a clinical not a laboratory diagnosis although may be confirmed by measuring the serum digoxin level. The toxic range for digoxin is greater than 2.5ng/mL, but around 10% of patients may show symptoms and signs of toxicity at levels below 2ng/mL, particularly in cases of concomitant hypokalaemia, hypomagnesaemia, hypoxia, heart failure, and hypercalcaemia. The serum digoxin level alone is therefore not a reliable indicator of the severity of toxicity.

In some patients, elevated digoxin concentration may be found in the serum without clinical manifestations of toxicity. In such cases, verification of the time when the laboratory sample was obtained is required, as a sample obtained less than 6 hours after the most recent dose of digoxin probably represents the distribution rather than plateau phase of its kinetics.

An apparently elevated digoxin serum level may be found in some uraemic patients, even if they are not taking digoxin, owing to endogenous production of digoxin-like substances. There have also been reports of elevated serum digoxin level in autopsy specimens of patients who did not show elevations ante mortem.

3 What factors may contribute to the development of this condition in older patients and what had probably happened in this case?

The following factors may contribute to the development of digoxin toxicity in older patients:

- Reduced renal function, since up to 75% of digoxin is excreted unchanged in urine. Physiological renal changes associated with ageing result in reduced renal blood flow by approximately 2% per year after the age of 40, reduced renal mass by approximately 10–20% between 40 and 80 years, and reduced glomerular filtration rate of about 50% between 50 and 90 years (see case 29). Routine formula calculations of renal function often overestimate actual renal function in older patients, owing to age-associated reductions in creatinine, secondary to reduced lean body mass.
- Coexisting conditions such as heart disease, chronic obstructive pulmonary disease, hypoxia, acute illness.
- Narrow therapeutic index; effective and toxic levels of digoxin are similar.
- Pharmacokinetic alterations owing to differences in the absorption and extra renal clearance of digoxin.
- Reduced hepatic function, although only small amounts are metabolized in liver and approximately 25% is bound to plasma proteins.
- Reduced lean body mass and therefore altered distribution of the drug.
- Dehydration that decreases glomerular filtration rate and clearance of digoxin.
- Drug interactions, e.g. affecting the reduction or elimination of digoxin, or causing electrolyte disturbances. Implicated drugs include, e.g. NSAIDs (indomethacin), macrolides (clarithromycin, erythromycin), amiodarone, diuretics (spironolactone, furosemide), quinidine, procainamide, beta-blockers, and calcium channel blockers. The introduction of laxatives (e.g. senna) to patients with heart failure taking digoxin was found to be associated with a 1.6-fold increased risk of digoxin toxicity, requiring hospitalization in one large population-based study owing to hypokalaemia.

In this patient, therefore, several factors may have contributed to digitalis toxicity, including: acute illness; dehydration; volume depletion (poor oral intake during the two weeks with cellulitis); decreased renal function; drugs (diuretics, laxatives, and erythromycin); hypokalaemia; and hypomagnesaemia. In particular, the introduction of a macrolide antibiotic was important owing to its effects on P-glycoprotein interaction, and possibly on gut flora, which normally account for about 10% of digoxin metabolism.

4 How would you treat this patient?

Treatment consists of discontinuation of digoxin and any drugs that might enhance its effects, supportive measures (intravenous fluids), correction of electrolytes, and consideration of digoxin-specific antibodies in cases of life-threatening arrhythmias. Arrhythmias should be closely monitored and treated if symptomatic with specific management (atropine, cardiac pacing, and antiarrhythmic drugs).

In acute ingestion/poisoning, gastric lavage, and active carbon should be considered. In the case of renal failure and hyperkalaemia, dialysis may be required to treat the hyperkalaemia although this will not remove digoxin significantly.

5 What other condition may cause a similar clinical picture and why is this alternative diagnosis more common in older people?

Acute poisoning caused by ingestion of plants including lily of the valley (*Convallaria majalis*), foxglove, or oleander may cause a similar clinical picture, as these contain cardiac glycosides with digitalis-like effects. In older patients, such ingestion is usually associated with cognitive impairment rather than suicidal intent. As with digoxin, the risk of symptomatic digitalis-like toxicity is increased with concurrent hypokalaemia. Patients ingesting large amounts will require hospitalization, treatment being as for digoxin intoxication with haemodynamic monitoring, correction of electrolyte abnormalities, consideration of digoxin-specific antibodies, but also gastric decontamination with activated charcoal.

Further reading

Alagiakrishnan K, Wiens CA (2004). An approach to drug induced delirium in the elderly. *Postgrad Med J*; **80**: 388–393.

Alexandre J, Foucault A, Coutance G, Scanu P, Milliez P (2012). Digitalis intoxication induced by an acute accidental poisoning by lily of the valley. *Circulation*; **125**: 1053–1055.

Ma G, Brady WJ, Pollack M, Chan TC (2001). Electrocardiographic manifestations: digitalis toxicity. *J Emerg Med*; **20**(2): 145–152.

Rathore SS, Wang Y, Krumholz HM (2002). Sex-based differences in the effect of digoxin for the treatment of heart failure. *N Engl J Med*; **347**: 1403–1411.

Schaeffer TH, Mlynarchek SL, Stanford CF, *et al.* (2010). Treatment of chronically digoxin-poisoned patients with a newer digoxin immune fab—a retrospective study. *J Am Osteopath Asso*; **110**(10): 587–592.

Wang MT, Li IH, Lee WJ, Huang TY, Leu HB, Chan AL (2011). Exposure to sennoside-digoxin interaction and risk of digoxin toxicity: a population-based nested case-control study. *Eur J Heart Fail*; **13**(11): 1238–1243.

Zapater P, Reus S, Tello A, Torrús D, Pérez-Mateo M, Horga JF (2002). A prospective study of the clarithromycin–digoxin interaction in elderly patients. *J Antimicrob Chemother*; **50**: 601–606.

Case 5

An 88-year-old woman was admitted directly to the acute geratology ward after a home visit by the GP. He had found the patient's home in disarray with rotting food in the fridge and a strong smell of urine throughout the house. The patient had been discharged from hospital two months previously, after a seven-month admission precipitated by pneumonia requiring ICU care. A fall and a fractured neck of femur, followed by non-ST-elevation myocardial infarction and subsequent heart failure, had complicated her recovery. The patient lived alone with no family nearby and was usually mobile short distances with a stick. A twice-daily care package had been arranged on discharge after the previous admission, but she had cancelled this within a month. Medications were paracetamol, aspirin, clopidogrel, atenolol, ramipril, simvastatin, codeine phosphate, omeprazole, furosemide, spironolactone, alendronate, vitamin D, plus calcium and digoxin.

On examination, she was tearful and extremely thin with BMI of 16. Observations showed normal temperature, heart rate of 68bpm (irregularly irregular), blood pressure of 112/68 mmHg, respiratory rate of 12 breaths per minute, and oxygen saturations of 97% on room air. The capillary refill was sluggish and the oral mucosa was very dry with a few ulcers associated with dentures. There was an ejection systolic murmur, which did not radiate. The lung fields were clear, and the abdomen was soft and non-tender with no palpable masses. There was bilateral lower limb soft tissue oedema. Transferring from bed to chair was difficult and required help from the nurses.

Investigations revealed the following:

- CXR: slightly enlarged heart; lungs clear
- ECG: 74bpm; AF; LVH
- Urine dip: negative nitrites; negative leucocytes, + protein
- Hb: 8.2g/dL; MCV 90fL; WCC 4.2×10^9/L; Neut 2.4×10^9/L; HCt 0.55L/L
- Na: 130mmol/L; K 3.1mmol/L; Urea 18mmol/L; Creat 240μmol/L
- ALT: 38IU/L; Bili 5μmol/L; Alp 267U/L; Albumin 18g/L
- Ca: 2.4mmol/L; TSH 2mU/L; free thyroxine 20pmol/L
- CRP: 6mg/L.

Questions

1 What are the features in this case that suggest a poor nutritional status in this patient? What is the meaning of the term 'malnutrition'? What are the causes of unintentional weight loss in older people and which are likely to be important in this case?
2 What is the prevalence of malnutrition in older people and how does this vary with place of residence/care setting?
3 Discuss the possible factors contributing to this patient's poor nutritional status.
4 How would you further assess her nutritional status?
5 How would you manage this patient?

Answers

1 What are the features in this case that suggest a poor nutritional status in this patient? What is the meaning of the term 'malnutrition'? What are the causes of unintentional weight loss in older people and which are likely to be important in this case?

The factors indicating poor nutritional state in this patient are:

- low BMI
- low albumin
- low Hb
- low Na, low K
- evidence of functional decline.

There is no universally accepted definition of malnutrition, but one that is commonly used identifies malnutrition as 'a state of nutrition in which a deficiency, or excess, of energy, protein and micronutrients causes measurable adverse effects on tissue/body form (body shape, size and composition) and function, and clinical outcome'.

Unintentional weight loss may occur because of:

- starvation
- sarcopenia
- cachexia.

Starvation is generally accepted to occur purely as a result of protein-energy deficiency and is synonymous with protein-energy malnutrition. The major factor that distinguishes starvation from other syndromes of unintentional weight loss is that it is reversed when adequate energy and protein intake is achieved.

Sarcopenia is associated with increased frailty, loss of strength, reduced physical function and diminished capacity for exercise as a result of decreased muscle mass and alterations to muscle structure at the microscopic level. The diagnosis relies on demonstrating reduced gait speed over 6 metres course (less than 1 m·s^{-1}) and objectively measured low muscle mass. Sarcopenia is thought to occur regardless of energy balance and may occur in obese patients. Recent evidence indicates that the most effective intervention is a combination of nutrition and resistance training.

Cachexia is mediated by pro-inflammatory cytokines and is associated with chronic conditions such as cancer, HIV/AIDS, heart failure, and chronic obstructive pulmonary disease. Cachexia is a complex metabolic syndrome associated with underlying illness and is characterized by loss of muscle with or without loss of fat mass. 'Geriatric cachexia' is proposed, by some, as being a consequence of ageing, independent of any underlying condition.

In practice it may be difficult to discriminate between the different syndromes underlying unintentional weight loss in an individual older patient as seen in the current case where there was likely predominantly protein-energy malnutrition (i.e. insufficient intake), but also possible contributions from sarcopenia and cachexia associated with heart failure. It is possible that poor nutrition and being underweight contributed to the extended length of stay and in-hospital complications on her previous admission, and that these in turn exacerbated the situation. Further research is required to validate proposed definitions and the criteria for sarcopenia and cachexia.

2 What is the prevalence of malnutrition in older people and how does this vary with place of residence/care setting?

Malnutrition is prevalent in older people, but varies according to setting, although estimates are conflicting owing to heterogeneity of assessment method and case-mix differences. Also, studies do not generally discriminate between the different aetiologies of malnutrition. A recent review of malnutrition rates in 4,507 patients, mean age 82.3 years, across 12 westernized countries, found the overall prevalence to be 22.8%. Among patients in rehabilitation, 50.5% were malnourished compared with 38.7% in hospital, and 5.8% in the community. In multicentre studies focussed in the acute care setting, 23–60% of older patients were malnourished and an estimated 22–28% were at nutritional risk (Table 5.1). Estimates from care homes vary from 15–70%, but there is a clear relationship between level of care required and prevalence of malnutrition.

Table 5.1 Prevalence of malnutrition in acute care settings

(Authors, year)	Number of hospitals; country	Total number of participants; age (years)	Number of participants	Nutrition screening/assessment method; stage of nutrition assessment	Malnutrition risk or prevalence
Agarwal et al., 2012	56 hospitals; Australia and New Zealand	$n = 3,122$; mean age: 65 ± 18 years	$n = 1,650$	SGA; during hospital admission	60% of elderly participants (≥65 years) were malnourished
Imoberdorf et al., 2010	Seven hospitals; Switzerland	$n = 32,837$; mean/median age not specified	Not specified	NRS-2002; on admission	Nutrition risk in 65–84-year-old participants: 22%; nutrition risk in participants aged >85 years: 28%
Pirlich et al., 2006	13 hospitals; Germany	$n = 1,886$; mean age: 62 ± 17 years	$n = 1,109$	SGA; during hospital admission	PEM prevalence in: 60–69 years: 23%; 70–79 years: 35%; ≥80 years: 55%
Correia and Campos, 2003	Hospitals from 13 countries in Latin America	$n = 9,348$; mean age: 52 ± 17 years	Not specified	SGA; during hospital admission	Protein-energy malnutrition prevalence in participants aged >60 years: 53%
Waitzberg et al., 2001	25 hospitals; Brazil	$n = 4,000$; mean age not specified	$n = 1,441$ (age >60 years)	SGA; during hospital admission	Protein-energy malnutrition prevalence in participants aged >60 years: 53%

NRS-2002, Nutrition Risk Screening 2002; PEM, protein-energy malnutrition; SGA, subjective global assessment. Adapted from Agarwal, 2013.

Reduced food intake in hospitals and care homes may be caused by:
- *Patient factors* including loss of appetite, acute illness, oral issues, low mood, dysphagia, confusion, isolation
- *Catering limitations* such as inflexible mealtimes, difficulty accessing food and beverage packaging, lack of menu variety, unappealing meals
- *Organizational barriers,* e.g. interruptions during mealtimes, inadequate feeding assistance, unpleasant smells, disruptive behaviour from staff members and other patients.

Concern about reports of poor hydration and nutrition of older people in hospital has prompted campaigns such as 'Hungry to be Heard' in the UK. Such campaigns attempt to raise awareness of the issues and encourage systems-level strategies, such as feeding assistance, use of red trays to identify those at risk, and protected mealtimes. There is increasing evidence that individualized nutritional support for malnourished elderly people during hospitalization, and post-discharge improves outcomes, and reduces complications.

3 Discuss the possible factors contributing to this patient's poor nutritional status.

There are several possible factors contributing to this patient's poor nutritional status:
- Depression (see case 18) as suggested by the tearfulness noted on admission, recent prolonged hospital admission, deterioration in functional ability, self-neglect (see case 13), and social isolation
- Social isolation as indicated by the lack of carer visits or nearby family
- Financial difficulties may be a factor
- Poor mobility and social isolation impacting on the ability to obtain food
- Poorly fitting dentures causing ulceration and making eating difficult
- Furosemide, digoxin, and spironolactone may alter the sense of taste and smell and long-term use of PPIs suppress gastric acidity and may predispose to small bowel bacterial overgrowth causing weight loss, and reduced micronutrient intake.

Cognition may be impaired and contribute to difficulties obtaining and preparing food or even recognizing the need to eat. Factors associated with poor food intake in older people are shown in Figure 5.1. As seen in the current case, protein-energy malnutrition in older patients is usually multifactorial comprising physiological, social, and economic elements. Risk factors for malnutrition are often referred to as 'the nine d's', many of which are potential contributors in the current case and include:

- dementia
- dysgeusia (change in the sense of taste)
- dysphagia
- diarrhoea
- depression
- disease, especially chronic illness, cancer
- poor dentition
- dysfunction, poor functional status
- drugs.

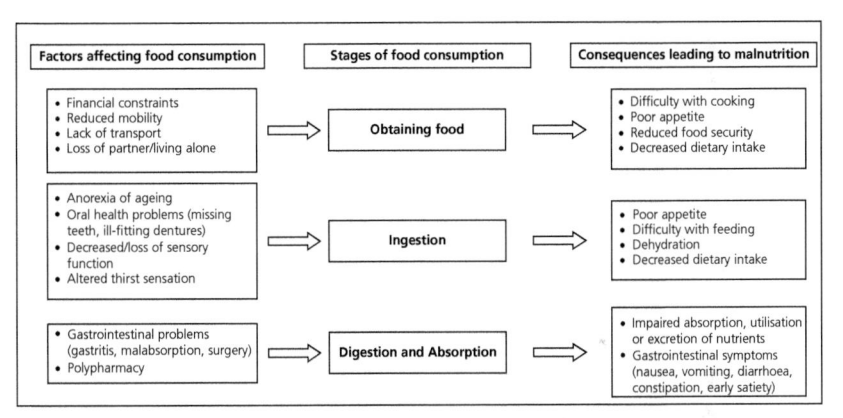

Fig. 5.1 Factors affecting food consumption in older people.

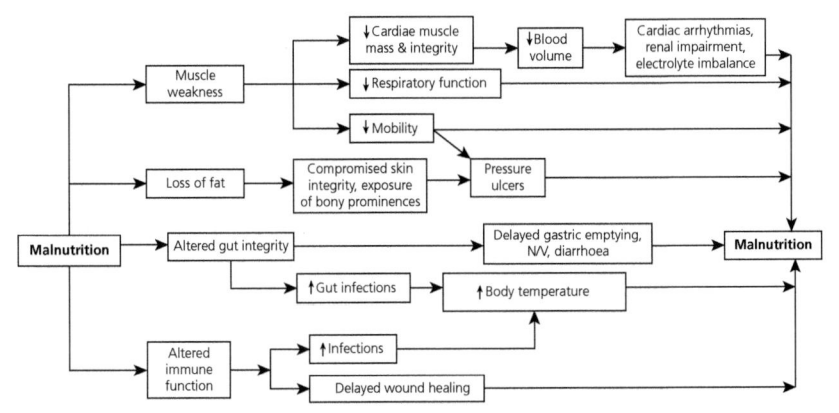

Fig. 5.2 Protein-energy malnutrition—a cause and consequence of adverse outcomes.
(Adapted from *Maturitas*, Vol 76, Issue 4, Agarwal et al., Malnutrition in the elderly: A narrative review, 296–302, Copyright (2013) with permission from Elsevier.)

Poor nutritional status is associated with functional decline, poor immune function, anaemia, impaired wound healing, decreased bone density, cognitive decline, increased length of stay, falls and higher mortality rates, and is a risk factor for delirium (see case 1). Figure 5.2 shows the factors contributing to malnutrition, and that in turn, malnutrition increases the vulnerability to conditions that lead to further malnutrition.

4 How would you further assess her nutritional status?

Formal assessment of the patient's nutritional status using a validated tool is required. Serum albumin is a commonly used biomarker in screening for malnutrition, but in acutely unwell patients it can be a poor reflection of nutritional status as it is also affected by infection and inflammation. Albumin also has a long half-life and is a poor indicator of recent change. Transferrin, although affected by a number of factors such as iron deficiency, hypoxia, chronic infection and liver disease, may be used as an early marker of protein and energy malnutrition.

A number of nutrition screening tools specific to the older adult population have been developed that contain different measured parameters:

- Biochemical and clinical indices: Nutritional Risk Index and the Geriatric Nutritional Risk Index (GNRI)
- Anthropometry; mobility; cognitive state; self-perceived health and nutrition; Mini Nutritional Assessment Screening Form (MNA-SF); Malnutrition Universal Screening Tool (MUST); and unintentional weight loss and poor intake (MST)
- Medical history, clinical and subjective evaluation: Nutrition Risk Screening 2002 (NRS-2002) (Table 5.2).

Table 5.2 Nutritional risk screening tool (NRS), 2002

Nutrition risk screening (NRS), 2002		
Step 1: Initial screening	Yes	No
Is BMI <20.5?		
Has the patient lost weight within the last three months?		
Has the patient had a reduced dietary intake in the last week?		
Is the patient severely ill? (e.g. in intensive therapy)		

Yes: If the answer is 'yes' to any question, the screening in step 2 is performed.

No: If the answer is 'no' to all questions, the patient is rescreened at weekly intervals. If the patient, e.g. is scheduled for a major operation, a preventive nutritional care plan is considered to avoid the associated risk status.

'MUST' Tool

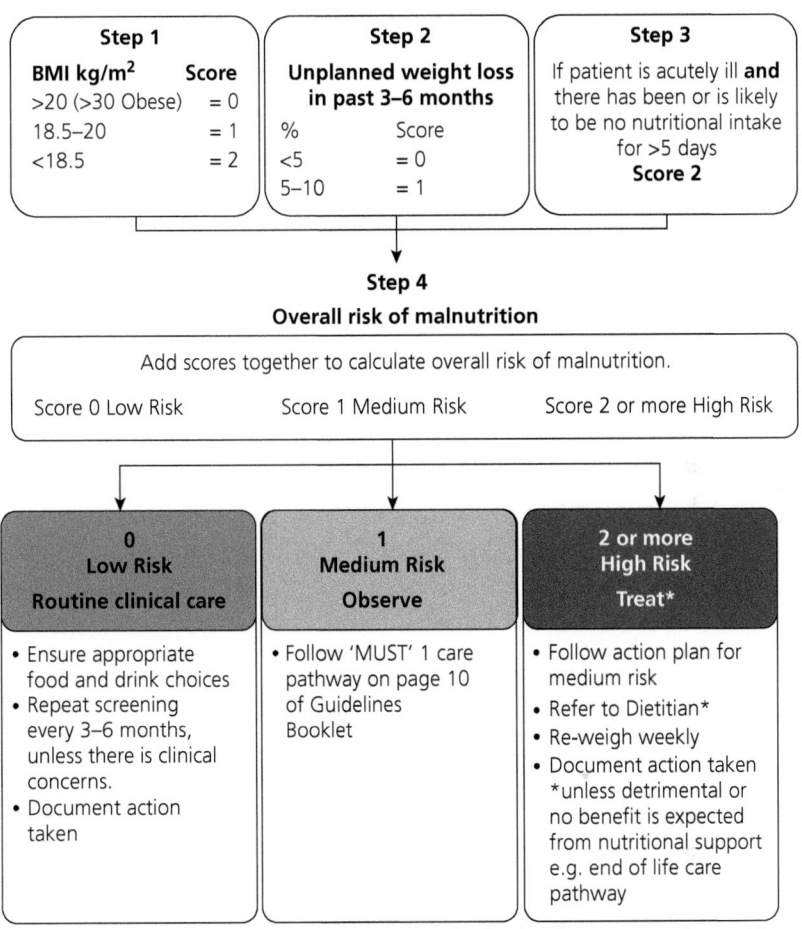

Step 1

BMI kg/m^2	Score
>20 (>30 Obese)	= 0
18.5–20	= 1
<18.5	= 2

Step 2

Unplanned weight loss in past 3–6 months

%	Score
<5	= 0
5–10	= 1

Step 3

If patient is acutely ill **and** there has been or is likely to be no nutritional intake for >5 days
Score 2

Step 4
Overall risk of malnutrition

Add scores together to calculate overall risk of malnutrition.

Score 0 Low Risk   Score 1 Medium Risk   Score 2 or more High Risk

0
Low Risk
Routine clinical care

- Ensure appropriate food and drink choices
- Repeat screening every 3–6 months, unless there is clinical concerns.
- Document action taken

1
Medium Risk
Observe

- Follow 'MUST' 1 care pathway on page 10 of Guidelines Booklet

2 or more
High Risk
Treat*

- Follow action plan for medium risk
- Refer to Dietitian*
- Re-weigh weekly
- Document action taken
*unless detrimental or no benefit is expected from nutritional support e.g. end of life care pathway

If unable to obtain height and weight use your professional judgement to estimate risk category (low, medium or high).

Fig. 5.3 The Malnutrition Universal Screening Tool (MUST).

(The 'Malnutrition Universal Screening Tool' ('MUST') is reproduced here with the kind permission of BAPEN (British Association for Parenteral and Enteral Nutrition). For further information on 'MUST' see http://www.bapen.org.uk.

The MUST score (Fig. 5.3) is pragmatic and is widely used in the UK hospital system to detect patients who are malnourished or at risk. Where a patient's height cannot be measured or the patient is unable to give this information, the ulnar length may be used to estimate height. If weight is unavailable, the mid upper arm circumference (normally around 23cm in men and 22cm in women) may be used as a rough estimate of BMI: if mid arm circumference is <23.5cm, BMI is likely to be <20 kg/m^2, if >32.0cm, BMI is likely to be >30 kg/m^2. The Mini Nutritional Assessment (MNA) combines anthropometric measurements, a questionnaire on diet characteristics, environment, and global health with a self-evaluation of nutritional state and health. The MNA has high specificity and sensitivity, and is a good predictor of mortality, increased length of hospital stay and discharge to nursing homes, but is relatively lengthy to apply routinely in the acute hospital environment. This patient's MUST score put her in the high-risk category (score >2).

5 How would you manage this patient?

In addition to formal nutritional assessment, this patient needs assessment of her mood and cognitive status (see case 18). Collateral history should be obtained from the GP and from the family or other informant with the patient's agreement An ongoing assessment and management plan should be instituted (Fig. 5.4)

Space for Patient Information Sticker

Oxford University Hospitals NHS Trust **ADL4**

Nutrition Risk Assessment and Management Plan

Date	Weight	Height	Step 1 BMI Score	Step 2 Wt loss Score	Step 3 Intake Score	Step 4 Total	Red Tray and/or lid?	Evaluation of previous intervention and/or on-going nutritional care plan	Completed by (initial):
Admission							Yes ☐ No ☐		
Week 1		See Above					Yes ☐ No ☐		
Week 2		See Above					Yes ☐ No ☐		
Week 3		See Above					Yes ☐ No ☐		
Week 4		See Above					Yes ☐ No ☐		

STEP 1: BMI Score

Weigh patient and find out patients height. Determine BMI Score (See BMI chart overleaf)

BMI kg/m2	Score
More than 20.1	=0
18.5-20	=1
18.4 or less	=2

(If unable to weigh patient or ask height seek alternative measurement guidelines)

→

STEP 2: Weight loss score

Unplanned weight loss in past 3-6 months (this includes obese patients)

% weight loss	Score
5% or less	=0
5.1-10%	=1
10.1% or more	=2

(If unable to weigh patient or ask height seek alternative measurement guidelines)

→

STEP 3: Nutritional Intake

Has there been or is there likely to be minimal nutritional intake for more than 5 days

	Score
If No	=0
If Yes	=2

i.e. Prolonged NBM/free fluids only, patient drowsy/confused and/or only managing a few spoonful's

→

STEP 4: Overall Score

Add all 3 scores together

Minimum = 0
Maximum = 6

See other side for action plan flow chart

Fig. 5.4 An example of a nutritional assessment and management plan based on the MUST as used at Oxford University Hospitals.

Reproduced here with kind permission of Oxford University Hospitals.

Specific management includes:

- Food charting. This enables assessment of calorie intake.
- Dietitian input.
- High calorie supplements.
- Help and encouragement with feeding.
- Trial of nasogastric tube feeding if necessary. This may be considered if the patient remains unable to increase food intake and weight despite the mentioned factors.
- Dentures refitting.
- Treatment of vitamin and/mineral deficiencies. Low levels of vitamin D, B_{12} and/or iron commonly occur in those with protein-energy malnutrition.
- Physiotherapist review. Improving mobility, muscle strengthening, and regular exercise will help improve appetite, mood, and is necessary for improving sarcopenia.
- Care needs assessment prior to discharge.
- Detailed handover to GP on discharge.

This patient was discovered to have early dementia and depression, which were managed appropriately. She did not have any close family. Her appetite and weight responded well to treatment, and she was discharged with a twice a day care package to help her with meals, medication, and personal care. Social services were engaged to clean her house (see case 13). The GP was telephoned prior to discharge to ensure continuity of care.

Further reading

Agarwal E, Miller M, Yaxley A, Isenring E (2013). Malnutrition in the elderly: a narrative review. *Maturitas*; **76**(4): 296–302.

Agarwal E, Ferguson M, Banks M, *et at.* Nutritional status and dietary intake of acute care patients: results from the Nutrition Care Day Survey 2010 . *Clinical Nutrition*. 2012; **31**: 41–47.

Ahmed T, Haboubi (2010). Assessment and management of nutrition in older people and its importance to health. *Clin Interv Aging*; **5**: 207–216.

Allen VJ, Methven L, Gosney MA (2013). Use of nutritional complete supplements in older adults with dementia: systematic review and meta-analysis of clinical outcomes. *Clin Nutr*; **32**(6): 950–957.

Correia MITD, and Campos ACL. Prevalence of hospital malnutrition in Latin America: the multicenter ELAN study. *Nutrition*. 2003; **19**: 823–825.

Cruz-Jentoft AJ, Landi F, Schneider SM, *et al.* (2014). Prevalence of and interventions for sarcopenia in ageing adults: a systematic review. Report of the International Sarcopenia Initiative (EWGSOP and IWGS). *Age Ageing*; **43**: 748–759.

Fearon K, Strasser F, Anker SD, et al. (2011). Definition and classification of cancer cachexia: an international consensus. *Lancet Oncol*; **12**(5): 489–495.

Fielding RA, Vellas B, Evans WJ, et al. (2011). Sarcopenia: an undiagnosed condition in older adults. Current consensus definition: prevalence, etiology, and consequences. International Working Group on Sarcopenia. *J Am Med Dir Assoc*; **12**: 249–256.

Imoberdorf R, Meier R, Krebs P, et al. Prevalence of undernutrition on admission to Swiss hospitals. *Clinical Nutrition*. 2010; **29**:38–41.

Kaiser MJ, Bauer JM, Rämsch C, et al. (2010), Mini Nutritional Assessment International Group. Frequency of malnutrition in older adults: a multinational perspective using the mini nutritional assessment. *J Am Geriatr Soc*; **58**(9): 1734.

Malnutrition Advisory Group (MAG) The 'MUST' explanatory booklet (2003). A guide to the 'Malnutrition Universal Screening Tool' ('MUST') for adults: a standing Committee of the British Association for Parenteral and Enteral Nutrition (BAPEN).

NICE guidelines (2006): Nutritional support in adults: http://www.nice.org.uk/guidance/cg32

Pirlich M, Schütz T, Norman K et al. The German hospital malnutrition study. *Clinical Nutrition*. 2006; **25**:563–572.

Van Nes M, Herrmann F, Gold G, Michael J, Rizzoli R (2001). Does the Mini Nutritional Assessment predict hospitalization outcomes in older people? *Age Ageing*; **30**(3): 221–226: http://www.scie.org.uk/publications/guides/guide15/files/hungrytobeheard.pdf

Waitzberg DL, Caiaffa WT and Correia MITD, Hospital malnutrition: the Brazilian national survey (IBRANUTRI): a study of 4000 patients. *Nutrition*. 2001; **17**: 573–580.

Young AM, Kidston S, Banks MD, Mudge AM, Isenring EA (2013). Malnutrition screening tools: comparison against two validated nutrition assessment methods in older medical inpatients. *Nutrition*; **29**(1): 101–106.

Case 6

A 74-year-old woman presented to the day hospital with difficulty walking, falls, dizziness, and urinary incontinence that had been gradually worsening over the previous 18 months. She had also become forgetful and was no longer able to manage her bank account. There was a past history of high blood pressure for which she was taking amlodipine. She was an ex-smoker and drank a moderate amount of alcohol.

On examination, she appeared well, and general systems were unremarkable. Blood pressure was 130/80mmHg without postural drop. Cranial nerves were normal. Tone was slightly increased in the arms, but power and sensation were normal throughout. Reflexes were symmetrical, but brisk in the lower limbs. Gait was slow, shuffling, wide-based, and unsteady. Plantar responses were thought to be upgoing.

MMSE was 19/30 and GDS was 4/15.

The investigations showed:

- Hb: 13.9g/dL; WCC 6.5 × 10^9/L; ESR 16mm/hr
- Glucose: 5.6mmol/L; cholesterol 4.6mmol/L; ESR 14mm/hr; CRP <8mg/L
- U&E, LFT, TFT, Ca, PO4, B$_{12}$, folate: all normal
- Urine dipstick: negative for blood; nitrites; leucocytes
- CXR: slightly enlarged heart
- ECG: sinus rhythm; heart rate 72bpm.

Questions

1 Give a differential diagnosis in this case. What is the most likely diagnosis?
2 Describe the symptoms and physical findings in this condition.
3 What further investigations might help confirm your diagnosis?
4 What is the pathogenesis of this condition?
5 Describe how you would manage this patient.
6 List complications of the treatment for this condition.
7 How are patients selected for intervention?
8 How good are the results of intervention?

Answers
1 Give a differential diagnosis in this case. What is the most likely diagnosis?

The differential diagnosis includes:

Normal pressure hydrocephalus, an idiopathic syndrome characterized by the triad of urinary incontinence, abnormal gait, and memory impairment. There is pathological enlargement of the cerebral ventricles, normal opening pressure on lumbar puncture, normal cerebrospinal fluid, and lack of a visible structural blockage of cerebrospinal fluid circulation within the ventricular system.

Secondary hydrocephalus caused by a prior precipitating factor, such as subarachnoid or intraventricular bleed, meningitis, neoplasm, trauma, or neurosurgery. Patients are generally younger than those with primary normal pressure hydrocephalus.

Cerebrovascular disease. Multiple strokes, small vessel disease, or extensive white matter disease may present with vascular parkinsonism, and cognitive impairment characterized by 'frontal features' including dysexecutive function, attentional deficits, urinary incontinence, apathy, and depression (see case 18).

Idiopathic Parkinson's disease, or atypical parkinsonian disorder (e.g. progressive supranuclear palsy or multiple system atrophy), although cognitive impairment would not usually be prominent in the early stages (see case 40).

Dementia including Alzheimer's dementia (AD) and dementia with Lewy bodies (DLB), although one would not expect such prominent gait difficulties and incontinence in early AD (see cases 25 and 46) and there were no typical features of DLB (see case 25).

Peripheral neuropathy may cause gait difficulty and falls, but is not usually associated with cognitive impairment (although this may be present, e.g. in vitamin B_{12} deficiency or alcohol excess). In the current case, the patient's sensation appeared normal, and reflexes were brisk.

Spinal cord compression may cause increased limb tone and falls. However, mechanical cord impingement does not affect cognition, although it may cause incontinence.

The most likely diagnosis is normal pressure hydrocephalus, as the patient had the Hakim–Adams triad of cognitive impairment, gait difficulty, and incontinence in the absence of other specific clinical features, suggestive of an alternative diagnosis. As normal pressure hydrocephalus is a potentially treatable (although rare at ~6% of cases) cause of dementia, it is important to recognize the condition. Diagnostic difficulty is however frequent, owing to overlap of the clinical and radiologic features with other neurological conditions as shown in the list of differential diagnoses above.

2 Describe the symptoms and physical findings in this condition.

Normal pressure hydrocephalus is characterized by:

Gait abnormality. The gait is typically shuffling, broad-based, bradykinetic or apraxic and may be termed 'magnetic', since the feet appear to be stuck to the floor. Patients are usually slow to rise from a chair and may walk with outwardly rotated feet and short steps. They may need to take several steps in turning. Abnormalities of gait are usually prominent in the early stages of the disease and usually respond better than the other abnormalities to treatment.

Cognitive impairment. Frontal and subcortical deficits are usually prominent (decreased attention and concentration, poor executive function, low verbal fluency, inertia, impaired abstraction), and there may also be disorientation, bradyphrenia, short-term memory deficit with retrieval difficulty, apraxia, and agnosia. The cognitive impairment is thus different from that seen in early AD in which short-term memory loss is prominent. More difficulty arises in distinguishing between normal pressure hydrocephalus and vascular dementia, in which the cognitive picture is similar, particularly when associated with subcortical vascular disease. This is compounded by the fact that radiological findings may also be similar in the absence of well-defined focal infarcts. The presence of early urinary incontinence favours a diagnosis of normal pressure hydrocephalus, as this is less common in vascular dementia.

Urinary incontinence. Urinary frequency or urgency from detrusor overactivity can precede incontinence and are caused by involvement of the sacral fibres of the corticospinal tract (see case 7). Impairment of gait and cognition can exacerbate urinary problems by causing difficulties with accessing the bathroom or failure to respond appropriately to incontinence.

The Hakim–Adams triad is not in itself diagnostic, since other conditions may produce similar features and not all patients with normal pressure hydrocephalus present with the full triad: in one study, all had gait impairment, but only around half were cognitively impaired and less than one third fulfilled the triad. Other possible features of normal pressure hydrocephalus are:

- lower limb spasticity, brisk reflexes without weakness, extensor plantar responses
- postural instability
- frontal signs, deteriorating to akinetic mutism in the later stages of the disease.

3 What further investigations might help confirm your diagnosis?

This patient had:

Further cognitive assessment by a neuropsychologist that showed impairments in processing speed, abstraction, verbal fluency, orientation, learning, and memory. Formal neuropsychological testing may be helpful in evaluating the effect of treatment, although short tests such as the 30-point Montreal Cognitive Assessment (MoCA) may suffice.

Brain imaging. Brain computed tomography is needed to exclude other conditions such as tumour, infarcts, subdural haematoma, and to look for evidence to support the diagnosis. In this patient, brain CT scan (Fig. 6.1) showed marked ventriculomegaly with dilatation of frontal and temporal horns, but without excessively widened cortical sulci.

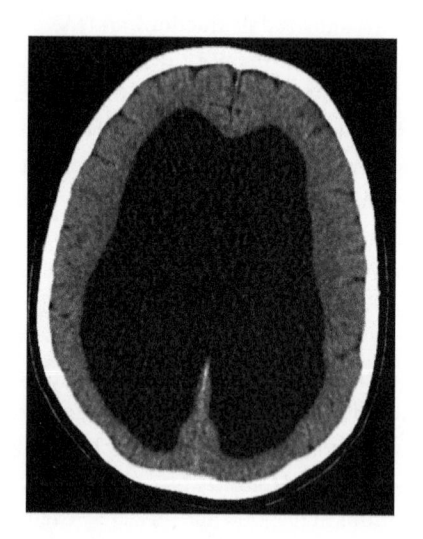

Fig. 6.1 CT scan of the brain, axial slice showing marked ventriculomegaly without periventricular density change or overt sulcal enlargement.

Magnetic resonance imaging may be considered. MRI is more specific and provides information on aqueductal stenosis if obstructive hydrocephalus is suspected, and may also show decreased attenuation in the aqueduct of Sylvius, rounding of frontal horns, thinning of the corpus callosum, and better visualization of cortical atrophy. Enlarged ventricles are diagnosed if the modified Evans ratio, derived from the maximum width of the cranial cavity at the inner tables of the skull and the maximal diameter of the frontal horns of the lateral ventricles, is >0.31. Compared with healthy controls, patients with normal pressure hydrocephalus have greater numbers of deep white matter lesions, with reduced regional peri- and paraventricular white matter cerebral blood flow, especially in frontal regions—but it is unclear whether this reduced blood flow is a consequence or a cause of neuronal dysfunction. Prominent white matter changes are thought to be a predictor of poorer response to shunting, possibly because such patients have primarily subcortical vascular dementia, or are in a late and irreversible stage of hydrocephalus. However, there are some reports of white matter changes improving after shunting.

Diffusion-weighted (magnetic resonance) imaging with quantification of intracranial apparent diffusion coefficient is emerging as a possible diagnostic marker in patients with normal pressure hydrocephalus, but further evaluation is needed.

Diffusion tensor (magnetic resonance) image analysis with semi-automatic methods is a promising method, but is still under evaluation.

Lumbar tap test. Removal of 30–50ml of cerebrospinal fluid by lumbar puncture, followed by assessment of clinical response is the most accepted diagnostic procedure with 90–100% positive predictive value. However, the negative predictive value is only 30–50%, as some patients without improvement after the procedure have nevertheless benefited from surgery. Measurement of gait speed, stride length (some clinicians videotape gait) and cognition should be undertaken before and 30–60 minutes (some authors advise 180 minutes) after the procedure. If the lumbar tap reveals elevated cerebrospinal fluid pressure, other diagnoses should be considered. Some centres offer intracranial pressure monitoring as a diagnostic test.

In this patient, opening pressure was not elevated and CSF laboratory tests were normal.

4 What is the pathogenesis of this condition?

Most patients with normal pressure hydrocephalus (NPH) are aged over 60 years, but incidence and prevalence rates are uncertain owing to conflicting reports, although both increase with age. One Norwegian study reported an annual incidence of 5.5 and prevalence of 21.9 per 100,000, and in another study, the incidence rate was 3.7/100 000/year for the total population, and 15/100,000/year for people aged over 50. The difference in reported rates is most likely to be related to methodological differences between studies in NPH diagnosis. Some studies have treated radiological appearances of ventricular dilatation, in association with gait impairment, cognitive impairment, and urinary incontinence, as diagnostic; others required full neurological evaluation. Cognitive impairment is believed to be caused by local pressure from the expanding ventricles, causing dysfunction of subcortical areas from mechanical stretching of nerve fibres and tracts. Secondary effects of distortion and impairment of the microcirculation may also be relevant.

Although normal cerebrospinal fluid pressure on lumbar puncture is a criterion for the diagnosis, the pathogenesis is thought to lie in intermittently high intraventricular pressure. Intracranial monitoring in some subjects has shown waves of high pressure reflecting temporary imbalance between rates of secretion and resorption of cerebrospinal fluid. The increase in capacitance provided by a shunt will damp the waves.

Defective resorption of cerebrospinal fluid rather than oversecretion is thought to be the key problem. While the conventional model is of cerebrospinal fluid being resorbed at the arachnoid granulations, some authors suspect that a substantial amount of resorption occurs in the brain parenchyma into capillaries or venules, and this may be the site of the problem in NPH. Some studies have found that arterial hypertension is more common in NPH than in age-matched healthy controls, and it is postulated that deep white matter ischaemia and small vessel arteriosclerosis play a role. Secondary NPH tends to present at earlier ages than the idiopathic form, and is caused by cerebral or subarachnoid haemorrhage, meningitis, neoplasm, trauma, or neurosurgery damage to the resorptive apparatus.

5 Describe how you would manage this patient.

The intervention of choice is a ventriculoperitoneal or, more rarely, ventriculoatrial shunt, to drain cerebrospinal fluid from the cerebral ventricles to be reabsorbed into the systemic circulation.

After removal of 50ml of CSF in this patient, there was immediate improvement in gait speed, but not in cognition. Patients who experience instant improvement in symptoms after the removal of a sample of 30–60 ml of cerebrospinal fluid, seem to have a better chance of a good response to shunt treatment, although the benefit may be only temporary. A ventriculoperitoneal shunt was therefore inserted (Fig. 6.2), and at the six-month follow-up her gait and urinary symptoms showed further improvement, but the MMSE remained unchanged at 19/30.

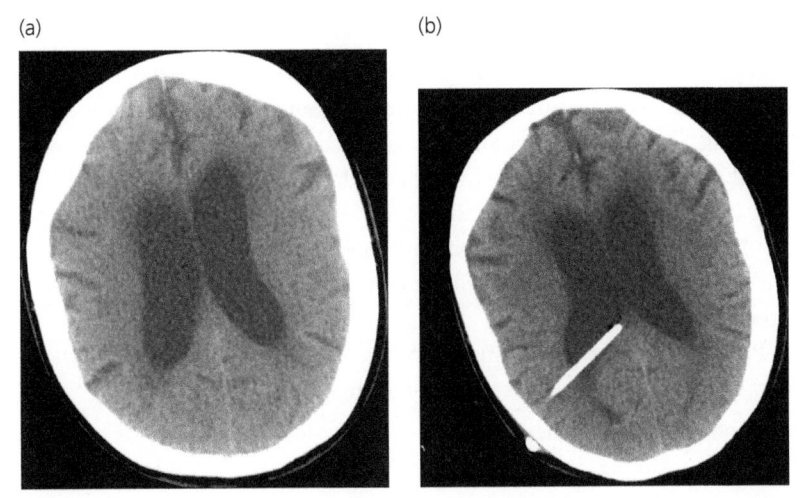

Fig. 6.2 CT scans of the brain: (a) axial slice, from a different patient, who presented with the triad of dementia, urinary incontinence and gait apraxia showing ventriculomegaly, and slight periventricular low attenuation. Image (b) shows the ventriculoperitoneal shunt in situ. There was no change in the radiological appearance (or the clinical status of the patient).

6 List complications of the treatment for this condition.

Shunt complications are common—at almost 40% in some series. Complications include:

- *Subdural haematoma and effusion*—most common during the first 12 months after operation, needing further surgical intervention in a small number of patients.
- *Infection*—usually in the first 30 days after intervention, with patients presenting with vomiting, nausea, headache, fever, and malaise.
- *Abdominal infections, viscus perforation, ascites in ventriculoperitoneal shunts.*
- *Blocked/malfunctioning shunts*—to be suspected if the patient fails to improve or maintain improvement after insertion of a shunt. This may occur at any time.
- *Seizures.*
- *Intracerebral haemorrhage*—according to some authors this is a complication in up to 6% of all patients, mainly presenting immediately after surgery.
- *Death*—perioperative or a consequence of another complication (e.g. postoperative pulmonary embolism).

7 How are patients selected for intervention?

Many centres recommend that a positive response to lumbar tap in the form of an objectively measured improvement in gait is the main indication for shunting. Some authors recommend a magnetic resonance scan with conventional spin echo, and if a prominent aqueductal void in cerebrospinal fluid flow is found, shunting is recommended. One report claims no false positive results with this technique. Patients with normal results needed further tests with a positive quantitative MR phase-contrast cerebrospinal fluid flow before proceeding to shunting.

Predictors for less successful shunting, although not sufficiently reliable alone to exclude shunting as a treatment, are:

- Moderate to severe dementia.
- Late presentation of abnormal gait.
- Advanced age (in some reported series).
- Postural instability if moderate or severe. In one small study it was found that a simple 'pull test' identifying patients unable to maintain posture after a sudden pull on their shoulders from behind while standing with feet slightly apart, was a good diagnostic predictor for poor shunt responsiveness. For most of these patients, an alternative neurological diagnosis was subsequently made.
- Concomitant disorders (e.g. cerebrovascular disorders, Alzheimer's disease).

8 How good are the results of intervention?

The evidence for effectiveness of shunting is poor and derived mainly from small numbers of patients selected through differing criteria, and without validated tools for the measurement of clinical response. Significant benefit from shunting seems to be achieved in only 30–50% of patients. Gait impairment usually shows the earliest and largest response to shunting since the corticospinal tracts supplying lower limb motor function pass close to the lateral ventricles in the corona radiata; one study found that 75% of patients had a positive response to shunting, but only one third maintained improvement over three years.

Urinary symptoms are reported to improve in up to half of cases, with complete remission for only a minority and reported rates of improvement in cognition are generally lower.

A handful of studies have reported better long-term results; the Dutch NPH trial reported that only a minority of patients who improved during the month following the operation declined over the year after the operation.

Further reading

Bradley WG (2000). Normal pressure hydrocephalus: new concepts on etiology and diagnosis. *AJNR Am J Neuroradiol*; **21**: 1586–1590.

Brean A, Eide PK (2008). Prevalence of probable idiopathic normal pressure hydrocephalus in a Norwegian population. *Acta Neurol Scand*; **118**(1): 48–53.

Hebb AO, Cusimano MD (2001). Idiopathic normal pressure hydrocephalus: a systematic review of diagnosis and outcome. *Neurosurgery*; **49**(5): 1166–1184.

Klassen BT, Ahlskog JE (2011). Normal pressure hydrocephalus: how often does the diagnosis hold water? *Neurology*; **77**: 1119–1125.

Marumoto K Koyama T, Hosomi M, Kodama N, Miyake H, Domen K (2012). Diffusion tensor imaging in elderly patients with idiopathic normal pressure hydrocephalus or Parkinson's disease: diagnosis of gait abnormalities. *Fluids Barriers CNS*; **9**: 20.

Momijan S, Owler BK, Czosnyka Z, Czosnyka M, Pena A, Pickard JD (2004). Pattern of white matter regional cerebral blood flow and autoregulation in normal pressure hydrocephalus. *Brain*; **127**(5): 965–972.

Ng SE, Low AM, Tang KK, Lim WE, Kwok RK (2009). Idiopathic normal pressure hydrocephalus: correlating magnetic resonance imaging biomarkers with clinical response. *Ann Acad Med Singapore*; **38**(9): 803–808.

Pujari S, Kharkar S, Metellus P, Shuck J, Williams MA, Rigamonti D (2008). Normal pressure hydrocephalus: long-term outcome after shunt surgery. *J Neurol Neurosurg Psychiatry*; **79**(11): 1282–1286.

Tanaka N, Yamaguchi S, Ishikawa H, Ishii H, Meguro K (2009). Prevalence of possible idiopathic normal-pressure hydrocephalus in Japan: the Osaki-Tajiri project. *Neuroepidemiology*; **32**(3): 171–175.

Case 7

A 76-year-old woman was reviewed in the follow-up clinic six weeks after an admission with heart failure. Following discharge, she had made good progress, and her exercise tolerance had increased steadily. She was now able to manage the stairs slowly without becoming short of breath. However, her daughter was concerned that she had developed urinary incontinence to the extent that she was now reluctant to leave the house.

The patient's past medical history included two myocardial infarctions, hypertension, hypercholesterolaemia, osteoarthritis, cholecystectomy, and occasional constipation. She lived alone in a two-bedroom house and walked using two sticks. Her daughter lived nearby and helped with shopping and cleaning.

Medications taken were aspirin 75mg od, ramipril 5mg od, furosemide 80mg bd, simvastatin 40mg on, amlodipine 5mg od, atenolol 25mg od, paracetamol, codeine phosphate, lactulose prn, senna prn.

On examination, she was able to lie flat, with a respiratory rate of 18 breaths per minute, heart rate 76bpm in atrial fibrillation, and oxygen saturation of 96% on air. There were some fine crepitations at the lung bases bilaterally, but JVP was within normal limits. There was mild pedal oedema bilaterally, but no sacral oedema.

Questions

1. Describe normal bladder physiology.
2. How does ageing affect the bladder?
3. Define and discuss the types of urinary incontinence.
4. How would you further assess this patient's urinary incontinence?
5. Describe the possible contributory causes to this patient's urinary incontinence.
6. Discuss management strategies for urinary incontinence.

Answers

1 Describe normal bladder physiology.

The maintenance of continence is complex. First, a patient must be mentally aware of the need to urinate and be physically able to reach the toilet. The neurological system, anatomy of the bladder, and urinary tract must be intact. Total bladder capacity is between 300–600ml, with the first urge to urinate occurring at 150–300ml. For urination to occur, the detrusor pressure increases to overcome the urethral resistance and the urethral muscle relaxes to facilitate this. Thus if intravesical pressure is greater than urethral resistance at times other than when voiding is desired, urinary leakage will occur. Intravesical pressure may be increased by intra-abdominal masses or by sneezing or laughing.

The bladder is composed of smooth fibres of detrusor muscle. As the bladder fills, there is an increase in sympathetic tone, closing the bladder neck, and causing contraction of the urethra while relaxing the dome of the bladder, thus decreasing parasympathetic activity. Somatic tone is also important in maintaining tone of the pelvic floor muscles especially through the sacral pudendal nerve. During micturition, there is a decrease in sympathetic and somatic tone alongside increasing parasympathetic activity, which causes the detrusor muscle to contract, causing urination. These processes are regulated by areas in the cerebral cortex and cerebellum, and thus can easily be affected by conditions such as dementia (see cases 6, 25, 43, 46), delirium (see case 1), and stroke (see case 19, 42).

2 How does ageing affect the bladder?

Bladder capacity decreases with increasing age, but there is an increase in post-voiding residual volume. There is also an increase in involuntary bladder contractions. While increasing age alone should not cause incontinence, bladder factors, combined with impaired mobility, multiple co-morbidities, and the polypharmacy common in later life, contribute to urinary incontinence.

3 Define and discuss the types of urinary incontinence.

There are four types of urinary incontinence with differing underlying pathogenesis:

Stress incontinence

Stress incontinence occurs when coughing, laughing, straining or lifting heavy objects increases the pressure in the bladder enough to overcome urethral resistance and cause leakage of urine. In women, it is frequently associated with weakened pelvic floor muscles and a history of difficult vaginal delivery. Symptoms often occur after the menopause when there is a decrease in oestrogenic stimulus to pelvic tissues. Stress incontinence is less frequent in men, but can occur after transurethral surgery and damage to the urinary sphincters.

Urge incontinence

Urge incontinence is involuntary leakage of urine accompanied or immediately preceded by urgency to micturate.

Mixed urinary incontinence

Mixed urinary incontinence is characterized by symptoms of both urge and stress incontinence. Treatment should focus on managing the predominant features.

Overactive bladder

In overactive bladder syndrome (OAB) symptoms of urgency occur with ('wet OAB') or without ('dry OAB') urge incontinence. OAB is usually associated with detrusor muscle instability and an increase of involuntary bladder contractions, resulting in increased frequency of voiding, nocturia, and urgency. Sometimes detrusor muscle instability is accompanied by impaired contractility resulting in inability to fully empty the bladder with only around one third of the volume being voided (detrusor hyperactivity and impaired contractility).

4 How would you further assess this patient's urinary incontinence?

In practice, it may be difficult to determine the predominant type of incontinence in a given patient and the symptom complexes frequently overlap. Therefore it is often helpful to adopt a more pragmatic approach in which a careful history and examination are accompanied by assessment for residual post-void volume with bladder ultrasound or in/out catheterization.

The patient or carer should be asked to keep a voiding diary over 4–7 days to establish the pattern of incontinence and the presence of any causative factors. It is important to also record the type and amount of fluid intake at different times throughout the day.

A full abdominal and neurological examination should be performed together with a cognitive screen. The abdominal examination should look for masses compressing the bladder and whether the bladder is palpable.

A digital rectal examination should be performed for sphincter tone and constipation. A vaginal examination should be considered in selected cases to look for atrophy, masses, rectocele, and vaginal prolapse. During vaginal examination, the 'cough test' may be used to assess stress incontinence: urine leakage immediately on coughing indicates weak pelvic floor muscles, whereas urinary leakage occurring a short while after suggests involuntary bladder contraction. The neurological examination should look for evidence of cognitive impairment (acute-delirium, or chronic—MCI or dementia), spinal cord lesions, or neuropathy.

Clinical investigations should include a clean-catch midstream urine sample to look for urinary tract infection, micro- and macroscopic haematuria (suggesting malignancy), and elevated glucose levels suggesting diabetes. A post-voiding residual bladder scan should be considered: a volume of greater than 100ml indicates incomplete bladder emptying. Causes of retention may include:

prostatic hypertrophy/carcinoma

severe constipation

urethral stricture

bladder diverticulum

urinary cystocoele

hypocontractile detrusor

spinal cord disease

bladder tumour.

Retention may present acutely with pain or if chronic, with abdominal mass, incontinence (dribbling overflow or urge from detrusor instability), infection, hydronephrosis, and renal failure, or with delirium (see case 1).

Further imaging studies may be appropriate, e.g. abdominal ultrasound to evaluate hydronephrosis or to assess abdominal masses. Urodynamic flow studies may be necessary where the sub-type of urinary incontinence remains uncertain. Rarely spinal MRI or other specialist imaging may be required.

5 Describe the possible contributory causes to this patient's urinary incontinence.

There are many possible contributing causes to this patient's urinary incontinence. Given the recent admission for heart failure, medications may have been added or altered. Furosemide may lead to urinary incontinence and ramipril may also contribute, since approximately 20% of patients taking ACE inhibitors develop a dry cough, which may worsen stress incontinence.

Constipation may have been exacerbated by codeine phosphate taken to relieve arthritic pain. In addition, the patient has limited mobility, requiring two sticks for walking and although her condition is improving, she can only manage stairs slowly. Perhaps she is unable to reach her bathroom in time, to which a simple solution would be to place a commode in an accessible area. A more detailed history and bladder diary revealed that the patient had symptoms of urgency and owing to her poor mobility was unable to reach the upstairs bathroom in her house. A commode was placed downstairs, and her furosemide was reduced to 80mg in the morning and 40mg at lunchtime. She was reviewed in clinic three months later and she had not had any further exacerbations of heart failure, and her symptoms of urinary incontinence had resolved.

6 Discuss possible management strategies for urinary incontinence.

First line management for stress incontinence or mixed symptoms should be pelvic floor exercises. Ideally these should be continued for at least three months before deemed ineffective. If unsuccessful, surgical intervention should be considered and suitable patients offered retropubic mid-urethral vaginal tape procedures, colposuspension, or injections of intramural bulking agents such as silicone, carbon-coated zirconium beads, or hyaluronic acid. However, it is important that women are made aware that they may require repeated injections to achieve efficacy, and that the effects can decrease over time. It also tends to be less successful than synthetic tapes or rectus fascia sling procedures.

For predominantly overactive bladder symptoms with or without urge incontinence, first line management is bladder retraining. For patients with cognitive impairment, carers should initiate regular toileting programmes. If this does not alleviate symptoms, then a trial of bladder stabilizing drugs (e.g. solifenacin, tolterodine) may be considered, although patients should be monitored for retention. Such drugs have anti-cholinergic effects and may cause dry mouth, constipation, postural hypotension, or exacerbation of cognitive impairment (see cases 6, 25, 43, 46). In patients with proven detrusor overactivity that has not responded to conservative management, bladder wall injection with botulinum toxin A can be considered after MDT review. This often has good clinical effect and results in the majority of women being symptom-free or having a large reduction in symptoms. However, the effects of the injection tend to wear off over time and this can mean repeated injections are required. This form of therapy can only be considered in women who are able and willing to be trained in intermittent self-catheterization as this can be required for variable lengths of time after the effects of the injections have worn off. In women who are unable to perform intermittent self-catheterization, or who have not responded to botulinum injections, then percutaneous nerve stimulation can be an option. Percutaneous sacral nerve stimulation is when the sacral nerve is stimulated by an implantable pulse generator via an electrode placed through the sacral foramen.

Alpha blockers (e.g. doxazosin, tamsulosin) may be used in benign prostatic hypertrophy to improve flow, although may cause hypotension. Double micturition (urinating twice within a few minutes) may help reduce residual volume and risk of UTI, although for atonic or hyponic bladders intermittent self-catheterization may be used in able patients.

Further reading

NICE Guidelines (Sept 2013). Urinary incontinence: The management of urinary incontinence in women.

Rogers RG (2008). Clinical practice: urinary stress incontinence in women. *N Engl J Med*; **358**: 1029–1036.

Shamliyan TA, Kane RL, Wyman J, Wilt TJ (2008). Systematic review: randomized, controlled trials of nonsurgical treatments for urinary incontinence in women. *Ann Intern Med*; **148**(6): 459–473.

SIGN guidelines (Dec 2004). 79: Management of urinary incontinence in primary care.

Wein AJ, Rackley RR (2006). Overactive bladder: a better understanding of pathophysiology, diagnosis and management. *J Urol*; **175**(3 pt 2): s5–s10.

Wood L, Anger J (2014). Urinary incontinence in women. *BMJ*; **15**: 349.

Case 8

A 72-year-old woman presented to the emergency department in a confused state with visual hallucinations. She had been found by her niece, still in bed in the afternoon in an unkempt state, talking to herself, and unable to recognize her niece. She appeared to have spent the past few days in bed and had not been seen by her neighbours or friends for several days. Approximately one week earlier, she had complained to her niece of some chest pain, and a cough. There was no past medical history other than hypertension.

She was a retired librarian living alone and was previously active and independent, playing golf weekly, and going for walks with friends almost every weekend. She did not smoke or drink. Her medications included ramipril and occasional paracetamol.

On examination, she was agitated and uncooperative with confused speech. Her AMTS was 0/10 and CAM was 4/4 consistent with delirium. Observations showed a temperature of 35.8° C, blood pressure 120/65mmHg, heart rate 90bpm, respiratory rate of 22 breaths per minute, and oxygen saturation 94% on 10L oxygen. There were coarse bilateral basal crepitations on auscultating the chest. The rest of the examination was unremarkable.

Investigations showed the following:

Hb 11g/dL; WCC 12.07 × 10^9/L; (neutroph.10.8 × 10^9/L); plt 356 × 10^9/L

Na: 135mmol/L; K 3.5mmol/L; urea 13.2mmol/L; creatinine 156mmol/L

CRP: >160mg/L

LFTs, TSH, and free thyroxine were normal

Calcium 4.45mmol/L; adjusted calcium 4.39mmol/L; phosphate 1.72mmol/L; PTH 0.4pmol/L

Arterial blood gas: pH 7.42, pCO_2 6.00kPa, pO_2 6.51kPa; lactate 3.2mmol/L;

ECG: sinus tachycardia

Chest X-ray: see Figure 8.1.

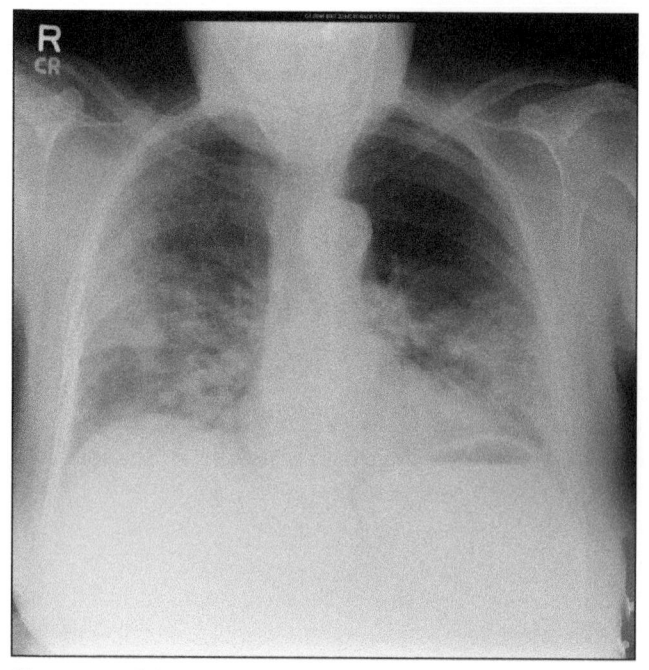

Fig. 8.1 Chest X-ray of the patient.

Questions

1 Describe the chest X-ray and state the most likely diagnoses in view of the clinical findings. What are the possible causes of hypercalcaemia in this case?
2 List the most common presenting features of hypercalcaemia.
3 How would you investigate this patient further?

Answers

1 Describe the chest X-ray and state the most likely diagnoses in view of the clinical findings. What are the possible causes of hypercalcaemia in this case?

The CXR shows extensive bilateral perihilar consolidation consistent with infection (Fig. 8.2). Pulmonary oedema could result in a similar appearance, but the heart size is within normal limits and the clinical picture is not consistent with this diagnosis.

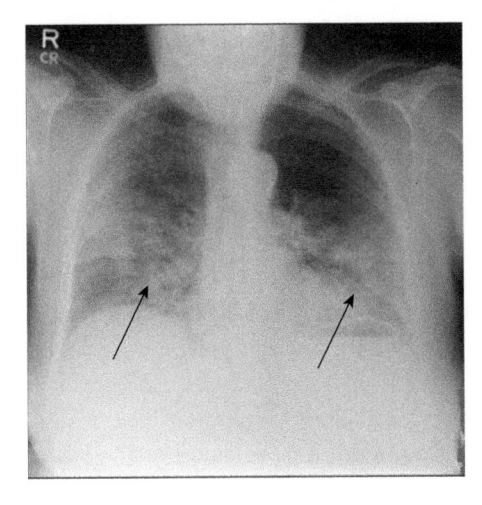

Fig. 8.2 The chest X-ray shows bilateral lung consolidations with a basal predominance (arrows).

The likely diagnoses include delirium (see case 1), secondary to chest infection, hypoxia, dehydration, and hypercalcaemia.

Hypercalcaemia is a relatively common clinical problem in older people and affects around 5% of hospitalized patients. The vast majority (~ 80%) are caused by primary hyperparathyroidism or malignancy. Primary hyperparathyroidism usually occurs in relatively well ambulatory patients, who are in the majority older than 65 years, three times more likely to be female, and calcium is not usually elevated above 3.25mmol/L. Parathyroid hormone level (PTH) is also important to exclude parathyroid crisis; patients may present with abdominal pain, coma, heart failure, and volume depletion. The current patient was unwell, had very abnormal calcium with a suppressed PTH and could thus not have had primary hyperparathyroidism. Causes of hypercalcaemia to consider in the current case are:

Malignancy: usually associated with osteolytic metastases that release local osteoclastic activating factors, production of calcitriol, ectopic parathyroid hormone, or PTH-related protein (a humoral factor that increases bone reabsorption in the skeleton and decreases renal excretion of calcium). Breast cancer is the most common cause, but others include ovarian, lung, oesophagus, kidney, cervix, and lymphoproliferative disorders (e.g. multiple myeloma, lymphomas). Malignant cause should be considered if hypercalcaemia is associated with rapid onset, systemic symptoms (e.g. loss of weight, poor appetite, malaise), and suppressed serum parathyroid hormone.

Infection and immobility. Immobilization causes osteoclastic bone resorption and release of calcium, suppression of PTH, and increased serum phosphate which reduces synthesis of 1,25-dihydroxy vitamin D. Hypercalcaemia occurs when bone resorption exceeds calcium excretion and this is more likely with concurrent infection including granulomatous disease (tuberculosis, leprosy), fungal illness (candidiasis, coccidiomycosis, histoplasmosis), cat scratch fever, and AIDS. Various humoral factors (PTH-like peptide, cytokines, interleukin-1, interleukin-6, tumour necrosis factor) produced during infection are thought to combine with the potentiating effects of acute illness on immobilization-induced bone resorption to raise calcium levels. Occasionally, immobilization may be associated with high calcium in the absence of infection, e.g. in long-term hospitalized disabled patients (e.g. post-stroke, polyneuropathy, hip fracture and spinal cord injury), and in very obese patients with critical illness and immobility in whom there is a sudden loss of weight-bearing effects on the bones.

There are many rare causes of hypercalcaemia of which the more common include:

- Drugs (e.g. thiazides [8% of such patients develop hypercalcaemia], lithium, calcium carbonate [antacid], vitamins D and A, theophyllines, methotrexate).
- Hyperproteinaemia (severe dehydration can cause hyperalbuminaemia with high protein binding of calcium).
- Paget's disease (see case 12).
- Milk-alkali syndrome.
- Familial hypocalciuric hypercalcaemia (usually long-standing and asymptomatic).
- Endocrinopathies of non-parathyroid origin, for example adrenal insufficiency. In Addisonian crisis, hypercalcaemia may occur from increased bone resorption, increased tubular calcium reabsorption, and increased binding to serum proteins. Hyperthyroidism causes mild hypercalcaemia in a minority of patients.

Rhabdomyolysis and acute renal failure. Hypercalcaemia can occur during the diuretic phase of renal failure and is common in patients with rhabdomyolysis owing to calcium release from injured muscle.

Sarcoidosis (due to calcitriol released from macrophages), Wegener's granulomatosis, acute granulomatous pneumonitis, granulomatous reaction to silicone injections.

Crohn's disease.

Renal insufficiency and high calcium intake.

2 List the most common presenting features of hypercalcaemia.

Patients with hypercalcaemia may present with confusion, lethargy, depression, stupor, coma, constipation, nausea, vomiting, peptic ulcer disease, muscle weakness (particularly proximal muscle weakness in the legs) and may have bony tenderness to palpation. There may also be polyuria, haematuria, or renal colic in cases of nephrolithiasis, hypertension, bradycardia, hyperreflexia, tongue fasciculation, and anorexia. The symptoms will depend on the rate and degree of rise of calcium: calcium levels of up to 3.5mmol/L can be well tolerated if developing gradually, but rapid elevation will cause symptoms.

3 How would you investigate this patient further?

Further investigations done in this patient included:

Blood and urine cultures, and serology for *Legionella*—all of which were negative.

Serum electrophoresis and urine electrophoresis to exclude multiple myeloma, results showed generalized proteinuria only.

PTH-related protein level (PTH-rp), which is usually increased in patients with humoral hypercalcaemia of malignancy. High levels indicate a poor prognosis and advanced disease. PTH-rp was negative in this patient.

Vitamin D metabolite levels (calcitriol and calcidiol). Calcitriol may be elevated in cases of primary hyperparathyroidism, lymphoma, and granulomatous disease; patients with high calcitriol should be investigated for these if no other cause of high calcium is apparent. Elevated calcidiol occurs in vitamin D intoxication. None was detectable in this patient.

Bone marrow aspirate/trephine, which did not demonstrate malignant cells.

Serum cortisol, adrenocorticotropic hormone (ACTH), Synacthen test: normal.

Bronchoalveolar lavage showed acute inflammation with no malignant cells; subsequent culture grew *Proteus mirabilis* and coliforms, but no mycobacteria.

HIV, syphilis: negative.

In most cases of hypercalcaemia, CXR (to look for evidence of malignancy or sarcoidosis), serum/urine electrophoresis for multiple myeloma and PTH level reveal the cause, and extensive investigation is not usually necessary.

Other helpful tests may be:

Urine calcium excretion level:

High or high-normal in malignancy and hyperparathyroidism, low in: (a) drugs, such as thiazide diuretics, which enhance calcium reabsorption in the distal tubule; (b) familial hypocalciuric hypercalcaemia and milk-alkali syndrome (the latter associated with metabolic alkalosis, mechanism unknown).

Serum chloride:

High (>103meq/L) in hyperparathyroidism and low in milk-alkali syndrome.

Serum phosphate:

Low level is common in hyperparathyroidism and malignancy due to inhibition of renal proximal tubular phosphate reabsorption, while high or normal levels are found in milk-alkali syndrome, immobilization, metastatic bone disease, granulomatous disease, thyrotoxicosis, and vitamin D intoxication.

CASE 8 | 81

Case progression

The patient continued to deteriorate and went on to have a CT scan of the chest (Fig. 8.3) together with the abdomen and pelvis, the latter being normal.

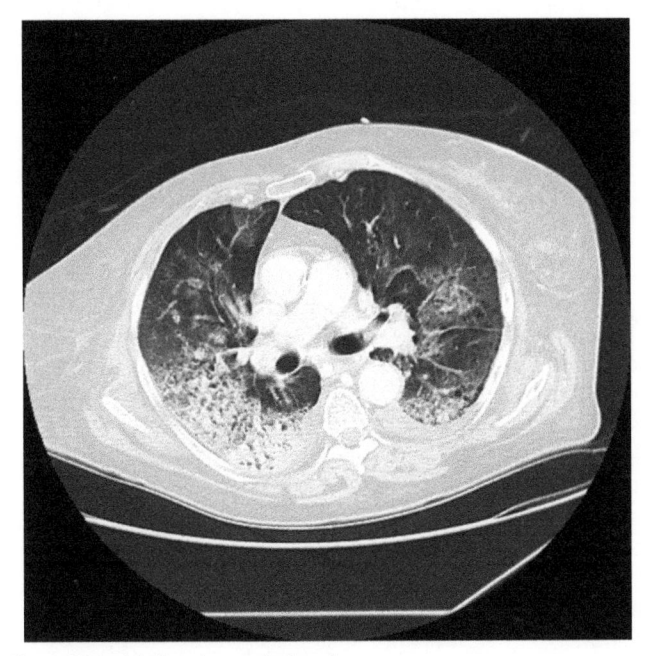

Fig. 8.3 Chest CT (axial slice, lung windows).

Questions continued

4 Describe the CT scan of the chest (Fig 8.3).
5 How would you manage this patient?
6 What do you think now to have been the cause of the hypercalcaemia, knowing that the CT of the abdomen and pelvis was normal?
7 What are the possible complications of hypercalcaemia?

Answers continued

4 Describe the CT scan of the chest (Fig 8.3).

The CT scan of the chest on lung windows shows extensive bilateral ground glass changes (large black arrows), posterior consolidations, with multiple bilateral small cystic/cavitating lung lesions (white arrow), and small pleural effusions (small black arrows) (Fig. 8.4). This was supportive of the diagnosis of chest infection. Bronchoalveolar lavage showed acute inflammation with no malignant cells, while subsequent culture grew *Proteus mirabilis* and coliforms, but no mycobacteria.

Fig. 8.4 The CT chest shows extensive bilateral ground glass changes (large black arrows), posterior consolidations and multiple bilateral small cystic/cavitating lung lesions (white arrow), and small pleural effusions (small black arrows).

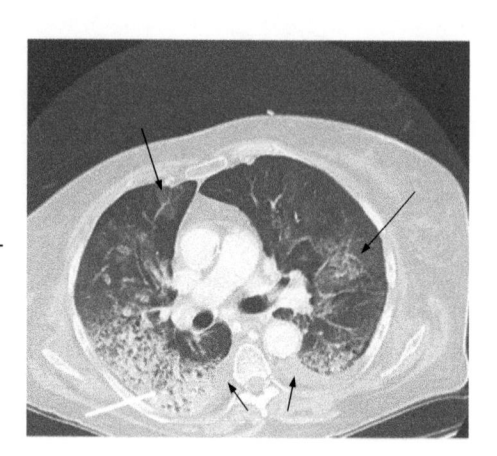

5 How would you manage this patient?

The patient was given fluids in order to restore extracellular fluid volume and reduce the inhibition of bone resorption together with calcitonin, intravenous bisphosphonates and antibiotics. She required ionotropic and ventilatory support in the intensive care unit. Calcium was normal on the third day after admission. Despite intensive treatment, she died on the tenth day of admission and the post-mortem examination revealed cavitating pneumonia, with no evidence of lung carcinoma, parathyroid tumours/hyperplasia, metastatic carcinoma, or multiple myeloma. The blood cultures subsequently grew Proteus.

In general, treatment of hypercalcaemia is through rehydration and diuresis to increase renal loss of calcium. In hypercalcaemia caused by immobility, contributing medications (e.g. vitamin D, calcium, thiazides) should be discontinued and volume repletion, antiosteoclastic agents, and passive mobility rehabilitation should be considered.

In mild hypercalcaemia (Ca <2.88mmol/L):

with mild symptoms, there is no need for urgent treatment, but the cause should be established, and the appropriate treatment started.

with significant symptoms immediate treatment is required, with intravenous fluids and loop diuretic, together with treatment of the underlying cause. Patients should be monitored for fluid balance, low potassium, and low magnesium.

Symptomatic hypercalcaemia or hypercalcaemia with serum adjusted Ca >3mmol/L) requires rapid correction of calcium with:

fluid replacement

agents that decrease bone resorption (e.g. bisphosphonates with osteoclast activity inhibition). Calcitonin can be used as an early treatment agent for severe hypercalcaemia, while the onset of action by other hypocalcaemic medications is awaited, as calcitonin works within two hours of administration. The disadvantage for its use is drug tolerance, which usually develops within two days.

haemodialysis (e.g. peritoneal dialysis) if there is a need for urgent lowering, if levels are refractory despite standard treatments (e.g. in parathyroid carcinoma) or if there is accompanying renal failure.

6 What do you think now to have been the cause of the hypercalcaemia, knowing that the CT of the abdomen and pelvis was normal?

The cause of hypercalcaemia was thought to have been severe community acquired pneumonia associated with sepsis and immobility. The high level of C-reactive protein indicated markedly increased circulatory pro-inflammatory cytokines. The very high level of calcium normalized with rehydration and bisphosphonates, suggesting that metastatic bone cancer, hematopoietic tumours, granulomatous disease, and solid tumours were unlikely. The abnormal renal function corrected with rehydration and normalization of calcium. The cause of death was multiple organ failure due to severe pneumonia and hypercalcaemia, associated with sepsis, and immobility.

Hypercalcaemia alone may induce acute renal failure as well as exacerbate chronic renal failure. Conversely, the presence of pre-existing renal failure in patients with new onset of immobilization is a high risk factor for the development of hypercalcaemia and rapid deterioration of renal function.

7 What are the possible complications of hypercalcaemia?

Complications of hypercalcaemia include:

- cardiovascular dysfunction: bradycardia, atrioventricular block, and arrhythmias
- hypertension
- hypercalcaemic crisis (Ca>4 mmol/L) leading to encephalopathy, acute renal failure, and death
- multiple organ failure, acute renal failure
- nephrocalcinosis.

Further reading

Gallacher SJ, Ralston SH, Dryburgh FJ, et al. (1990). Immobilization-related hypercalcaemia- a possible novel mechanism and response to pamidronate. *Postgrad Med J*; **66**(781): 918–922.

Jacobs TP, Bilezikian JP (2005). Rare causes of hypercalcaemia. *J Clin Endocrinol Metab*; **90**(11): 6316–6322.

Jeffries CC, Ledgerwood AM, Lucas CE (2005). Life-threatening tertiary hyperparathyroidism in the critically ill. *Am J Surg*; **189**: 369–372.

Loh HH, Noor NM (2014). The use of hemodialysis in refractory hypercalcemia secondary to parathyroid carcinoma. *Case Rep Crit Care*; 140906.

Minisola S, Pepe J, Piemonte S, Cipriani C (2015). The diagnosis and management of hypercalcaemia. *BMJ*; 350: h2723.

Nierman DM, Mechanik JI (2000). Biochemical response to treatment of bone hyperresorption in chronically critical ill patients. *Chest*; **118**: 761–766.

Sugimoto T, Sakaguchi M, Ogawa N, et al. (2007). Marked hypercalcaemia in sepsis-induced multiple organ failure. *Nephrol Dial Transplant*; **22**: 1272–1273.

Case 9

A 72-year-old Afro-Caribbean man was reviewed in the follow-up clinic six weeks after hospitalization for heart failure, during which his treatment was changed. Following discharge, his breathing had improved such that he was able to walk at least half a mile before becoming short of breath. However, he had lost a stone in weight and complained of poor appetite, nausea, and a rash that had developed shortly after discharge and was worsening despite prescription of an emollient cream. There was no change in bowel habit. He also complained of left knee discomfort.

He lived with his wife and nephew in a three-bedroom house, and had been a UK resident since emigrating from Trinidad 47 years earlier. He had given up smoking after his first myocardial infarction at age 41, although still drank a shot of rum each night. He had had a further myocardial infarction two years before and the past history also included hypertension, hypercholesterolaemia, asthma, hypothyroidism, gastric ulcer, and diverticular disease.

Medications taken were aspirin 75mg od, omeprazole 20mg od, simvastatin 20mg od, hydralazine 50mg bd, ramipril 10mg od, isosorbide dinitrate 80mg bd, bisoprolol 2.5mg od, paracetamol 1g qds, codeine phosphate 30mg qds, and levothyroxine 75mcg od.

On examination, observations were stable, but temperature was 37.8°C. The jugular venous pressure was not raised. The apex beat was displaced laterally and there was a quiet pansystolic murmur. There were a few bibasal crepitations and some mild pitting pedal oedema of the ankles. The abdomen was soft and non-tender with normal bowel sounds. There was an erythematous maculopapular rash on the trunk with some surrounding excoriation marks. The patient had some difficulty in getting on and off the examination couch owing to left knee pain, but the joint did not appear to be swollen or erythematous.

Investigations showed the following:

- Hb: 9.6g/dL
- MCV: 79fL
- WCC: 13.1×10^9/L
- Neut: 6.7×10^9/L

- Na: 133mmol/L
- K: 4.2mmol/L
- Urea: 10mmol/L; baseline 8mmol/L
- Creat: 122μmol/L; baseline 116μmol/L
- ALT: 26IU/L
- Bili: 14μmol/L
- Alp: 240U/L
- Albumin: 27g/L
- CRP: 38mg/L.

Questions

1 What is the most likely explanation of this patient's symptoms and how would you confirm the diagnosis?
2 What are the other clinical features of this condition?
3 How would you manage this patient?

Answers

1 What is the most likely explanation of this patient's symptoms and how would you confirm the diagnosis?

The most likely diagnosis is drug-induced systemic lupus erythematosus. This Afro-Caribbean man presented with weight loss, nausea, and a low-grade fever, rash, and joint pain. Investigations showed microcytic anaemia, elevated white cell count, and mildly raised CRP. These features are consistent with systemic lupus erythematosus (SLE), secondary to hydralazine. Other implicated drugs include methyldopa, minocyline, diltiazem, quinidine, the oral contraceptive pill, and sulphonamides. Risk of hydralazine-induced SLE is dose related and symptoms may occur weeks to years after initiation of the drug causing diagnostic difficulty.

The exact mechanism by which hydralazine causes SLE is unclear, but it has been linked to HLA—DR4 in those who are 'slow acetylators'. The prevalence is also higher in older patients because of decreased drug clearance and the increased likelihood of polypharmacy, which can interfere with the metabolism of the drug resulting in higher serum levels. There are no established criteria for the diagnosis of drug-induced SLE, but there should be at least one clinical feature of SLE with positive antinuclear antibodies (ANA) and clinical improvement is usually rapid after withdrawal of the responsible medication. Antihistone antibodies are present in over 90% of cases, but are rarely accompanied by the presence of other non-ANA autoantibodies, in contrast to idiopathic SLE where antihistone antibodies (present in 80%) are accompanied by anti-dsDNA antibodies in 80%, anti-sm antibodies in 20–30%, and anti-RNP antibodies in 40–50%.

2 What are the other clinical features of this condition?

Drug-induced SLE has many clinical features in common with idiopathic SLE, but tends to run a milder clinical course with less severe multisystem involvement. It affects males and females equally in comparison to SLE, which has a strong female preponderance. Arthralgias and myalgias are prominent features, although rashes are seen less frequently affecting only 10–20% of patients, compared with around 70% in idiopathic SLE. Chest pain secondary to pleurisy and pericarditis may occur, but involvement of the central nervous system is rare. Necrotizing glomerulonephritis is the most common form of renal disease in drug-induced SLE, with immune-complex mediated glomerulonephritis being less common. In hydralazine-induced nephritis anti-MPO and atypical ANCA antibodies, such as anti-lactoferrin and anti-elastase, are found.

3 How would you manage this patient?

The most important management step is to recognize the condition and to withdraw the hydralazine. Symptoms should resolve within weeks and rarely is any other intervention required. In cases of disabling polyarthropathy, a short course of low dose corticosteroid therapy may be used. Occasionally, cytotoxic therapy such as cyclophosphamide is required. Where blood pressure has been well controlled by hydralazine, there is some evidence to suggest that cadralazine, another vasodilator metabolized via a different pathway, may offer good hypertensive control without the side effects of hydralazine. In case reports where patients have been switched from hydralazine to cadralazine, there has been resolution of lupus symptoms, and ANA titres have returned to negative within months. It should be noted that this patient is not on spironolactone, which has been shown to reduce symptoms and mortality in patients with severe heart failure, and might obviate the need for hydralazine-type medication.

Further reading

Finks SW, Finks AL, Self TH (2006). Hydralazine-induced lupus: maintaining vigilance with increased use in patients with heart failure. *South Med J*; **99**(1): 18–22.

Mulder H (1990). Conversion of drug induced SLE syndrome by the vasodilating agent cadralazine. *Eur J Clin Pharmacol*; **38**: 303.

Sarzi-Puttini P, Atzeni F, Capsoni F, Lubrano E, Doria A (2005). Drug-induced lupus erythematosus. *Autoimmunity*; **38**(7): 507–518.

Case 10

A 68-year-old woman presented to the rapid access geratology clinic with a four-week history of malaise, lethargy, and loss of appetite. Over the preceding two weeks, she had developed night sweats, and frequent episodes of rigor. There was a past history of a fall, and right arm fracture 10 years earlier, together with osteoporosis. She suffered from chronic left shoulder pain, and four weeks previously had had an intra-articular shoulder injection as a day-case procedure in a local hospital. She lived with her husband and was taking calcium, vitamin D, and risedronate.

On examination, she was alert and orientated, but her temperature was 38.5°C with a tachycardia of 140bpm regular, and a blood pressure of 105/70mmHg. There was a systolic murmur at the left sternal border and at the apex, radiating to the neck, and to the axilla. There were a few basal crepitations bilaterally and oxygen saturation was 95% on air. The abdomen was unremarkable, neck stiffness was absent, and examination of the cranial nerves and limbs was normal.

Investigations showed the following:

- Hb 10.2g/dL; MCV 94.8fL; WCC 28.37 × 10^9/L (polymorphs 24.68 × 10^9/L; lymphocytes 2.27 × 109/L; monocytes 1.42 × 109g/L); platelets 150 × 10^9/L
- Prothrombin time 13.5s; APTT 34s
- Na 141mmol/L; K 4.3mmol/L; Cr 120μmol/L; glucose 6mmol/L; bili 18μmol/L; alb 35g/L; ALT 45 IU/L; alk phos 330IU/L
- ESR 110mmH; CRP 70mg/L
- Urinalysis: blood +, no protein, no nitrites
- Chest X-ray: see Fig. 10.1
- ECG: sinus rhythm; occasional ventricular extrasystoles
- Urine dipstick: trace of protein and blood; urine culture: negative
- Blood culture (sample taken in the community): *Staphyloccocus aureus*.

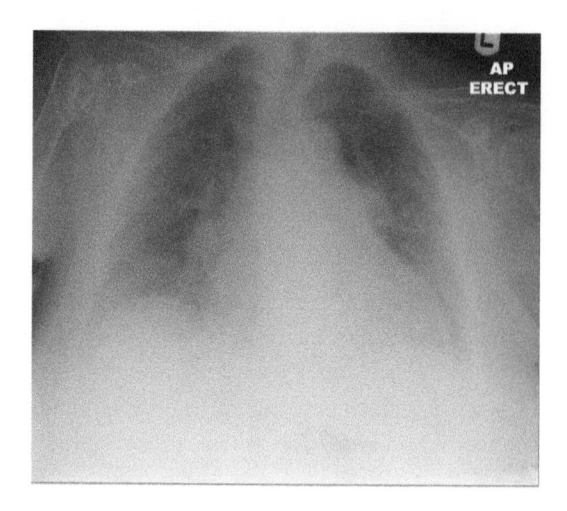

Fig. 10.1 Chest X-ray of the patient.

Questions

1. What does the chest X-ray show (Fig.10.1)? What is the most likely underlying diagnosis and when should you suspect it in older patients?
2. How would you confirm the diagnosis in this patient? List the diagnostic criteria.
3. List the most common risk factors for this condition in developed countries.
4. How may the clinical features of this condition differ in older versus younger patients?
5. How would you manage this patient?

Answers

1 What does the chest X-ray show? What is the most likely underlying diagnosis and when should you suspect it in older patients?

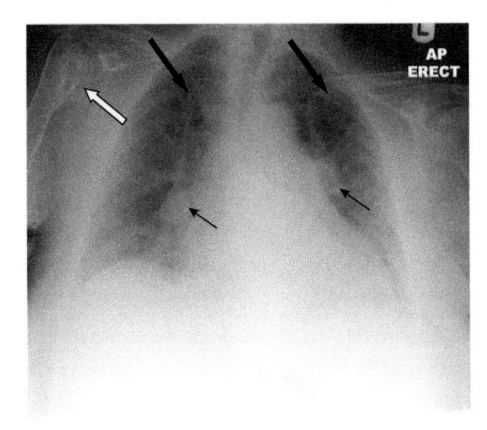

Fig. 10.2 The patient's chest x-ray with arrows indicating abnormalities (see text).

The chest X-ray (Fig10.2) shows an enlarged heart, large bulky hila (small black arrows) and upper lobe vein diversion (large black arrows) consistent with left ventricular volume overload. An old fracture of the right shoulder with secondary osteoarthritis (OA) is also noted (white arrow).

The history of intra-articular injection followed by malaise, lethargy, loss of appetite, night sweats and rigors, together with the examination findings of systolic murmur and cardiomegaly, suggests the diagnosis of infective endocarditis. The intra-articular injection is assumed to have been the portal of entry of infection. Infective endocarditis may be more common after invasive procedures in older patients (>70 years), or following previous hospitalization. Older patients are also more likely to have cardiac structural changes, including valvular sclerosis and prosthetic heart valves, and thus greater susceptibility to endocarditis. Young people in contrast, are more likely to develop endocarditis following intravenous drug use, with higher incidence of right-sided endocarditis.

Infective endocarditis is an incompletely understood, heterogeneous disease, caused by microbial infection of the endocardial surface, or prosthetic material in the heart. It has an incidence of between 1.4–6.2 per 100,000 people a year. If not treated, infective endocarditis is almost always fatal and has a significant mortality rate even with treatment. The mean age of patients with infective endocarditis has risen to over 60 years since the 1990s, owing to a significant decline in the prevalence of chronic rheumatic heart disease in industrialized societies (the mean age was 30 years in the 1950s). The overall incidence of infective endocarditis has however remained the same over the past 30 years owing to changes in the nature of the associated risk factors.

Infective endocarditis can present as an acute, subacute, or chronic disease. Some patients may only have low-grade fever or other non-specific symptoms and up to 25% of older patients may have symptoms for over one month before diagnosis. The differential diagnosis often includes chronic infection, malignancy, autoimmune, or rheumatological disease (see cases 16, 39).

Infective endocarditis should be suspected if the patient has:

- A new regurgitation murmur.
- Temperature of >38°C accompanied by previous infective endocarditis, degenerative, or congenital valvular heart disease, intracardial prosthetic devices, recent intervention with bacteraemia, positive blood cultures typical for infective endocarditis, systemic abscesses (e.g. spleen, cerebral, pulmonary embolism/infiltration), new conduction abnormalities, congestive heart failure, Osler nodes, Roth spots, Janeway lesions (only found in around 5% of patients), or splinter haemorrhages. It should be noted that fever may be absent in older patients, the immunocompromized, or in those on antibiotic treatment.
- Fever or sepsis of unknown origin (see case 16).
- Systemic embolic state of unknown origin.

The most common organisms in infective endocarditis are:

- *Staphylococcus aureus* (most common). All patients found to have Staphylococcal bacteraemia, should be clinically evaluated for infective endocarditis.
- Viridans group streptococci (becoming less common).
- *Streptococcus bovis* (especially common in Europe).
- Entercocci.
- Around 10% of patients with infective endocarditis have negative bacterial cultures owing to inadequate microbiological techniques, administration of antimicrobials before sampling, or the presence of nonbacterial, fastidious, or slow-growing microorganisms including fungi, *Chlamydia spp*, *Bartonella spp*, *Coxiella burnetii*, Brucella *spp*, mycobacteria, viruses, *Tropheryma whipplei* or HACEK organisms (*Haemophilus spp, Actinobacillus actinomycetemcomitans, Cardiobacterium hominis, Eikenella spp, Kingella*). Such patients need serological tests or cell cultures, depending on history and exposure to risk factors.

It remains unclear why gram-negative aerobic bacilli seldom adhere to vegetations.

2 How would you confirm the diagnosis in this patient? List the diagnostic criteria.

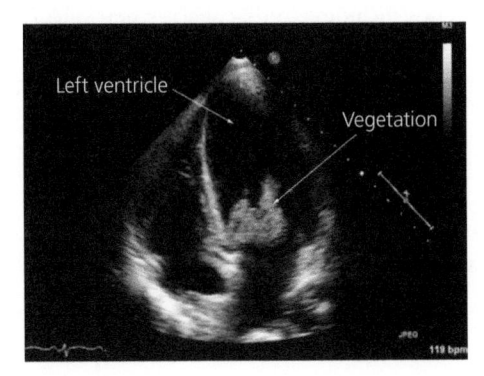

Fig. 10.3 Transthoracic echocardiograph from the patient, showing a large vegetation on the mitral valve.

This patient had three blood cultures taken from different sites, which were all positive for *Staphyloccocus aureus*. Transthoracic echocardiography was performed which revealed a large vegetation over the mitral valve (see Fig. 10.3).

Transthoracic echocardiography has a sensitivity for vegetations in infective endocarditis of around 60% and specificity of 100%. Transoesophageal echocardiography (which may not be readily available in many clinical settings) is more sensitive (approaching 100%) without a loss of specificity and is particularly good at visualizing cardiac abscesses, for evaluating prosthetic valves, severe valvular regurgitation, and aortic valve pathology.

Repeated ECGs should be performed to look for conduction abnormalities indicating infection-abscess extending to the valvular annulus, or new ischaemia resulting from emboli to the coronary circulation. The chest X-ray may reveal heart failure (as shown in Fig. 10.1) and focal infiltrates with/or without cavitations from septic pulmonary emboli. Early cerebral MRI scanning to look for ischaemic stroke and mycotic aneurysms is controversial, but may lead to a change of therapeutic strategy (e.g. valve replacement versus conservative management).

In this patient, the diagnosis was confirmed with positive major blood and ECHO Duke criteria, with additional positive minor criteria for the diagnosis of infective endocarditis.

The revised Duke criteria for the diagnosis of infective endocarditis are*:

Major criteria

- Three positive blood cultures for organisms consistent with endocarditis
- Two positive blood cultures for organisms typical of endocarditis
- One positive blood culture or serologic evidence for *Coxiella burnetii*
- Echocardiographic evidence, including cardiac abscess, new valvular regurgitation, new dehiscence of prosthetic valve, oscillating intracardiac mass (e.g. on implanted material, on a heart valve, or supporting structures).

Minor criteria

- Vascular lesions (e.g. Janeway lesions, conjunctiva, or intracranial haemorrhages, arterial embolism, mycotic aneurysm, septic pulmonary embolism)
- Temperature >38°C
- Intravenous drug abuse
- Serologic evidence of infection with organisms consistent with infective endocarditis
- Predisposing cardiac condition
- Immunological phenomena such as rheumatoid factor, Roth's spots, Osler nodes, glomerulonephritis (usually with positive red cell casts in urine)
- Blood cultures consistent with, but not meeting the major criteria listed.

Definite clinical diagnosis:

Histological tissue showing microorganism or microorganisms cultured from intracardiac abscess, vegetations or tissue, or two major criteria, or one major and three minor criteria, or five minor criteria.

Possible diagnosis:

- One major and one minor criterion, or three minor criteria.

The diagnosis of infective endocarditis is rejected in cases of:

- symptom resolution in ≤ four days of antibiotic use
- alternative diagnosis

(*Adapted from Li JS, Sexton DJ, Mick N, *et al.* (2000). Proposed modifications to the Duke criteria for the diagnosis of infective endocarditis. *Clin Infect Dis;* 30: 633–638, American Heart Association.)

- insufficient criteria for the diagnosis of possible infective endocarditis
- no pathological evidence of infective endocarditis at autopsy or surgery in cases with ≤ four days of antibiotic

3 List the most common risk factors for this condition in developed countries.

Risk factors for infective endocarditis include:

- history of a hospital-based invasive procedure with risk of bacteraemia within three preceding months (as seen in the current patient)
- a pre-existing valve lesion (congenital or more frequently degenerative)
- older age (ECHO detects degenerative valve lesions in up to 50% of asymptomatic patients aged over 60 years probably accounting for the increased risk of infective endocarditis in the older population)
- intracardiac devices, e.g. pacemaker
- intravenous drug usage (rarer in older patients)
- prosthetic valve
- previous history of endocarditis
- diabetes mellitus
- bacteraemia with particularly virulent microorganisms
- haemodialysis.

4 How may the clinical features of this condition differ in older versus younger patients?

Older patients with degenerative and prosthetic valvular disease are now the most vulnerable to infective endocarditis. The mitral valve is affected in up to 50% and the aortic valve in around 40% of patients; other sites such as the tricuspid or pulmonary valve, pacemaker leads, and mural endocardium are less frequently affected.

Infective endocarditis in older versus younger patients has the following characteristics:

- Patients more commonly present only with confusion, fever of unknown origin (see case 16), weight loss, or anorexia.
- Fever may be less frequent or even absent.
- Diagnosis is more frequently delayed.
- The clinical course may be more severe (related to insidious initial symptoms, delayed diagnosis, and higher incidence of more aggressive microorganisms).

- Less likely to have splenomegaly and cutaneous lesions.
- More likely to have cardiomegaly and pleural effusion.
- Increased risk of nosocomial infections.
- Increased risk of in-hospital death and poorer general prognosis.
- In some studies, smaller vegetations, and lower embolic risk.
- Greater likelihood of anaemia.
- Greater likelihood of infection with *Enterococci, Streptococcus bovi,* and methicillin-resistant *Staphylococcus aureus*.
- Higher rate of predisposing disease (degenerative valvular disease, diabetes mellitus, and cancer).
- Lower rate of intravenous drug use and HIV infection.
- Higher rate of negative blood cultures owing to more frequent use of empirical antibiotic therapy before hospital admission.
- Less likely to be surgically treated (possibly owing to co-morbidities or frailty).
- Less likely to develop valvular insufficiency or perforation.
- More likely to have mitral valve involvement (possibly because of degenerative mitral disease).

5 How would you manage this patient?

This patient was admitted to hospital and three sets of blood cultures were taken. Treatment with intravenous antibiotics was initiated according to local guidelines and with input from microbiology, cardiology, and cardiothoracic specialists, with close monitoring for complications and response to treatment.

When patients are acutely ill, three sets of blood cultures should be obtained over one hour, before starting empirical antibiotic therapy. In non-critically ill patients, blood cultures, and further investigations may be obtained over one to three days pending definitive diagnosis. There is no evidence for the initiation of antithrombotic drugs in the active phase of infective endocarditis and systemic embolism is best treated through rapid initiation of appropriate antibiotics. However, there is some evidence that early rather than later surgical intervention is better for preventing embolic events. Patients with a source of bacteraemia must have appropriate management, (e.g. removal of an infected device, abscess drainage).

Development of the case:

On the second day of admission, the patient suddenly became more unwell, confused, and complained of left-sided abdominal pain. On examination, she was delirious with left-sided weakness. Abdominal CT and brain scanning were performed (Figs 10.4 to 10.6).

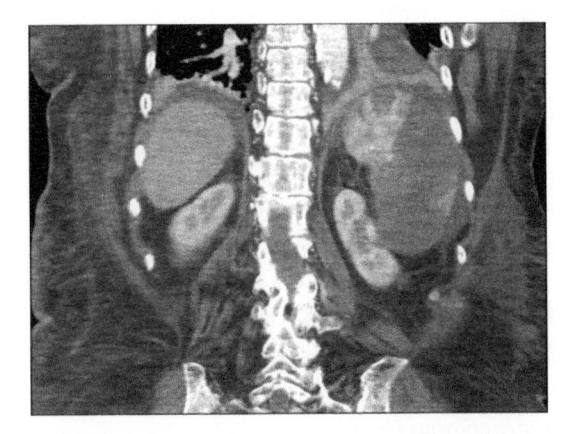

Fig. 10.4 Coronal CT image of the abdomen.

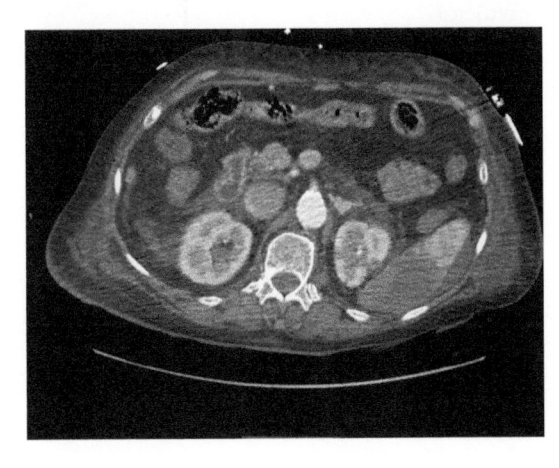

Fig. 10.5 Axial CT image of the abdomen.

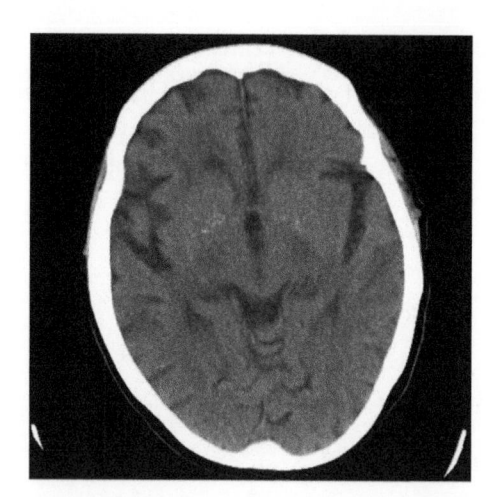

Fig. 10.6 Axial non-contrast CT brain slice at the level of the basal ganglia.

Questions continued

6 Describe the findings in Figures 10.4 to 10.6. What complications have occurred and are these more common in older patients?
7 List the poor prognostic predictors.
8 Is older age a contraindication for surgical treatment? List at least five indications for surgery.

Answers continued

6 Describe the findings on Figs.10.4 to 10.6. What complications have occurred and are these more common in older patients?

The CT images show small renal and large splenic infarcts (white arrows on Fig. 10.7a and b), bibasal atelectasis (stars), small effusion, and a little ascites (Fig 10.7a and b). There is also a brain infarct visible on the CT brain scan (Fig. 10.8).

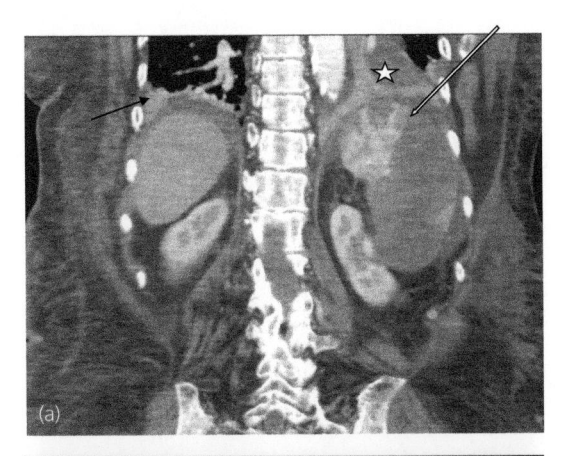

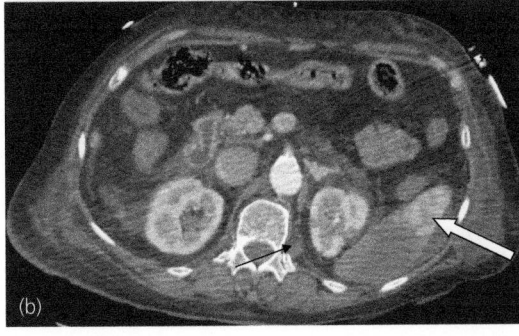

Fig. 10.7 The coronal and axial abdominal CT slices show small renal and large splenic infarcts (white arrows). There is also atelectasis (stars) (a) and a small effusion (b) black arrow.

This patient therefore developed renal, splenic, and brain embolic infarcts. The risk of embolism in infective endocarditis is estimated at between 30 and 50%, being highest immediately after starting antibiotics and falling thereafter. The brain and spleen are the most common sites of embolism in left-sided infective endocarditis, and pulmonary embolism is most common in right-sided and pacemaker-lead endocarditis.

There appears to be a lower frequency of embolic events in infective endocarditis affecting prosthetic valves, the reasons for which are not completely understood. Possible explanations include generally smaller vegetation size and ongoing anticoagulation treatment with warfarin.

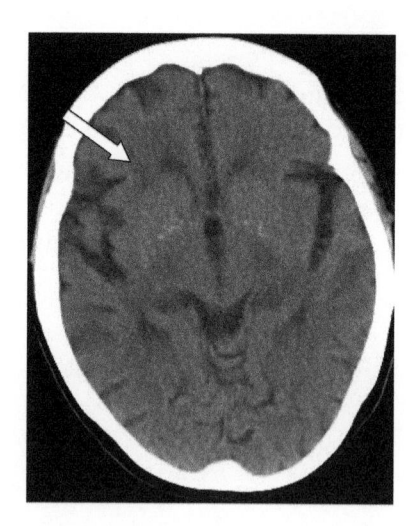

Fig. 10.8 The CT brain axial scan slice shows an area of hypodensity in the right frontal lobe (arrow).

The risk of embolism is increased with:

- younger age
- high CRP
- increased size of vegetations (>10–15 mm)
- mobile vegetations
- multivalvular involvement
- low albumin
- mitral valve vegetations (particularly if infected with *Staphylococcus*)
- *Staphylococci, Streptococcus bovis, Candida spp* infective endocarditis.

7 List the poor prognostic predictors.

Poor prognostic predictors for infective endocarditis are:

- older age
- increased co-morbidities
- prosthetic valve involvement
- mitral valve vegetations
- paravalvular complications
- heart failure
- hospitalization in previous three months
- pulmonary oedema
- staphylococcus aureus infection

- diabetes mellitus (insulin-dependent)
- stroke.

Early valve replacement was scheduled but the patient had a catastrophic embolic stroke and died four days after admission.

8 Is older age a contraindication for surgical treatment? List at least five indications for surgery.

Age alone is not a contraindication for surgery. However, older patients less frequently undergo surgery because of:

- co-morbidities
- lower rate of endocarditis due to *S aureus*
- lower rate of valvular impairment (insufficiency, perforation).

The individualized decisions for surgical intervention should be made after multi-disciplinary discussion (e.g. in cases of infection caused by an antimicrobial-resistant organism, valvular dysfunction precipitating heart failure, valve dehiscence on a paravalvular abscess, recurrent emboli). Poor surgical outcome is more likely in patients with preoperative:

- renal insufficiency
- advanced age, frailty (see case 35) and co-morbidities
- persistent infection
- heart failure with NYHA III, or IV, or who have been previously hospitalized for heart failure.

Surgery is generally not indicated for right-sided infective endocarditis (tricuspid or pulmonary valve).

Emergency surgery (within 24 hours) is recommended in cases of heart failure and there is:

- aortic or mitral infective endocarditis causing severe acute regurgitation, or valve obstruction, with refractory pulmonary oedema, or cardiogenic shock.
- aortic or mitral infective endocarditis causing refractory pulmonary oedema or shock, due to fistula into chamber, or pericardium.

Urgent surgery (within a few days) is recommended in cases with:

- heart failure and aortic or mitral severe acute regurgitation, or valve obstruction and persisting heart failure, or ECHO signs of poor haemodynamic tolerance (early mitral closure or pulmonary hypertension)
- fungal infections

- fever >7–10 days and positive blood cultures
- abscess, fistula, enlarging vegetation, false aneurysm
- aortic or mitral disease with vegetations of >10mm and, despite appropriate antibiotic, one or more embolic events
- aortic or mitral endocarditis with vegetations of >10mm and presence of other predictors of complications (abscess, persistent infection, or heart failure)
- isolated large vegetations >15mm.

Further reading

Baddour L, Wilson WR, Bayer AS, *et al.* (2005). American Heart association. Scientific statement. Infective endocarditis. Diagnosis, antimicrobial therapy and management of complications. *Circulation*; **111**: e394–e434.

Connaughton M, Rivett JG (2010). Easily missed? Infective endocarditis. *BMJ*; **341**: c6596.

Duval X, Iung B, Klein I, *et al.* (2010) Effect of early cerebral magnetic resonance imaging on clinical decisions in infective endocarditis: a prospective study. *Ann Intern Med*; **152**: 497.

Fedeli U, Schievano E, Buonfrate D, Pellizzer G, Spolaore P (2011). Increasing incidence and mortality of infective endocarditis: a population-based study through a record-linkage system. *BMC Infect Dis*; **11**: 48.

Habib G, Hoen B, Tornos P, *et al.* (2009). Guidelines of the prevention, diagnosis, and treatment of infective endocarditis (new version 2009): Task Force on the prevention, diagnosis, and treatment of Infective Endocarditis of the European Society of Cardiology (ESC). *Eur Heart J*; **30**: 2369–2413.

Hill E, Herijgers P, Herregods MC, Peetermans WE (2006). Evolving trends in infective endocarditis. *Clin Microbiol Infect*; **12**: 5–12.

Hill EE, Vanderschueren S, Verhaegen J, *et al.* (2007). Risk factors for infective endocarditis and outcome of patients with Staphylococcus aureus bacteremia. *Mayo Clin Proced*; **82**(10): 1165–1169.

Li JS, Sexton DJ, Mick N, *et al.* (2000). Proposed modifications to the Duke criteria for the diagnosis of infective endocarditis. *Clin Infect Dis*; **30**: 633–638.

López J, Revilla A, Vilacosta I, *et al.* (2010). Age-dependent profile of left-sided infective endocarditis: A 3-center experience. *Circulation*; **121**: 892–897.

Murdoch DR, Corey GR, Hoen B, *et al.* (2009) Clinical presentation, etiology and outcome of infective endocarditis in the 21st century. *Arch Intern Med*; **169**(5): 463–473.

Prendergast BD, Tornos P (2010). Surgery for infective endocarditis: who and when? *Circulation*; **121**: 1141–1152.

Ramin B, Malhotra J, Schreiber Y, Macpherson P (2013). Infective endocarditis in a new immigrant. *Can Fam Physician*; **59**(6): 644–646.

Tleyjeh IM, Abdel-Latif A, Rahbi H, *et al.* (2007). A systematic review of population-based studies of infective endocarditis. *Chest*; **132**: 1025–1035.

Case 11

A woman was brought in by ambulance after collapsing at a family lunch organized to celebrate her 78th birthday. On arrival in the emergency department, she was anxious, and had little memory of the collapse. She could remember the meal and recalled feeling light-headed shortly after coffee. Her daughter reported that her mother had said she felt unwell at the end of the meal while still seated at the table, and had then collapsed onto the floor where she remained unconscious for approximately five minutes. She had been well prior to the meal. Past medical history included gastro-oesophageal reflux disease, TIA six months earlier, hypertension, and mild osteoarthritis. Medications taken were omeprazole, aspirin, ramipril, amlodipine, and paracetamol. She was a carer for her frail 84-year-old husband and was still driving.

On examination, she was warm and well perfused, with a blood pressure of 132/90mmHg, heart rate 78bpm regular, and a respiratory rate of 18 breaths per minute. Cardiovascular, respiratory, abdominal, and neurological examination did not reveal any abnormalities. There was a superficial cut on the right forearm, which was washed and dressed by nursing staff.

Investigations showed the following:

- Blood results: Hb 11.2g/dL; WCC 5.1 × 10^9/L; neut 3.2 × 10^9/L; plt 350 × 10^9/L; Na 140 mmol/L; K 4.1mmol/L; urea 9mmol/L; creat 111µmol/L
- CXR: mild blunting of the costophrenic angles bilaterally
- ECG: normal sinus rhythm
- Urine dip: unremarkable.

Questions

1 What is the most likely cause for this patient's collapse? List other possible causes.
2 Describe further assessments you would consider.
3 Discuss the management of the condition that you gave as the answer to Question 1.
4 What advice would you give regarding driving?

Answers

1 What is the most likely cause for this patient's collapse? List other possible causes.

The most likely cause for this patient's collapse is postprandial syncope. Syncope is the sudden temporary loss of consciousness caused by impaired flow of blood to the brain (reduced cerebral perfusion). The patient becomes unresponsive with a loss of postural control, e.g. slumping or falling. Consciousness usually returns within minutes. Syncope is a common cause of emergency referral of older people and is associated with significant morbidity and mortality (e.g. hip fracture), anxiety, and social isolation.

Postprandial syncope occurs as a result of increased blood flow to the gut vasculature after a meal. This results in a drop in systemic blood pressure and temporary cerebral hypoperfusion in individuals unable to compensate haemodynamically. Peak reductions in blood pressure occur at around 75 minutes after eating. Although minor postprandial decreases in blood pressure are thought to occur in the majority of nursing home residents, and approximately one third of community dwelling older people, most remain asymptomatic. Decreases of greater than 20mmHg may result in syncope. The diagnosis may be made on the basis of the history and exclusion of other causes, and is supported by the finding of postural hypotension, particularly following a meal.

Other possible causes of syncope include:

Cardiac pathology. This includes acute cardiac ischaemia or arrhythmia, e.g. heart block. In the current case, the normal ECG made a rhythm disturbance unlikely.

Postural hypotension. This is the most common cause of syncope in older people and may be exacerbated by dehydration, drugs, or intercurrent illness—particularly sepsis. This patient was taking two antihypertensive medications, which may have increased her susceptibility.

Vasovagal syncope (faint). This is common in young as well as older people and is usually precipitated by fright or emotion. There are usually prodromal symptoms of light-headedness, nausea, and the patient may become pale. The diagnosis should be made with caution in older people in whom other causes of syncope are more common.

Carotid sinus syndrome. Carotid sinus baroreceptor stimulation causes an exaggerated response, with drop in blood pressure, and marked bradycardia often precipitated by head turning.

Cough, micturition, or defaecation syncope. In the current case, coughing may have been precipitated by choking on food, but the history was not suggestive. Also the patient was taking ramipril, which may cause cough.

Outflow obstruction. In older people this is most commonly caused by aortic stenosis (see case 35). Syncope typically occurs in the context of exertion. In the current case, the clinical features did not suggest this diagnosis.

The diagnosis of the underlying cause of a syncopal episode requires careful questioning regarding possible precipitants, e.g.

- standing – orthostatic hypotension
- sitting, or lying – seizure
- eating/coughing/straining – postprandial/cough/mictutrition/defaecation syncope exertion–outflow obstruction, or ischaemia.

Prodromal symptoms should be sought, e.g. palpitations and it should be noted that not all cerebral hypoperfusion will result in complete loss of consciousness, some patients will have pre-syncope and not black out completely. Conversely, many patients will be unaware or unable to remember that they lost consciousness, and will instead report a 'fall' (see case 27), denying blackout. The history from the patient is therefore often unclear and it is extremely important to obtain a witness account wherever possible, by telephone if necessary. In the absence of a witness account, it may be difficult to be certain of the diagnosis.

The major differential diagnosis for syncope is seizure (see cases 25, 44). In the current case it would appear highly unlikely given the short-lived episode of loss of consciousness, lack of typical features, and absence of a postictal phase of confusion.

2 Describe further assessments you would consider.

A thorough history should be taken as stated earlier. Any previous similar episodes should be recorded since these may help identify the cause. The timing of antihypertensive medications should be determined and the possibility of medication error should be considered, e.g. excess dosage. A history of head turning before the collapse should prompt consideration of carotid sinus hypersensitivity. Although the patient had had a recent TIA, it is most unlikely that the collapse was caused by a cerebrovascular event: loss of consciousness is not a feature of TIA and although brain stem stroke may cause collapse, rapid recovery after minutes would not be expected.

All patients with syncope should have routine blood tests to look for anaemia, sepsis, myocardial ischaemia, as well as an ECG. Other tests will be guided by the clinical history and may include echocardiogram, and prolonged

ECG monitoring. Less commonly, ECG monitoring during carotid sinus massage (carotid sinus hypersensitivity), or tilt table testing for suspected orthostatic hypotension not demonstrated by postural blood pressures may be required. Brain scan and electroencephalography (EEG) should be considered where seizures are a possibility. In the current case, the patient had had a similar episode with near collapse after a meal a few months earlier, and was found to have postural hypotension.

In many older people with syncope, the cause remains uncertain despite full investigation, or the cause appears to be multifactorial. In such cases, any reversible cause should be addressed although it may be difficult to be certain of the balance of risks and benefits, for example in stopping antidepressant medication, which may be contributing to postural hypotension.

3 Discuss the management of the condition that you gave as the answer to Question 1.

The treatment of postprandial hypotension can be difficult. Carbohydrate load increases the risk of postprandial hypotension and smaller meals with a low carbohydrate load should be advised. Dehydration should be avoided and patients should drink plenty of water with meals and avoid excessive alcohol. Coffee at the end of the meal may help. Antihypertensive drugs should be taken such that the peak effect of the medication does not coincide with meal times. This patient's ramipril was stopped and she was given advice about meals.

4 What advice would you give regarding driving?

Driving restrictions for syncope vary according to the underlying diagnosis and in the UK can be found at http://www.dvla.gov.uk/at_a_glance. This patient would be allowed to continue driving, as the collapse would be classified as a 'simple faint' with provocation (heavy meal) and prodromal symptoms. In syncope of unknown cause, patients who are low risk (no structural heart disease or ECG changes) driving can be resumed after four weeks from the incident. In high risk patients (structural heart disease, ECG changes, injury caused during previous episode, syncope occurring while driving or sitting) where the cause of the syncope is unknown or has occurred more than once over a six-month period, patients should be advised not to drive for six months, or until four weeks after a cause has been identified and treated.

Further reading

Chen L, Chen MH, Larson MG, Evans J, Benjamin EJ, Levy D (2000). Risk factors for syncope in a community-based sample (the Framingham Heart Study). *Am J Cardiol*; 85(10): 1189–1193.

For Medical Practitioners. At a glance guide to current medical standards of fitness to drive. http://www.dft.gov.uk/dvla/~/media/pdf/medical/at_a_glance.ashx

Jansen R, Lipsitz L (1995). Postprandial hypotension: epidemiology, pathophysiology and clinical management. *Ann Intern Med*;**122**(4): 286–295.

Parry SW, Steen N, Bexton RS, Tynan M, Kenny RA (2009). Pacing in elderly recurrent falls with carotid sinus hypersensitivity: a randomised, double-blind, placebo controlled crossover trial. *Heart*; **95**(5): 405–409.

Seifer C (2013). Carotid sinus syndrome. *Cardiol Clin*; **31**(1): 111–121.

Soteriades ES, Evans JC, Larson MG, *et al.* (2002). Incidence and prognosis of syncope. *N Engl J Med*; 19; **347**(12): 878–885.

Case 12

An 86-year-old woman, previously well and independent, was admitted with left hip and leg pain, which had come on gradually over several months. The pain had recently begun to wake her during the night. Two weeks before admission, she had had a urinary tract infection treated by her GP, but she had remained unwell, and her mobility had decreased such that she was almost immobile owing to hip and leg pain, only managing transfers between chair and bed. There was no weight loss and functional inquiry revealed nil else of note.

There was a past medical history of hypertension. She was a non-smoker and drank little alcohol. Medications taken were ramipril and paracetamol.

On examination, she looked well, temperature was 36.4°C, pulse was 72bpm regular, and blood pressure was 140/70mmHg. Passive movements of the left leg joints including the hip were normal, but she was unable to mobilize owing to left leg pain. Examination was otherwise normal.

Initial investigation showed the following:

- Hb 13.0g/dl; WCC 6.5 × 10^9L; plt 350 × 10^9/L
- Albumin 35g/L; alk phos 420iU/L; bilirubin 8μmol/L; ALT 14 IU/L; γ-glutamyl-transpeptidase 20IU/L; glc 5mmol/L
- U&E, TFTs, CK, B_{12}, folate, clotting: normal
- Adjusted Ca 2.7mmol/L, serum/urine electrophoresis: normal
- CRP <2mg/l; ESR 35mm/h
- Urine dipstick and microscopy: no protein, blood, or casts seen
- Blood and urine culture: negative
- CXR: normal
- X-rays of pelvis and left hip (Figs. 12.1 and 12.2).

110 | CASE HISTORIES IN GERIATRIC MEDICINE

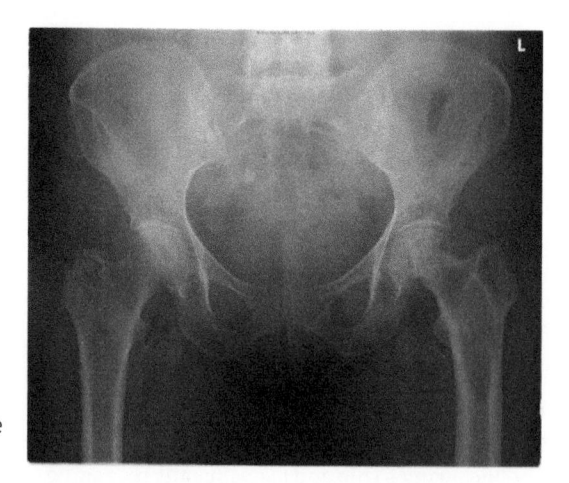

Fig. 12.1 Plain X-ray of the patient's pelvis.

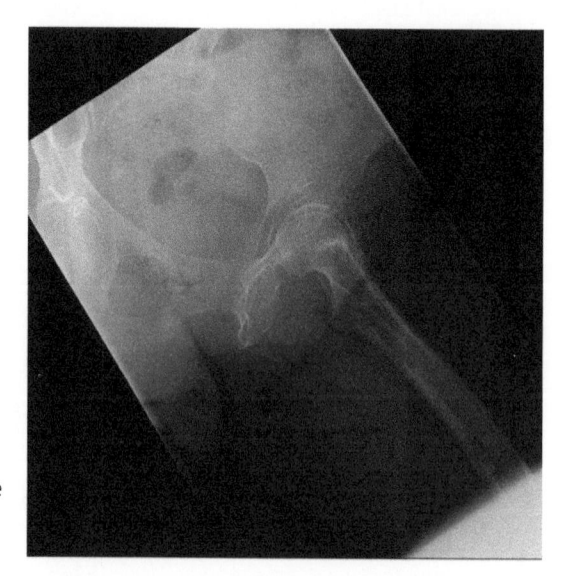

Fig. 12.2 Plain X-ray of the patient's left hip, lateral view.

Questions

1 What do the pelvis and hip X-rays show? Give a differential diagnosis.
2 What further investigations would you consider for this patient?

Answers

1 What do the pelvis and hip X-rays show? Give a differential diagnosis.

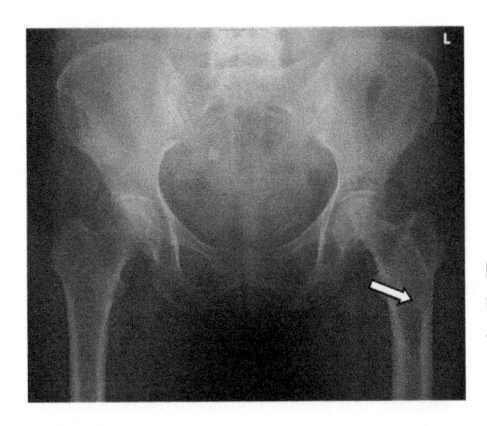

Fig. 12.3 Plain X-ray of the pelvis with small white arrow showing a focal lesion in the left femoral neck and proximal shaft.

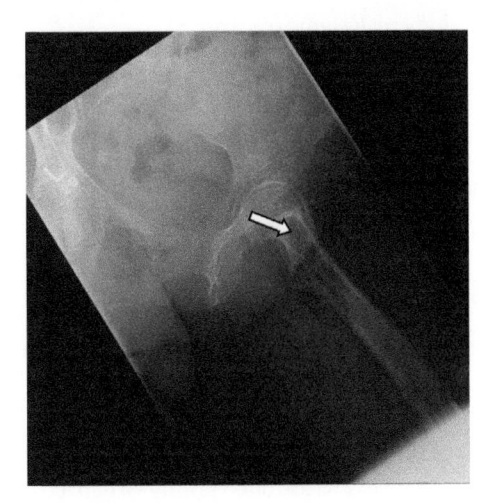

Fig. 12.4 Plain X-ray of left hip, lateral view with white arrow demonstrating two distinct lesions in the left femoral neck and proximal shaft.

The pelvis and hip X-rays show (Fig. 12.3, small white arrow) several lytic lesions in the left proximal femur—two distinct lesions in the left femoral neck and proximal shaft (Fig. 12.4, white arrow). The differential diagnosis is thus for the cause of lytic bone lesions associated with pain, difficulty mobilizing, and raised calcium and alkaline phosphatase, and includes:

- *Multiple malignant deposits.* The diagnosis of malignancy is supported by the radiological findings, history of new and increasing hip and leg pain especially at night, and abnormal biochemistry results (elevated calcium and alkaline phosphatase). In older patients, the most common sources of bone infiltration are secondary tumours (in women frequently of the breast and in men of the prostate or bronchus), multiple myeloma, haematological malignancies, and primary bone tumours. The spine, followed by the pelvis, ribs, skull, and long bones, are most commonly affected in metastatic bone disease.

- *Paget's disease.* Except for pain, the patient was well with no history of weight loss, anaemia, or prior malignant disease, which would make malignancy less likely. Severe pain, nocturnal pain, and pain worsening on mobilizing could be consistent with Paget's disease, in which elevated serum calcium and alkaline phosphatase may be present. Paget's disease is less likely to be the cause of lytic bone lesions if elevated alkaline phosphatase of bone origin has been present for less than a year.

- *Granulomatous lesions* (sarcoidosis, tuberculosis, coccidiomycosis) may cause osteolytic lesions, mimicking metastatic tumour, or myeloma, and occasionally are associated with hypercalcaemia (see case 8).

2 What further investigations would you consider for this patient?

Further investigations to consider include:

- Radionuclide bone scan
- CT scan of the pelvis and hip
- MRI scan of the pelvis and hip.

As plain X-rays (in combination with blood tests, history, and clinical findings) were not diagnostic in this case, a Technetium-99 radionuclide bone scan was organized to visualize the whole skeleton. The take-up of Technetium-99 is related to the intensity of osteoblastic activity thus metastatic tumour, metabolic bone disorders, and myeloma are often poorly visualized. In the current case, the bone scan showed the lesions identified on plain X-rays as 'hot' so supporting, but not confirming, a diagnosis of Paget's disease (Figure 12.5). The plain X-ray of the skull (Figure 12.6) may also show thickening of the skull vault.

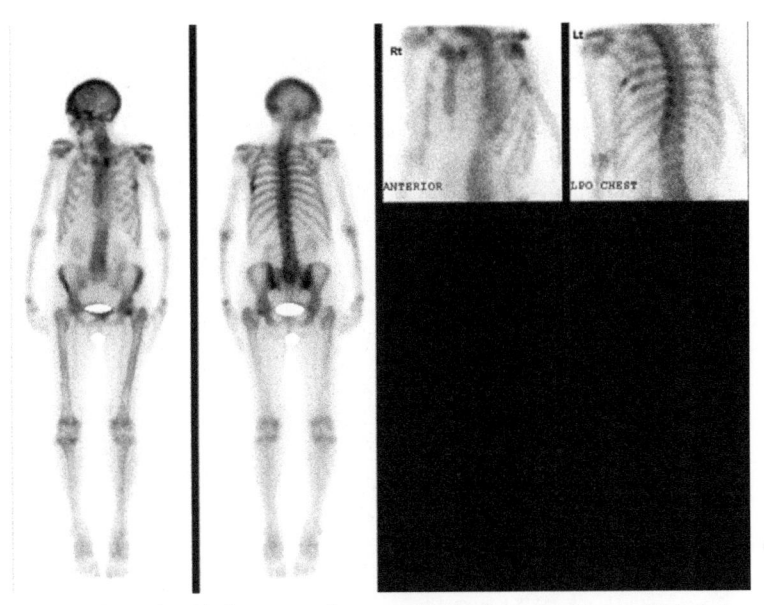

Fig. 12.5 Radionucleotide bone scan from another patient showing multiple hot spots in the skull, upper humerus, ribs, spine, and pelvis.

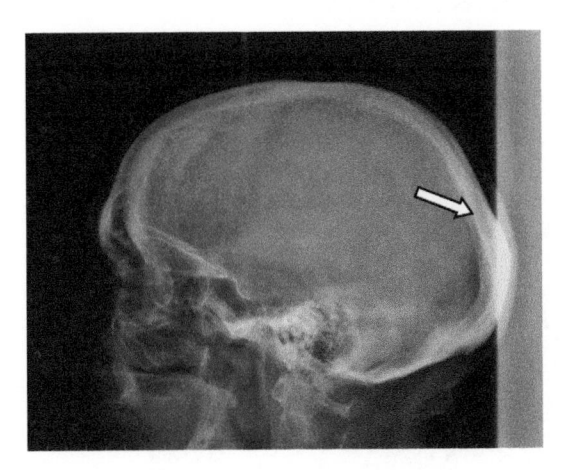

Fig. 12.6 Plain X-ray of the skull from the same patient as Figure 12.5, showing thickening and enlargement of the skull vault (arrow).

Case continuation

The bone scan was not diagnostic and further imaging was organized including CT (Fig. 12.7) and MRI bone scan of the pelvis and hip (Figs. 12.8 and 12.9).

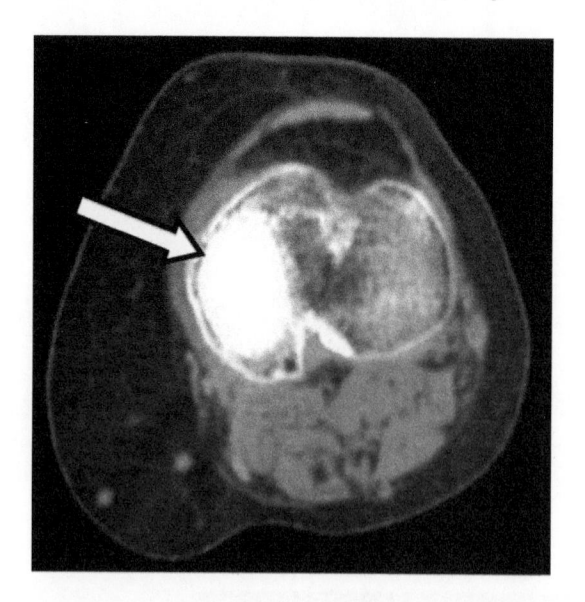

Fig. 12.7

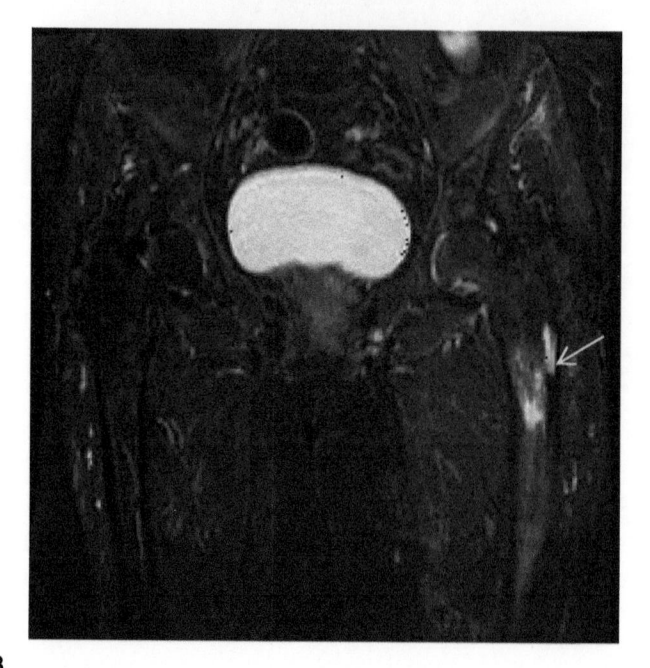

Fig. 12.8

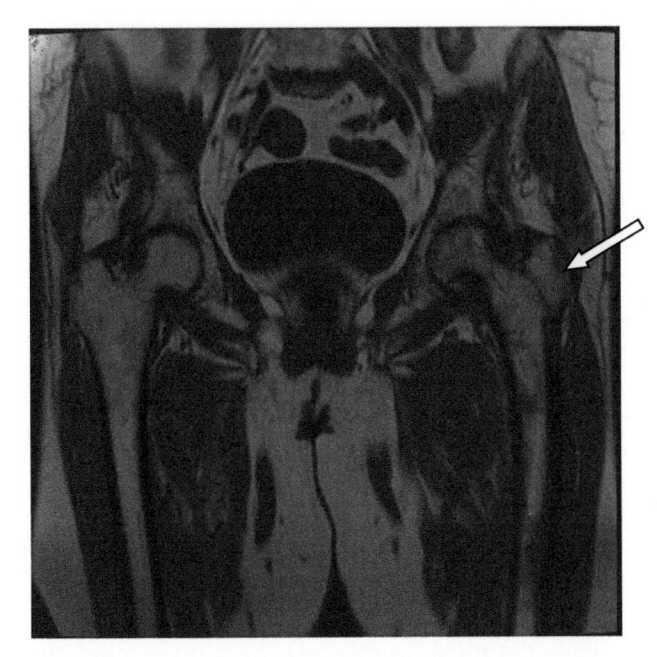

Fig. 12.9

Questions continued

3 Describe Figures 12.7, 12.8 and 12.9.
4 What is the most likely diagnosis in this case, bearing in mind all the clinical features? How could you confirm the diagnosis?
5 Describe the aetiology and main presenting characteristics of this condition.
6 What treatments may be considered for this condition?
7 What are the indications for treatment in older patients?

Answers continued

3 Describe Figures 12.7, 12.8 and 12.9.

Figure 12.7 shows a CT image with a lytic lesion in the posterior aspect of the proximal femur. CT is helpful in demonstrating internal skeletal structure (particularly if a high-resolution technique is used), but was felt not to be diagnostic in this case. A magnetic resonance imaging scan was therefore performed which has ~90% specificity and 100% sensitivity for the identification of bone metastases.

Figure 12.8 shows a coronal T1-weighted MRI scan of the pelvis with a high signal lesion in the posterior aspect of the proximal femur with two distinct components and cortical penetration, white arrow).

Figure 12.9 shows coronal T-weighted MRI scan of the pelvis with a lesion in the inferior aspect of the left femoral head and neck, and lesions in the femoral shaft inferior to the trochanters.

Both the CT and MR images are compatible with malignancy but also with Paget's disease.

4 What is the most likely diagnosis in this case, bearing in mind all the clinical features? How could you confirm the diagnosis?

Although it was not possible to make a definitive diagnosis even with the information from multi-modal bone imaging, Paget's disease was considered the most likely diagnosis as the patient was well with no history of weight loss,

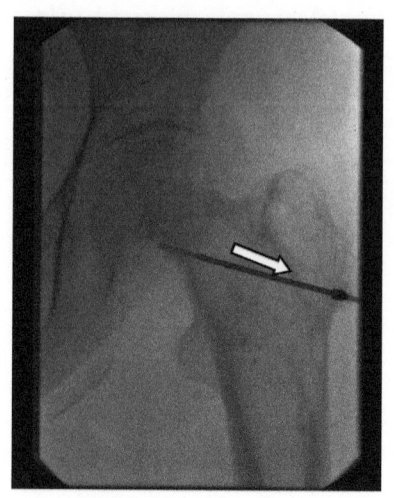

Fig. 12.10 Plain X-ray, showing the bone biopsy needle in situ in the left femur.

anaemia, or previous malignant disease, and the elevations in levels of alkaline phosphatase and calcium were mild. However, a bone biopsy was undertaken to confirm the diagnosis, which confirmed Paget's disease (Fig. 12.10).

5 Describe the aetiology and main presenting characteristics of this condition.

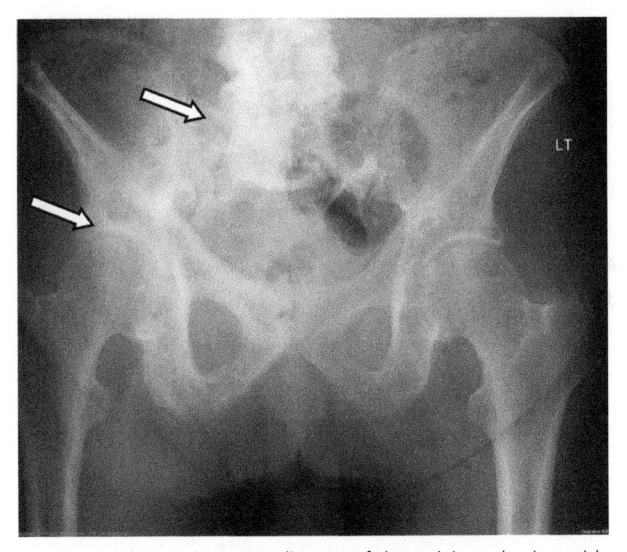

Fig. 12.11 Plain X-ray, showing Paget's disease of the pelvis and spine with patchy sclerosis and thickening of the pelvic bones and vertebrae (arrows).

The aetiology of Paget's disease is not known, although viral infections (paramyxovirus, measles virus, or canine distemper virus) have been postulated. Genetic factors are also thought to be significant. A seven- to ten-fold increase in risk of developing Paget's disease has been estimated for first-degree relatives and 30% of patients with familial Paget's disease carry mutations of the sequestosome -1 gene. Paget's disease is uncommon in Africans, Scandinavians, and Asians, being commonest in Western Europe and in British migrants. The disease usually presents in late life; it is rare before the age of 40 and the mean age of diagnosis is around 70 years. UK prevalence is 8% for men and 5% for women in their seventies, and approximately 10% for the general population aged over 85 years. The prevalence and severity of Paget's disease have declined over the past 25 years in UK, but not in the USA, Spain, or Italy, for reasons that are not yet clear.

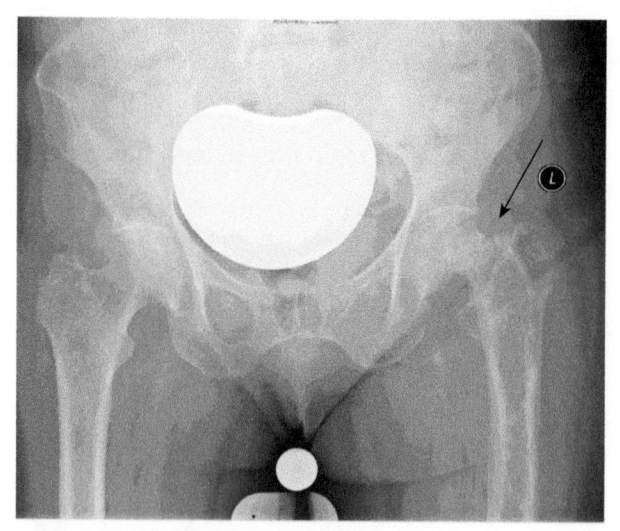

Fig. 12.12 Plain X-ray of the same patient as Fig. 12.10 some six months later, showing a fracture of the left neck of femur (arrow).

Paget's disease is associated with excessive osteoclastic and osteoblastic activity, and increased bone turnover. Most cases are asymptomatic at the time of diagnosis. More than 70% of cases involve the pelvis, and other commonly affected sites include the spine and the femur (Fig. 12.11). The tibia, fibula, skull, (Fig. 12.6) and face bones may also be involved, but other sites are rare. Disease may involve one or multiple bones in an individual. Complications occur in around 30% of cases. Modes of presentation include:

- *Incidental finding*. Paget's disease may be diagnosed during radiological procedures done for other reasons, or from routine blood tests revealing raised alkaline phosphatase. Alkaline phosphatase activity is elevated in around 50% of cases of untreated Paget's disease.

- *Pain* is the most common presenting symptom and ranges from a slight ache to a deep unpleasant pain that is usually worse on movement. Pain may be caused directly by the bone lesion, by nerve compression, or by degenerative arthritis secondary to bone abnormality. If pain becomes suddenly severe, the possibility of sarcomatous transformation or fracture must be considered. Improvement in pain after bisphosphonate treatment is supportive of a diagnosis of Paget's disease.

- *Osteosarcoma* has an annual incidence of around 1% in patients with Paget's disease, and in cases of extensive disease, the cumulative incidence has been estimated at 10%. Osteosarcoma should be considered in patients with Paget's disease who develop swelling or severe pain.
- *Fractures (fissure fractures and pathological fractures)* (Fig. 12.12). The most commonly affected sites include the femur and pelvis. Fractures may be associated with significant extravasation of blood (see case 24) and may occur following minimal or no trauma. Malunion may ensue.
- *Bone deformities* may cause a variety of problems depending on the affected bones. Bowing of the legs may alter the gait and cause secondary back pain. Skull enlargement, usually in the occipital and frontal regions is common, as is kyphosis of the trunk and loss of body height.
- *Increased warmth* of the skin over lesions.
- *Secondary osteoarthritis* due to bone remodelling next to joints producing abnormal anatomy and changes in joint biomechanics.
- *Gout.*
- *Deafness* can occur from cochlear capsule dysfunction owing to loss of bone mineral density as well as from eighth nerve compression.
- *Neurological complications* include nerve compression causing visual disturbance, facial palsy, or spinal nerve symptoms. Central nervous problems can include spinal cord compression, distortion of the base of the skull (platybasia) leading to blockage of the aqueduct of Sylvius, as well as hydrocephalus and cerebellar dysfunction, due to cervicomedullary junction compression.
- *High-output heart failure* (risk has been estimated to be 3–4%).
- *Dental malocclusion,* due to jaw deformity.
- *Dilated scalp veins.*
- *Hypercalcaemia* can develop in older patients particularly after periods of immobility, probably because of a shift in the balance of bone formation and resorption in the context of high bone turnover (see case 8).
- *Retinal angioid streaks* are probably not a true association of Paget's disease, although often quoted in textbook descriptions of the disease.

6 What treatments may be considered for this condition?

Treatments for Paget's disease include:
- *Bisphosphonates* are drugs of first choice. Their mechanism of action is not completely understood and levels of calcium should be monitored during

treatment. Trials of bisphosphonates for the treatment of pain in Paget's disease showed significant superiority over placebo. There are no significant clinical differences between the different bisphosphonates, although one trial found zolendronic acid to be more effective in some aspects of quality of life and in pain control.

- *Calcitonin* may be considered if there is intolerance of, or lack of benefit from bisphosphonates. However, there are no randomized controlled trials demonstrating efficacy in controlling pain.
- *Analgesia*. Patients usually need analgesic medication in addition to other treatments.
- *Surgery* may be indicated for fractures, replacement of severely osteoarthritic joints adjacent to Pagetic bone, decompression in spinal stenosis, or nerve entrapment, and rarely for osteosarcoma (6% survival over five years).
- *Physiotherapy* to encourage mobilization and weight bearing.
- *Orthotics* for established deformity.
- *Occupational therapy* to support activities of daily living.

7 What are the indications for treatment in older patients?

Patients with asymptomatic Paget's disease do not benefit from treatment as confirmed in recent trials. The two main indications for treatment are pain and hypercalcaemia:

- *Pain*. It may be difficult to elucidate the cause of pain in older patients with Paget's disease and co-morbidities, and so a trial of treatment for Paget's-related pain may be required. In our patient, the biopsy results were diagnostic and there was also little in the way of co-morbidity to cause uncertainty regarding the origin of the pain. She responded well to bisphosphonates and analgesia (following the 'analgesic ladder', see case 41), including non-steroidal anti-inflammatory drugs.
- *Hypercalcaemia*. Bisphosphonates are usually given, although there are no convincing trials establishing benefit. Hypercalcaemia in Paget's disease is usually associated with immobility, so alternative causes of hypercalcaemia such as hyperparathyroidism should be considered if the patient is mobile.

Other reported indications for treatment, but with lack of evidence for benefit, are:

- *Fractures.* There are no studies that show improvement in fracture healing and there are conflicting results from studies of the effect of antipagetic therapy on the risk of developing fractures.
- *Neurological complications.* There has been interest in ways of preventing or slowing the development of neurological complications in patients with Paget's disease. There is only case report evidence for calcitonin and bisphosphonates reducing spinal cord dysfunction, as well as other neurological problems in patients with Paget's disease, while surgical interventions have been reported not to be of benefit. Current recommendations are to offer medical treatment initially, with surgery being considered when medical therapy fails.
- *Blood loss.* During preparation for elective orthopaedic surgery involving Pagetic bone, bisphosphonates are given to reduce operative bleeding, although efficacy has not been established by adequate controlled trials.
- *Sarcoma.* There is no evidence that any medical treatment prevents sarcomatous change or slows progression of established disease.
- *Bony deformities and involvement of weight-bearing bones.* There is no evidence for benefit from any treatment.

Further reading

Bastin S, Bird H, Gamble G, Cundy T (2009). Paget's disease of bone-becoming a rarity? *Rheumatology*; **48**(10): 1232–1235.

Jacobs TP, Bilezikian JP (2005). Rare causes of hypercalcaemia. *J Clin Endocrinol Metab*; **90**: 6316–6322.

Ralston SH, Langston AL, Reid IR (2008). Pathogenesis and management of Paget's disease of bone. *Lancet*; **372**: 155.

Reid IR, Brown JP, Levitt N, et al. (2013). Re-treatment of relapsed Paget's disease of bone with zoledronic acid: results from an open-label study. *Bonekey Rep*; **6**: 442.

Siris ES, Lyles KW, Singer FR, Meunier PJ (2006). Medical management of Paget's disease of bone: indications for treatment and review of current therapies. *J Bone Miner Res*; **21**(Suppl 2): 94–98.

Wang PL, Meyer MM, Orloff SL, Anderson S (2004). Bone resorption and relative immobilization hypercalcemia with prolonged continuous renal replacement therapy and citrate anticoagulation. *Am J Kidney Dis*; **44**(6): 1110–1114.

Case 13

Case 13.A

A 76-year-old woman was admitted as an emergency having fallen after tripping over her cat. She had been unable to get up and her 84-year-old husband, who was himself disabled, called the ambulance. The GP letter stated that 'this patient lives in a house which is unsafe owing to subsidence, there is no central heating and there is evidence of hoarding. It is very dirty and cluttered with traces of animal and human excrement on the carpets and furniture' (see Fig. 13.1). The patient was admitted to the acute medical ward where she was found to be constipated and dehydrated.

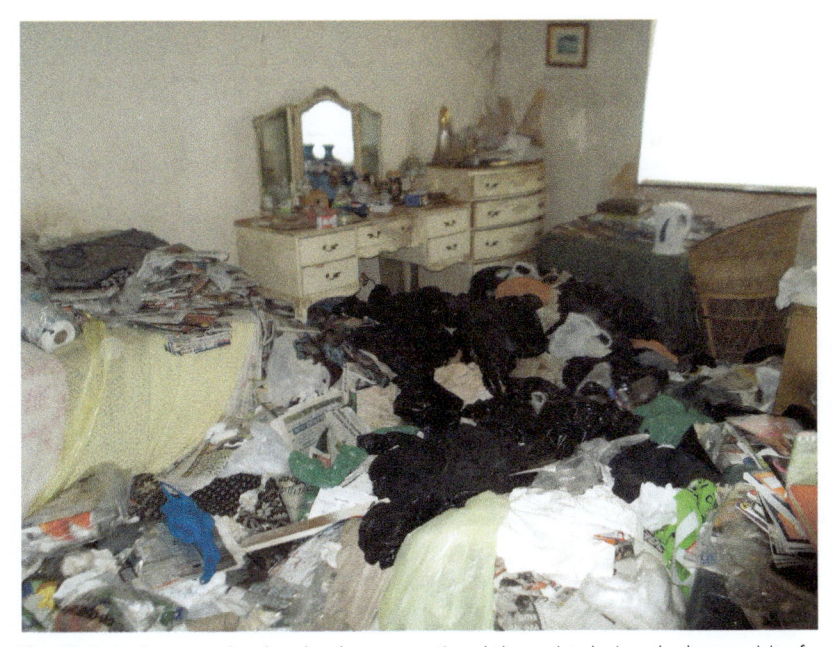

Fig. 13.1 A photograph taken by the occupational therapist during the home visit of patient A.

The past medical history included idiopathic Parkinson's disease diagnosed 15 years earlier, long-standing urinary incontinence, and constipation. She and her husband had no children, nor any friends. Medications were entacapone, co-careldopa, rasagiline, and paracetamol. Ropinirole had been stopped about six months previously because of frequent hallucinations, which had subsequently improved. This was the third hospital admission within six months.

On examination, she was unkempt with dirty hair, nails, and clothes. She had a stooped posture, spoke in a quiet voice and was dribbling. BMI was 17, temperature was 36.8°C, pulse was 72bpm regular, and blood pressure was 105/70mmHg without significant postural drop. MMSE was 22/30 (losing points on recall and praxis) and GDS was 3/15. She had an expressionless face, reduced blinking, and tremor in both hands, more prominent on the right. Initiation of movement was slow and there was prominent bradykinesia. She walked slowly with a Zimmer frame and her gait was shuffling.

During admission, she was given laxatives and rehydration, had a medication review, physiotherapy and occupational therapy input, but refused a suggested home visit. She also refused a formal package of post-discharge care despite not having been able to wash and dress herself, or prepare food for the preceding eight months. She was determined to leave hospital as soon as possible.

Case 13.B

A 79-year-old man was brought to the emergency department with shortness of breath and left-sided weakness, and was diagnosed with right lower lobe pneumonia and ischaemic stroke, with dysphagia. While the weakness improved rapidly, his swallowing impairment remained unchanged. In preparation for discharge, he was advised a soft diet of puréed food and thickened fluids of double cream consistency, as thin fluids made him cough and he was at high risk of aspiration. He refused these dietary modifications and also rejected any suggestion of possible future PEG tube insertion. He had one child, an estranged daughter in South Africa, whom he refused to contact.

On examination prior to discharge, MMSE was 26/30 and GDS was 4/15. General system examination was unremarkable, but on CNS examination he had left arm and leg weakness with power of 4/5, with left-sided increased reflexes, and up-going plantar reflex.

Questions

1 What assessment would you need to make first for both these patients prior to further discharge planning?
2 How would you proceed in making this assessment?
3 In what circumstances would these two patients fail the assessment?
4 What difficulties are commonly encountered while conducting this assessment?
5 What are the most common reasons for making this assessment in older people?

Answers
1 What assessment would you need to make first for both these patients prior to further discharge planning?

In both cases, there was a conflict between what the health team thought was in the best interests of the patients (beneficence), and the patients' own wishes (autonomy). Both patients refused what the health team saw as necessary treatment to provide as part of their 'duty or standard of care' before discharging them.

In order to ensure that these patients were making decisions on the basis of understanding the issues and implications, their competence or mental capacity needed to be assessed. Such assessment may be complex and difficult, and is usually undertaken in cases when important issues are under consideration, often complicated by contention or conflict (for example, when a will needs to be written, or discharge destination decided). In cases A and B, both patients needed assessment of their capacity to make relevant decisions as they had declined what the medical team felt were the most reasonable and least risky management options.

According to the Mental Capacity Act, the assessment of a patient's mental capacity has two stages:

i. The first stage addresses the question of whether the patient is suffering from brain (mind) impairment, or any kind of disturbance that affects the way that the brain (mind) works. This may involve, for example, the presence of severe pain, dementia, delirium, or other physical or medical conditions that cause confusion, drowsiness, or loss of consciousness.

ii. If the answer to the previous question is yes, then the second stage addresses the question of whether this impairment (disturbance) interferes with the patient's ability to make the specific decision in question.

Affirmative answers to these questions should not lead automatically to the conclusion that the patient has no capacity to make any decision; rather, it should trigger further assessment of the impact on the patient's ability to decide on the specific issue under consideration. It is usually helpful to explore whether the patient's decision-making capacity is impaired by such factors as poor cognition, disordered thinking, or emotional disorder. One of the assessment aims is to establish the distinction between these factors and the impairment of decisional capacity. Such assessment is individually based and achieved, and relates to the specific decision that needs to be made at the specific time.

2 How would you proceed in making this assessment?

In order to assess mental capacity, further principles need to be followed:

i. The starting point is the assumption that an adult person is competent, unless there is evidence to the contrary (in other words decision-making capacity should be presumed).

ii. Every patient must be treated equally, with fairness. No one should be labelled 'incapable' as a consequence of age. The majority of older people will have no problems with decision-making. Several studies, however, have found cognitive function to be associated with lower scores in assessments of capacity. This was confounded in some studies by factors such as level of reading skills, education, and verbal reasoning, or by a particular diagnosis, medical condition, appearance, or behaviour; all of these may lead to unjustified assumptions about capacity.

In case A, the history of occasional hallucinations was not sufficient grounds for deciding that she had no capacity. It was, however, necessary to establish whether the hallucinations or cognitive impairment interfered with her decision-making. Impaired mental status does not automatically equate to incompetence.

iii. All practical steps have to be taken to help someone to make a decision before they may be treated as having lack of capacity. As far as possible, support should be given to the patient to participate in the decision-making process or to decide for him or herself. If needed, information should be given in the form of non-verbal communication, i.e. drawings or photographs. With appropriate advice, the majority of older patients will have no problem in understanding the nature of the proposed treatment/procedure/discharge plan, and the associated risks.

iv. Patients have autonomy to make an unwise decision if they possess capacity to make that decision, even if their decisions are not sensible in the judgement of others; the patient may not share the same priorities. An unwise or eccentric decision as made by both patients above does not constitute evidence that the person lacks mental capacity.

During this assessment it is important to keep in mind that:

- Capacity may change over time and also rapidly (e.g. with acute illness).
- Capacity can be situation-dependent.
- The patient should be given time to absorb and discuss the facts. Several sessions may be needed for this, and it may also be beneficial if other health professionals and relatives are encouraged to discuss the topic in question with the patient.

- Capacity relates to the patient's ability to understand the relevant information and to relate the significance of the relevant information to the choice offered to him or her.
- It is crucial to be certain that the patient is aware of the nature and the consequences of a decision. The patient's understanding must be checked by asking questions related to that decision.
- A second opinion, perhaps from a psychogeriatrician, should be sought in borderline or contentious cases.
- The results of the assessment, including verbatim statements by the patient, must be documented.
- The threshold of declaring a patient incompetent can be relatively low if a beneficial, low-risk treatment is refused.

The assessment is not to be carried forward and is not generalizable; it is a decision about a person's capacity to make a particular decision at a particular time.

3 In what circumstances would these two patients fail the assessment?

Both of these patients would have lacked capacity if they were not able to:

i. Understand the information (medical facts) relevant to the decision, and the consequences. For example, the patient in case B needed to understand (in broad terms) that his swallowing difficulties were caused by stroke, creating the need for specially prepared food and thickened fluids in order to minimize the risk of aspiration pneumonia possibly leading to re-admission to hospital or death.

ii. Retain the information relevant to the decision and appreciate its relevance by demonstrating the ability to recognize that it applies personally to him/her. In many circumstances, clinicians may confuse a patient's ability to express a choice (often relatively eloquently), with their ability to use and weigh information sufficient to make an informed decision.

iii. Use, apply, or weigh the information relevant to the decision as part of making that decision, in order to consider different options, with the ability to balance the risks and benefits in making a choice.

iv. Communicate their decision to express their choice. For some patients, this may entail the use of blinking, shaking or nodding the head, the use of communication aids, interpreters, or family members, and others who know how the patient communicates.

For instance, a patient may express at length that they wish to return home because no one is able to look after their cat, but fail to realize that they are unable to adequately care for themselves. It is the using and weighing of the information that should be most robustly scrutinized in the medical setting.

The clinical team should ask questions to check the patient's understanding, as well as to determine whether his/her mood or thinking is affected by illness. It is good practice to ask the patient to repeat the information that the clinician has provided in relation to the decision in question. Thus, the patient should be able to answer such questions as: 'Can you please tell me what I've told you about . . . ?', and 'What do you think will happen if you decide to do X, or if you decide to refuse X?'. Competence for each relevant decision should be assessed separately.

If the patient fails one or more parts of this test, s/he lacks the relevant capacity. Clinicians should be aware, however, that patients might refuse to make a choice/decision, despite being able to reason, understand, and retain the relevant information.

In cases A and B, the assessment confirmed that they had capacity to make the decisions in question. The patient in case A remained adamant about going home to be looked after by her husband, understanding clearly all the consequences of her decision. The patient in case B was similarly competent, and stated that 'food and drink are my last pleasures and I am going to take all risks attached to taking it as I wish'.

4 What difficulties are commonly encountered while conducting this assessment?

The evidence suggests that on the whole, operationalized capacity assessments performed by different interviewers, or by different raters of the same interview are highly reliable with high levels of agreement, being consistent across very divergent clinical groups, including those in whom problems with capacity will largely be due to cognitive impairments (e.g. dementia, delirium, and learning disability).

However, when the judgement of a clinician is compared with that of an assessor using a capacity measurement tool, the results are different. Clinicians are less likely to state that the patient lacks capacity, and reliability estimates are generally in the 'slight' to 'fair' range, which could be that unless the patient is actively refusing treatment, there is little reason for the clinician to question the patient's capacity, reflecting the legal position that mental capacity is presumed. Secondly, clinicians may lack knowledge and training in assessing mental capacity. Some studies indicate that clinicians in many different specialities systematically underestimate the extent of cognitive impairments or miss mental disorders, and that mental capacity is widely misunderstood. Clinicians must avoid conflating a patient's ability to 'express a choice' with a capacitous decision. For example, a patient who is able to clearly verbalize a desire to go home, with a stated reluctance to go to a nursing home, may be perceived as someone who has capacity. In fact, they may have no recognition of their physical disabilities and needs for care, which can no longer be provided in the home environment (e.g. because of double incontinence, immobility, their home being too small for necessary equipment). In other words, while they passed one of the four domains of a capacity assessment, they have an inability to 'use and weigh' pertinent information to make a fully capacitous choice.

5 What are the most common reasons for making this assessment in older people?

Not much research has been conducted into mental capacity in older people, and evidence-based knowledge is scarce. The most common reasons for mental capacity assessments in older people are related to specific decisions about:

- Discharge planning. A psychiatric assessment of mental capacity in older people is mostly requested in cases when the avoidance of institutionalization is an issue.
- Treatment, especially where formal written consent is required.
- Finances.

One recent survey found that issues regarding capacity may arise in approximately 40% of medical in-patients.

Case 13.A—developments

Two months after her discharge, she and her husband had a fall on the stairs while he was helping her, and she sustained a hip fracture. A few days after this event, her husband was admitted to another hospital with myocardial infarction and died.

On this occasion, her recovery was complicated by severe anaemia requiring blood transfusion, two episodes of chest infection, double incontinence, and poor mobility. She had several episodes of delirium and was keen to leave hospital at all times. After spending six months in hospital, she was only able to transfer from a bed to a chair with the assistance of two carers and a frame, remained doubly incontinent, and her memory had deteriorated from when she was first admitted. At this stage, her MMSE was 15/30. When discharge planning was discussed, she wanted to go home, and was not keen on any care package. She was convinced that she could look after herself.

Questions continued

6 How would you proceed with her further management and what would you do next, if she lacked capacity for further decisions about her care and discharge plans?

7 How was she managed during the spells of delirium and wanting to leave the hospital? How could you keep a patient like this in hospital against her will?

Answers continued

6 How would you proceed with her further management and what would you do next, if she were assessed as lacking capacity for further decisions about her care and discharge plans?

The patient required a new assessment of mental capacity, which showed that this time she could not understand, retain, and weigh the relevant information regarding her discharge plans and further care. Consequently, she was assessed as lacking capacity to make such decisions. In her further assessment, the following questions were considered:

- Will the patient have capacity in the future in relation to this matter and if so, when? (i.e. might there be a change in the patient's communicative, physical, and cognitive ability?)
- Might her mental capacity fluctuate?
- Does the decision have to be taken at this time or can it be delayed?

In this case it was thought that the answers were negative to all questions. She recovered from the infection, but her mobility and her memory had deteriorated significantly. She tried to wander at night and remained doubly incontinent.

If the patient had previously appointed a Lasting Power of Attorney, granting decision-making authority over her financial, health, and social care decisions to a named person in the event of her losing mental capacity, that person could now advocate on her behalf regarding the discharge arrangements. The attorney is required to act as proxy in the patient's best interests and may seek support from the healthcare team. For patients without Lasting Power of Attorney, application to the Court of Protection can be made to request the appointment of a Court Appointed Deputy to act as his or her agent (a friend or relative). However, this patient had no next-of-kin and was therefore referred to the Independent Mental Capacity Advocacy Service (IMCAS), and an IMCA (Independent Mental Capacity Advocate) was appointed.

The 'best interest' decision checklist was applied to the patient's management as follows:

- Have all relevant circumstances/factors been considered, including the patient's previous written statements, wishes, values, religious/cultural beliefs, when she had capacity? Has the effect of the decision on other people been taken into account?
- Has the patient's involvement in the decision been encouraged? While a patient may not be able to take the actual decision, his or her views and values are still relevant in making a 'best interest' decision.

- Were the opinions of others, such as family members, unpaid carers, friends, lawyers, district nurses, and anyone else involved in his or her care, taken into consideration? Were all relevant circumstances investigated? Did everyone contribute to identifying relevant options?
- Were the risks and benefits of the treatment/procedure balanced?
- Was the decision based only on age, appearance, behaviour, or condition of this patient?
- Is the patient's carer/family (where applicable) wellbeing and level of distress taken into account in the decision-making process?
- Based on the risks and benefits of the relevant options, has the least restrictive option for the patient, in terms of rights and freedom of action been selected?
- Has care been taken to ensure that any act or decision taken on her behalf was in her best interest?

The most common reasons for referral to the IMCAS in patients lacking capacity who are without friends or relatives, or for those at risk of abuse (see case 3), are for:

- Placement in a care home for more than eight weeks.
- Hospital admission longer than 28 days.
- Accommodation change to a different care home or different hospital.
- A decision concerning high risk or contentious medical treatment.
- In case of safeguarding concerns (e.g. related to family and friends).

The role of the IMCA (who is not a decision maker) is to:

- Obtain all information (e.g. from social care notes and medical notes) relating to the relevant circumstances and factors, such as the patient's previous and present wishes, values and beliefs, or written statements, religious, and cultural values.
- Provide an independent safeguard for important decisions.
- Find out the opinion of others (e.g. family, carers, friends), and the effect of the decision on other people.
- Support the patient in the decision-making process.
- Challenge the social care or medical decision (if necessary).
- Request a second opinion (if necessary).
- Consider the least restrictive option for the patient, in terms of rights and freedom of action.

- Make a submission to a local authority or NHS body, which is taken into account if needed.
- Ensure that any act or decision will be in the patient's best interest.
- Remember that the patient's best interest may not be identical with his or her best interest in purely medical terms.
- Write a report.

In the event of a dispute (e.g. if someone challenges a recommendation by the IMCA and a consensus cannot be reached), the Court of Protection makes the final decision. It has jurisdiction as a final arbiter for all capacity issues. This patient had regular reviews, with careful record-keeping in her medical notes. The IMCA appointed in this case and other members of the team had 'a best interest meeting', and judged that it was in the patient's best interest to be discharged from the hospital to a care home.

As the patient did not have an Advanced Directive, no appointed attorney, and no relatives or close friends, it was necessary to apply for the IMCA appointment, and afterwards the following 'best interest' decision checklist was applied:

- Will this patient have capacity in the future in relation to this matter?
- Does the decision have to be taken at this time or can it be delayed?
- Does mental capacity fluctuate?
- Have all relevant circumstances/factors been considered, including the patient's previous written statements, wishes, values, religious/cultural beliefs, when she had capacity? Has the effect of the decision on other people been taken into account?
- Has the patient's involvement in the decision been encouraged? While a patient may not be able to take the actual decision, his or her views are still relevant in making a 'best interest' decision.
- Were the opinions of others, such as family members, unpaid carers, friends, lawyers, district nurses (who will probably know the patient better than does the GP) and everyone else involved in his or her care, taken into consideration? Were all relevant circumstances investigated? Did everyone contribute to identifying relevant options?
- Were the risks and benefits of the treatment/procedure balanced?
- Was the decision based only on age, appearance, behaviour, or condition of this patient?
- Is the patient's carer/family wellbeing and level of distress taken in to the decision-making process?

- Based on the risks and benefits of the relevant options, has the least restrictive option for the patient, in terms of rights and freedom of action been selected?
- Has care been taken to ensure that any act or decision taken on behalf of the patient was in her best interest?

This patient had regular reviews, with careful record-keeping in her medical notes. The IMCA appointed in this case and other members of the team had 'a best interest meeting' and judged that it was in the patient's best interest to be discharged from the hospital to a care home.

7 How was she managed during the spells of delirium and wanting to leave the hospital? How could you keep a patient like this in hospital against her will?

This patient lacked capacity owing to acute illness and delirium, and was unable to understand, retain, and use information relevant to the decision about her further treatment. It was therefore necessary to find out as soon as possible from the patient's GP whether she had made an Advance Directive refusing relevant treatment, or if she had drawn up a Lasting Power of Attorney in the past. She had done neither. She did not improve and persistently attempted to climb out of bed and to leave the ward, at times needing to be restrained by the nursing staff. Sedation was administered on occasions in order to calm her verbal and physical aggression, and distress. Care in hospital while she was delirious and unable to give consent was provided under the Mental Capacity Act. Section 5 of the Mental Capacity Act states that it is to be presumed that a person has consented to care or treatment where they lack mental capacity and that the decision maker (in this case the consultant for the patient's care) acts in the best interests of the patient. Section 5 protects the physician from legal liability in a situation where treatment might be interpreted as inappropriate, neglectful, or interfering, and might otherwise be grounds for civil or even criminal charges, e.g. through interfering with the patient's body.

At times, it was only possible to take blood samples or give antibiotic using restraint. This was justified under the Mental Capacity Act 2005, since:

- reasonable steps were taken first to establish that she lacked capacity in relation to the matter in question
- it was in her best interests for the act to be done
- it was reasonably believed that it was necessary to do the act to prevent harm to her

- the act in question was a proportionate response to the likelihood of her suffering harm
- the act in question was a proportionate response to the seriousness of that harm and was judged to be in her best interests.

A full exploration of alternative ways of providing the care and/or treatment was undertaken, in order to identify any less restrictive ways of providing care, which would avoid a deprivation of liberty.

As it was judged that antibiotic treatment, fluid replacements, and hospital care were in her best interests, but would result in a deprivation of liberty, her medical team applied for deprivation of liberty (applies to England and Wales only) from a supervisory body. The necessary preconditions for this application included the following conditions:

- she was older than 18 years and of unsound mind
- lack of capacity was not subject to the Mental Health Act 1983
- the deprivation of liberty would be in her best interest
- the deprivation of liberty did not conflict with any valid advanced decisions made by her (e.g. under an Lasting Power of Attorney).

The deprivation of liberty was granted. This has maximum duration of 12 months and is valid if it is in writing, if it describes the purpose of the deprivation of liberty, the time period, any conditions attached, and the reasons that each of the qualifying criteria are met. Appeals against decisions can be made to the Court of Protection. The Deprivation of Liberty Safeguards was made as an amendment to the Mental Capacity Act 2005 and has been in use since 1 April 2009. It is designed as a protection from the unlawful deprivation of a person's liberty (in a hospital or care home). In cases with approved 'standard authorization', the person concerned will be given a relevant representative (usually a family member or a friend), or access to an IMCA.

In 2014, after the Supreme Court handed down its judgement in the case of 'P vs. Cheshire West and Chester Council and another' and 'P and Q vs. Surrey County Council', to determine 'whether arrangements made for the care and/or treatment of an individual lacking capacity to consent to those arrangements amount to a deprivation of liberty', resulted in a revised test for deprivation of liberty, regarding the following:

1. The person lacks capacity to consent to the arrangements of continuous supervision and control, which s/he requires and is not free to leave.
2. The person's lack of objection, compliance, or the reason or purpose behind a placement is not relevant for that decision.

3 Given the person's needs, the relative normality of the placement is not relevant for that decision.
4 Only the Court of Protection can authorize a deprivation of liberty in domestic settings (e.g. a placement in a supported living arrangement in the community).

Case 13.B—developments

After two months at home, this patient was readmitted to hospital, after he had been found on the floor by his carers. He was diagnosed with aspiration pneumonia, sepsis, and delirium. Overnight, he pulled out his intravenous access several times. He refused blood tests and asked repeatedly for a drink of water, but the admitting team assessed him as unsafe to have any oral intake. The following morning his GP provided a copy of his Advance Directive, which had been signed a month before with instructions that if he lost competence and was unwell, he wished to be given only oral food and fluids, even if these were deemed to be unsafe. He had also made a decision that he did not want to be considered for resuscitation or to be given any further active treatment, specifically antibiotics or parenteral fluids. He wanted to be 'kept comfortable' only.

His daughter arrived from abroad and insisted that he should be given intravenous fluid and antibiotics, as well as to be considered for resuscitation. She stated: 'You have to give him everything as he is confused and not in his right mind.'

Questions

1 What would you do next in this case?
2 What do you need to have in mind when deciding about his cardiopulmonary resuscitation (CPR)?
3 Summarize the evidence about the survival of older people following CPR.
4 How would you proceed in managing this case?

Answers

1 What would you do next in this case?

It is first necessary to find out whether his Advance Directive is valid. If it is valid, it needs to be respected. A valid Advance Directive satisfies the following conditions:

- It is in writing.
- It is signed by the patient or someone else at the patient's direction.
- The signature has been witnessed and the witness has also signed it.
- The patient was not under pressure when making the Advanced Directive.
- The patient was able to envisage his or her future clinical circumstances.
- The circumstances specified in the Advanced Directive are now actual and ongoing.
- The directive specifies the treatment.
- It states that it applies to life-sustaining treatment and that the decision stands even if life is at risk.
- It has authority over all other views (including relatives and friends).
- It does not request treatment that is illegal, or not clinically indicated.
- It cannot refuse basic care (e.g. to be kept comfortable), but may include refusal of hydration and artificial nutrition, which are classed as treatments.

Advance directives may be changed or withdrawn by a patient at any time, if s/he still has capacity to do so. It is also important that the patient has acted consistently with the directive prior to losing mental capacity. The Advance Directive may become invalid if it takes no account of circumstances that were not anticipated at the time of its preparation, but are now present.

From discussion with this patient's GP and on checking the Advance Directive, it was clearly valid.

2 What do you need to have in mind when deciding about his cardiopulmonary resuscitation (CPR)?

As the formal assessment of his capacity at the time of writing the Advance Directive showed that the patient possessed the relevant decision-related capacity, his decision against resuscitation had to be respected, despite his daughter's wishes.

Decisions in geriatric practice often concern the withholding or withdrawal of treatment, which can present very difficult challenges. When making or discussing cardiopulmonary resuscitation decisions, it is helpful to consider that:

- It is not always appropriate to proceed with resuscitation.
- Discussion with a competent patient is necessary, but only if the patient is willing to discuss the matter.
- Discussion with the relatives and with the team involved in the care of an incapacitated patient is necessary.
- A decision about attempting CPR mostly hinges on the patient's realistic chances of survival, and the specific risks and benefits of resuscitation.
- It is often difficult to predict the chance of survival and this should be discussed.
- Clinicians act in the best interest of incapacitated patients and should discuss this problem with relatives or people close to the patients, mainly to find out about the patient's previous wishes.
- It should be explained that decisions about Do Not Attempt Resuscitation are separate from decisions about other treatments.
- A competent patient's decision to refuse resuscitation must be respected.
- For patients with a foreseeable risk of cardiac arrest, it is recommended that the decision should be made in advance.
- Resuscitation should not be attempted if the benefit would be outweighed by the expected burdens.
- Resuscitation should not be attempted if the medical team involved in the patient's care is certain, to the extent possible, that it will not be successful.
- All discussion and decisions should be fully documented.

3 Summarize the evidence about the survival of older people following CPR.

Little is known about survival of older people after CPR, but age alone is not a good predictor. Some authors suggest that when clinicians discuss CPR with older patients, it is much better to say 'resuscitation attempt', as the word resuscitation somehow implies success. The best survival rate in the older population occurs in cases with:

- witnessed arrests
- ventricular tachycardia or fibrillation

and outcomes are notably poor in cases of patients with:

- pneumonia
- electromechanical dissociation (pulseless electrical activity)
- asystole
- coma
- cancer
- housebound status
- hypotension
- renal failure.

4 How would you proceed in managing this case?

In this case, a careful and candid discussion with the patient's daughter was necessary, on the basis that her father had had capacity to decide about these issues and that the wishes stated in his Advance Directive should therefore be respected. It may be helpful in such cases to explore the relative's reasoning and motives, and s/he might benefit subsequently from bereavement counselling, especially if there is an element of guilt. This was particularly relevant in this case, as the daughter had been noted as 'estranged' from her father.

If a difference of opinion between clinicians and relatives over a CPR decision persists, the following steps are recommended:

- Obtain a second clinical opinion (especially if no Advance Directive is available).
- Seek medico-legal advice.
- Obtain a clinical ethics team opinion. Some UK NHS trusts have clinical ethics committees (include lay and professionals as members), and provide ethical support for clinicians in assessing capacity, consent issues, refusal of treatment issues, do not resuscitate orders, etc.

In practice, a difficult situation commonly arises when a patient with decision-related capacity becomes unwell, with very poor chance of surviving cardiopulmonary resuscitation, yet still insists on resuscitation. In such cases, the current guidance (in the UK) is not to make a decision until arrest occurs. However, if the request comes from relatives of an incapacitated patient in such circumstances and who has made no Advance Directive decision on resuscitation, there are no guidelines. It is important to know that doctors are not obliged to offer treatment that is unlikely to be beneficial.

The patient in case B was managed according to his wishes and instructions from his Advance Directive. His daughter accepted the situation after several discussions with the medical team, the patient's GP, and the hospital's legal advisor.

Further reading

BMA (2008). Mental Capacity Act Tool Kit.

Flegel KM, MacDonald N (2008). Decision-making capacity in an age of control. *CMAJ*; Jan 15; **178**(2): 127.

Gould M (2013). MPs call for investigation into how psychiatric patients are being detained. *BMJ*; **347**: f5135.

Harwood DM, Hope T, Jacoby R (2005). Cognitive impairment in medical inpatients. II: Do physicians miss cognitive impairment? *Age Ageing*; **26**: 37–39.

Hassan TB, MacNamara AF, Davy A, Bing A, Bodiwala GG (1999). Managing patients with deliberate self harm who refuse treatment in the accident and emergency department. *Br Med J*; 319: 107–109.

Jackson E, Warner J (2002). How much do doctors know about consent and capacity? *J R Soc Med*; **95**: 601–603.

McCartney JR, Palmateer LM (1985). Assessment of cognitive deficit in geriatric patients. A study of physician behavior. *J Am Geriatr Soc*; **33**: 467–471.

Mujic F, Von Heising M, Stewart RJ, Prince MJ (2009). Mental capacity assessments among general hospital inpatients referred to a specialist liaison psychiatry service for older people. *Int Psychogeriatr*; **21**:4; 729–737.

NHS guidelines on Deprivation of Liberty Safeguards: http://webarchive.nationalarchives.gov.uk/20130107105354/http://www.ic.nhs.uk/webfiles/Services/Omnibus%20Guidance/Collection%20Guidance/DOLS/DoLS_2012_13_validation_guidance.doc

Office of Public Sector Information. Mental Capacity Act Code of Practice. Ref: ISBN 9780117037465. Ref: ISBN 9780117037465. PDF, 952KB, 301 pages

Office of Public Sector Information. Mental Capacity Act 2005(c9). http://www.opsi.gov.uk/ACTS/acts2005/

Okai D, Owen G, McGuire H, Singh S, Churchill R, Hotopf M (2007). Mental capacity in psychiatric patients: systematic review. *Br J Psychiatry*; **191**: 291–297.

Owen GS, Richardson G, David AS, Szmukler G, Hayward P, Hotopf M (2008). Mental capacity to make decisions on treatment in people admitted to psychiatric hospitals: cross sectional study. *BMJ*; **337**: a448.

Slowther A, Johnston C, Goodall J, Hope T (2004). Development of clinical ethics committees. *BMJ*; **328**: 950–952. http://supremecourt.uk/decidedcases/docs/UKSC_2012_0068_Judgment.pdf

Case 14

An 82-year-old man was admitted from a nursing home generally unwell with a temperature of 38.6°C. The staff at the nursing home reported a gradual decline in the patient's mobility following a fractured neck of femur six months previously with a more abrupt decline over the preceding three days. The past medical history included hypertension, myocardial infarction, type 2 diabetes, and stroke resulting in mild right-sided weakness.

Examination showed atrial fibrillation at 110bpm, with a respiratory rate of 22 breaths per minute, and oxygen saturation of 96% on air. Respiratory system examination was unremarkable, but cardiovascular examination revealed a pansystolic murmur radiating to the axilla. The abdomen was soft and non-tender with no palpable masses. At the base of the sacrum, there was a pressure sore with surrounding erythema (Fig. 14.1).

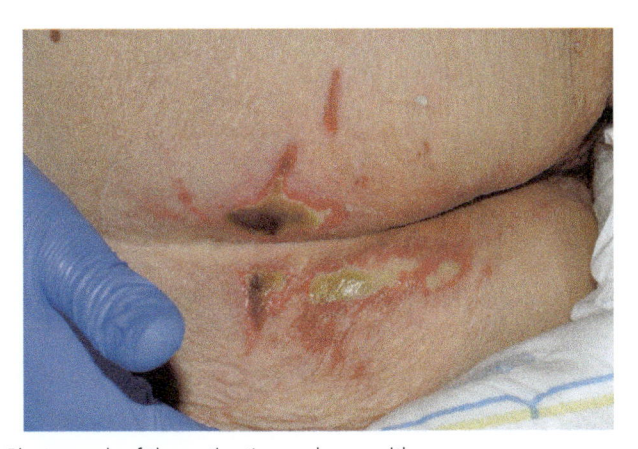

Fig. 14.1 Photograph of the patient's sacral area with pressure sore.

Investigations showed the following:
- Hb: 13.3g/dL
- WCC: 19.8×10^9/L
- Neutrophils: 12×10^9/L

- Sodium: 149mmol/L
- Potassium: 4.7mmol/L
- Urea: 9mmol/L
- Creatinine: 149μmol/L
- CRP: 128mg/L
- Random glucose: 13mmol/L
- CXR: slightly enlarged heart with blunting of the costophrenic angle (Fig. 14.2)
- ECG: rate 116bpm, AF, left axis deviation.

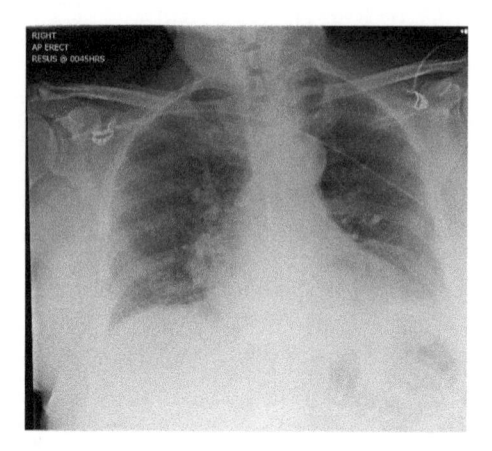

Fig. 14.2 Chest X-ray showing enlarged heart.

Questions

1. What grade (European Pressure Ulcer Advisory Panel Grading) is the pressure sore shown in Fig. 14.1?
2. List the key features of the pressure sore that should be documented.
3. Which areas of the body are commonly affected by pressure sores?
4. Describe the three main mechanical factors that contribute to the development of pressure sores. What are the important intrinsic physiological factors?
5. Discuss the management strategies for pressure sores and for this patient in particular.

Answers

1 What grade (European Pressure Ulcer Advisory Panel Grading) is the pressure sore shown in Figure 14.1?

The pressure sore shown in Figure 14.1 is grade 3.

The European Pressure Ulcer Advisory Panel Grading system is as follows:

Grade 1 (Fig. 14.3)

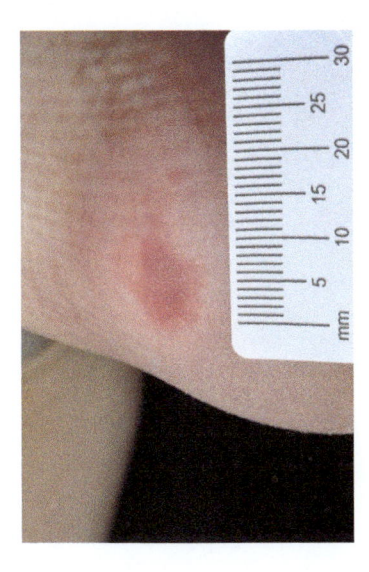

Fig. 14.3 A Grade 1 pressure sore presenting as an area of non-blanchable erythema on intact skin.

An area of non-blanchable erythema on intact skin. In darker-skinned patients discolouration may appear blue or purple. There may also be thickening, warmth, or oedema of the skin.

Grade 2 (Fig 14.4a and 14.4 b)

A superficial ulcer involving loss of either, or both the epidermis and dermis. It may present as a blister with surrounding erythema Figures 14.4 a and b.

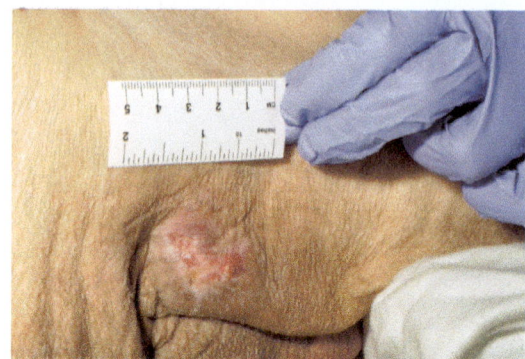

Fig. 14.4 A Grade 2 pressure sore (a and b).

Grade 3 (Fig 14.5)

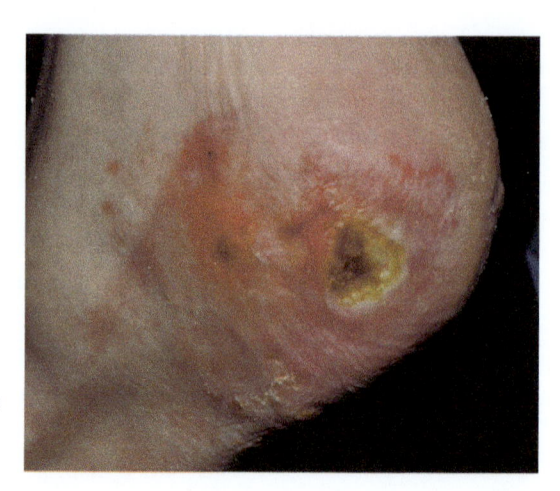

Fig. 14.5 Grade 3 pressure sore with necrosis of the underlying tissue.

Full-thickness skin loss with necrosis of the underlying subcutaneous tissue, which does not penetrate the fascia.

Grade 4 (Fig. 14.6)

Severe tissue necrosis involving the muscle and/or bone, and surrounding fascia. These ulcers are particularly prone to infection and are very difficult to heal.

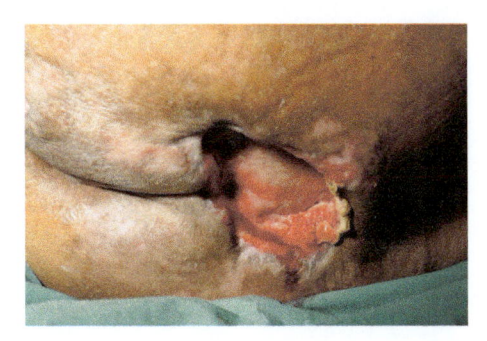

Fig. 14.6 A Grade 4 pressure sore with severe necrosis.

Documentation of the grade and any progression of pressure sores is mandatory, especially on admission to hospital or a care home. Pressure sores are a common cause of complaints against care homes and hospitals, and it is important therefore to be able to establish their origin. It is important to note that sores may not become apparent until sometime after a precipitating event (e.g. prolonged immobilization during surgery) when the patient has moved to a different clinical area, or has even been discharged.

2 List the key features of the pressure sore that should be documented.

Photographs or tracings of the pressure sores should be included in the notes. Key features that should be described include:

a. The grade
b. Date of diagnosis
c. Size—length, width, and depth (Fig. 14.7)
d. Colour—erythema, granulation tissue, yellow or clear exudate, and areas of necrosis (black) (Fig. 14.8)
e. Odour

148 | CASE HISTORIES IN GERIATRIC MEDICINE

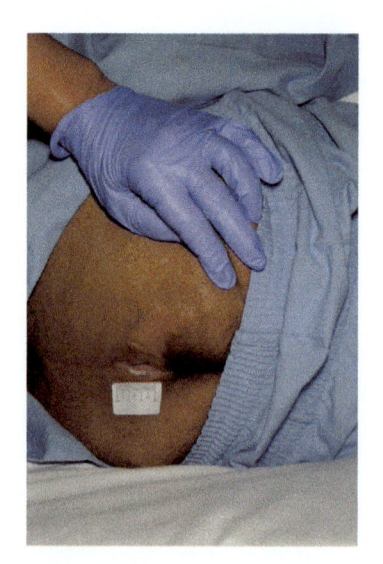

Fig. 14.7 The dimensions of the patient's pressure sore are measured.

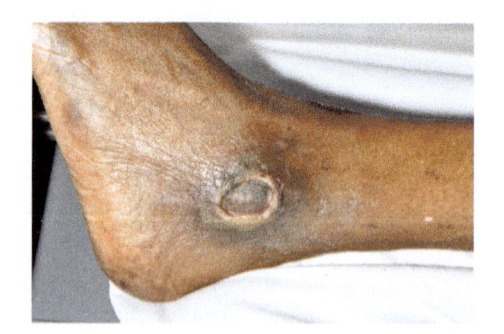

Fig. 14.8 The colour of a pressure sore is noted.

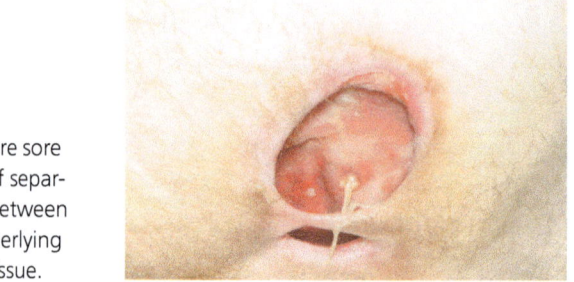

Fig. 14.9 Pressure sore with evidence of separation of tissue between surface and underlying subcutaneous tissue.

f. State of surrounding tissue
g. Evidence of separation of tissue between the surface and underlying subcutaneous tissue (Fig. 14.9).

3 Which areas of the body are commonly affected by pressure sores?

Areas commonly affected by pressure sores are:
a. Ischial tuberosity
b. Sacrum
c. Trochanter
d. Heel
e. Bony spinous processes in patients with kyphosis.

4 Describe the three main mechanical factors that contribute to the development of pressure sores. What are the important intrinsic physiological factors?

The mechanical factors that contribute to pressure sores include pressure, friction, and shearing forces.

Pressure

As the name suggests, pressure is of paramount importance in the development of pressure sores. Even young healthy individuals will develop sores if left immobile in the same position for long enough. External pressure occludes the small capillaries of the skin, preventing adequate supply of oxygen and nutrients, and leads to irreversible ischaemia, tissue damage, and necrosis. A constant pressure of greater than 32mmHg (average arteriolar capillary bed pressure) applied for sufficient time will impede blood flow sufficiently to cause irreversible ischaemic damage in normal skin. However, the pressure and time required for arteriolar occlusion will be less in those with peripheral artery disease, or who are otherwise vulnerable. In such patients, sores may develop over short (one hour or less) time periods, hence the importance of avoiding trolley waits in emergency departments, care during long operations, the use of pressure relieving mattresses, and regular turning.

Friction

Frictional damage may result from skin movement over bed sheets and against clothing that damages the superficial skin layer including the blood capillaries and may cause thrombosis. Dampness of the skin from sweat, washing, or urinary incontinence increases frictional force and exacerbates damage.

Shearing force

Shearing forces occur for instance, when a patient positioned upright in bed slumps downwards, stretching and distorting the skin, subcutaneous tissues, and blood vessels. This is a key factor in sacral pressure sore development.

Both frictional and shearing forces are exacerbated by loose folds of skin, which are common among older people owing to loss of subcutaneous tissue, poor hydration, and nutrition.

Intrinsic physiological factors

Intrinsic physiological factors that are important in pressure sore development include:

- Nutritional status
- Anaemia
- Hydration status
- Fever
- Infection
- Hypoxia
- Hypotension
- Ischaemic heart disease
- Peripheral neuropathy
- Spinal cord damage
- Immobility
- Incontinence
- Obesity.

Susceptibility to pressure sores is probably a good proxy measure of frailty with which the aforementioned factors are frequently associated (see cases 5, 7, 13, 15, 19, 21, 24, 25, 32, 41, 46, 47).

5 Discuss the management strategies for pressure sores and for this patient in particular.

The most important factor in pressure sore management is prevention. On admission to hospital or care home, patients should undergo a pressure sore risk assessment and this should be reviewed regularly. Common risk assessment tools include the Braden, Norton, Waterlow, and Pressure Sore Prediction Score scales.

Sites of potential skin breakdown should be monitored and checked daily. The forces and physiological factors leading to the development of a pressure sore will vary between individuals, and although frequently multifactorial, attempts should be made to identify and address the key precipitating or exacerbating factors (e.g. nutrition, incontinence, seating, or bed type).

This patient has a grade 3 pressure sore. In such cases, necrotic tissue should be debrided by autolytic, chemical, mechanical, or surgical means, and ulcers should be regularly cleaned and inspected to look for signs of infection. Modern hydrocolloid, hydrogels, and foam dressings are preferred over traditional paraffin and simple gauze dressings. Air mattresses, which alternate levels of pressure over vulnerable areas, should be used. Expert advice from tissue viability nurses should be sought when available. If there is suspected systemic infection, cellulitis or osteomyelitis, wound, and blood cultures should be taken, and appropriate antibiotics initiated. This patient was systemically unwell and improved with intravenous flucloxacillin. The pansystolic murmur raised the possibility of endocarditis (see case 10), but this was not confirmed.

Surgery may be considered for grade 3–4 ulcers if conservative measures fail. Procedures range from superficial debridement in which the wound is left open to heal, abscess drainage, bone removal, and skin flap repair. However, surgery is more commonly performed on younger patients with poor mobility from, e.g. multiple sclerosis, who tend to be less frail with fewer co-morbidities than older patients in whom surgery may be considered high risk.

Further reading

Royal College of Nursing Guidelines (September 2009). The management of pressure ulcers in primary and secondary care.
NICE Guidelines (2005). The prevention and treatment of pressure ulcers.
European Pressure Ulcer Advisory Panel (2003). Pressure ulcer treatment guidelines.
European Pressure Ulcer Advisory Panel (2003). Pressure ulcer grading system.

Case 15

A 78-year-old man was seen in the rapid access clinic with a six-week history of shortness of breath on exertion, tiredness, and lethargy. His feet were swollen and he had noticed a recent gain in weight. Several nights earlier, he had had to sleep in a chair, as lying in bed even with three pillows exacerbated the shortness of breath and he had also had episodes of waking up during the night gasping for breath. There was a past history of high blood pressure (although he did not take his prescribed amlodipine regularly as it made his feet and legs swollen), diet controlled diabetes mellitus, and deep vein thrombosis of the right leg following a flight from China two months previously, for which he was taking warfarin. He had never smoked and did not consume any alcohol.

On examination, he was apyrexial with regular pulse of 72bpm, blood pressure of 150/80mmHg and oxygen saturation on room air was 96%. The jugular venous pressure was elevated and there were bilateral basal lung crepitations, pitting oedema to the knees, and sacral oedema. The rest of the examination was unremarkable.

The GP had organized tests for FBC, U&E, TFT, LFT, fasting glucose, cholesterol, and C-reactive protein, all of which were normal and B-type natriuretic peptide (BNP), which was raised at 600pg/mL (normal—up to 100pg/mL).

Further investigations showed the following:

- INR: 3.5
- CXR: see Figure 15.1a
- ECG: left axis deviation; sinus rhythm; heart rate 72bpm
- Urine dipstick and microscopy: no blood or protein; no cells; no casts.

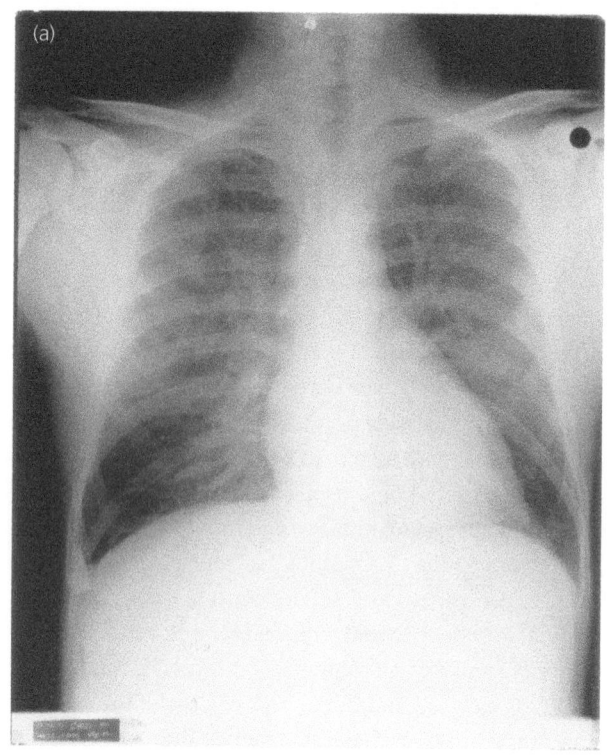

Fig. 15.1a Plain X-ray of the patient's chest (posteroanterior view).

Questions

1 What is the most likely syndrome illustrated by this case and what is the prevalence in older patients?
2 How would you further investigate this patient?
3 What is the significance of the elevated BNP?

CASE 15 | 155

Answers

1 What is the most likely syndrome illustrated by this case and what is the prevalence in older patients?

The syndrome, indicated by the symptoms, clinical signs, and investigations (chest X-ray, see Fig.15.1b and elevated BNP) is heart failure.

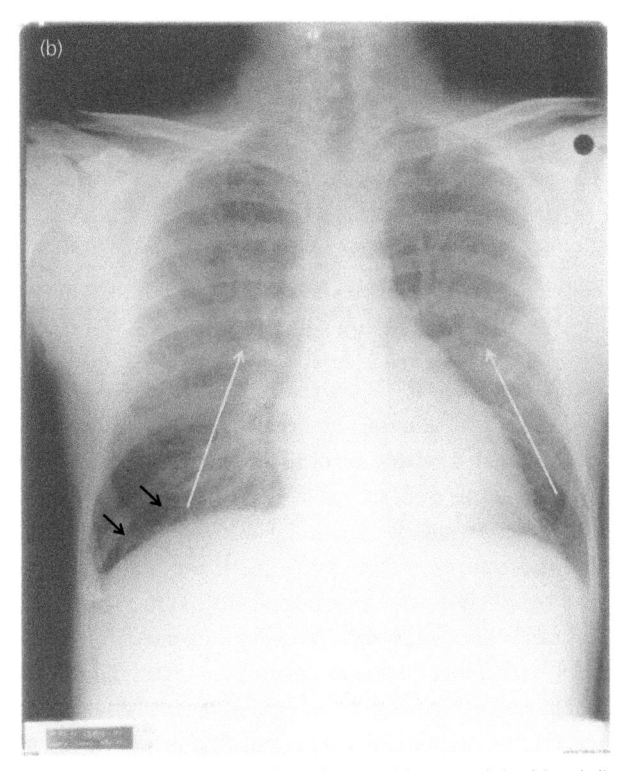

Fig. 15.1b Chest X-ray showing normal size heart with upper lobe blood diversion (white arrows) and curly B lines at the bases (small black arrows)

Heart failure can be defined as an abnormality of cardiac structure or function leading to failure of the heart to deliver oxygen at a rate commensurate with the requirements of the metabolizing tissues, despite normal filling pressures (or only at the expense of increased filling pressures). Patients can be classified by ejection fraction into two groups: heart failure with reduced ejection fraction (EF <50%) (HFrEF) and heart failure with preserved ejection fraction (EF ≥50%) (HFpEF).

Many of the symptoms and signs of HF are nondiscriminating and therefore of limited diagnostic value although some are more specific (at the expense of a reduced sensitivity—see Table 15.1).

Table 15.1 More sensitive versus more specific signs in heart failure

More sensitive Less specific	More specific Less sensitive
Leg oedema, lung crackles	Dyspnoea on exertion
ECG changes, e.g. left axis deviation; heart block; infarct; left bundle branch block; ST-changes; and left ventricular hypertrophy	Paroxysmal nocturnal dyspnoea
	Orthopnoea
	Raised JVP

This patient therefore had several of the more specific signs of heart failure (orthopnea, paroxysmal nocturnal dyspnoea and raised jugular venous pressure) as well as several of the more sensitive but less specific signs including lung crepitations and leg oedema, making the diagnosis relatively straightforward. Severity of symptoms may be classified using the New York Heart Association system (see Box 15.1).

Many of the signs of heart failure result from sodium and water retention, and resolve quickly with diuretic therapy, i.e. may be absent in patients receiving such treatment. Demonstration of an underlying cardiac cause is therefore central to the diagnosis of heart failure, e.g. this may be myocardial disease causing systolic ventricular dysfunction. However, abnormalities of ventricular diastolic function or of the valves, pericardium, endocardium, heart rhythm, and conduction, can also cause heart failure, and more than one abnormality can be present. Identification of the underlying cardiac problem is also crucial for therapeutic reasons, as the precise pathology determines the specific treatment used (e.g. valve surgery for valvular disease, specific pharmacological therapy for left ventricle systolic dysfunction, etc.).

Approximately 1–2% of the adult population in developed countries has heart failure, with the prevalence rising to ≥10% among persons 70 years of age or older. In older people, the diagnosis of heart failure is often more difficult because of non-specific or misleading symptoms including general deterioration in function, fatigue which may be attributed to 'normal ageing', co-morbidities, swollen legs, and obscuring of symptoms due to cognitive impairment, functional limitations, or communication difficulties. Heart failure is associated with a fatality rate of around 30–40% within a year of diagnosis and around 10% will die annually. Heart failure accounts for 5% of all hospital admissions in the UK and from 1999 to 2000, admission rates for people aged over 85 years increased by over 50% for men and around one third for women, and it has been predicted that hospital admissions resulting from heart failure will continue to rise over the next 25 years, as the population ages.

Box 15.1 New York Heart Association functional classification based on severity of symptoms and physical activity

Class I

No limitation of physical activity. Ordinary physical activity does not cause undue breathlessness, fatigue, or palpitations

Class II

Slight limitation of physical activity. Comfortable at rest, but ordinary physical activity results in undue breathlessness, fatigue, or palpitations

Class III

Marked limitation of physical activity. Comfortable at rest, but less than ordinary physical activity results in undue breathlessness, fatigue, or palpitations

Class IV

Unable to carry on any physical activity without discomfort. Symptoms at rest can be present. If any physical activity is undertaken, discomfort is increased

(Source: American Heart Association, Inc.)

2 How would you further investigate this patient?

Further investigations should include:

- Echocardiogram (ECHO)
- Specific tests to establish the underlying cause of the heart failure if the ECHO is inconclusive.

Numerous guidelines exist regarding the diagnosis, investigation and management of heart failure (e.g. European Society of Cardiology, the Scottish Intercollegiate Guidelines Network, and the National Institute of Clinical Excellence). Detailed history and examination is followed by investigations targeted where necessary to determine the underlying cause, as well as to quantify the degree of failure, and whether or not there is LV dysfunction.

Investigations to consider in all patients

The ECG and ECHO are the most useful tests for suspected heart failure.

A 12-lead ECG is recommended to determine heart rhythm, electrical conduction abnormalities, heart rate, QRS morphology, and QRS duration, and to detect evidence of LV hypertrophy or Q waves. The ECG has prognostic importance (e.g. indicating loss of viable myocardium), and may indicate the aetiology of HF, e.g. from a previous infarct.. The ECG findings are also important for decisions about treatment (e.g. rate control and anticoagulation for atrial fibrillation, pacing for bradycardia, or if criteria for cardiac resynchronization therapy are met). Heart failure is very unlikely (likelihood <2%) in patients presenting acutely with a completely normal ECG. In patients with a non-acute presentation, a normal ECG has a somewhat lower negative predictive value (likelihood ~10–14%).

Transthoracic echocardiography is recommended to evaluate cardiac structure and function, including diastolic function, and to measure left ventricular ejection fraction to confirm the diagnosis of HF, assist in the planning and monitoring of treatment, and to obtain prognostic information. This information is crucial in determining appropriate treatment (e.g. an angiotensin-converting-enzyme inhibitor and beta-blocker for systolic dysfunction, or surgery for aortic stenosis).

Routine biochemical and haematological investigations are recommended in order to:

i. Evaluate patient suitability for diuretic, renin–angiotensin–aldosterone antagonist, and anticoagulant therapy (and monitor treatment).
ii. Detect reversible/treatable factors exacerbating or causing heart failure (e.g. thyroid dysfunction) and co-morbidities (e.g. iron deficiency anaemia).
iii. Obtain prognostic information (e.g. reduced creatinine clearance and anaemia, which are associated with a poorer prognosis).

Measurement of natriuretic peptide (BNP, NT-proBNP, or MR-proANP) should be considered to:

i. Exclude alternative causes of dyspnoea (if the BNP level is below the exclusion cut-point, heart failure is very unlikely)
ii. Obtain prognostic information—BNP levels correlate with the severity of heart failure. In addition, the prognosis is better if the BNP level falls significantly (>30%) after treatment.

A chest X-ray should be considered to detect/exclude lung disease, e.g. cancer (but does not exclude asthma/COPD). It may also identify pulmonary congestion/oedema/upper lobe diversion/pleural effusions (as seen in Fig. 15.1) and is more useful in patients with suspected heart failure in the acute setting.

Investigations to consider in selected patients

Magnetic resonance imaging may be recommended to evaluate cardiac structure and function, to measure LVEF, and to characterize cardiac tissue, especially in subjects with inadequate echocardiographic images, or where the echocardiographic findings are inconclusive or incomplete.

Exercise testing should be considered in physically fit patients to detect reversible myocardial ischaemia, as well as myocardial perfusion imaging.

Coronary angiography is recommended in patients with angina pectoris, who are considered suitable for coronary revascularization, to evaluate the coronary anatomy.

3 What is the significance of the elevated BNP?

This patient's BNP level was 600pg/mL, which is consistent with a diagnosis of heart failure and also suggests a poor prognosis.

A normal natriuretic peptide level in an untreated patient virtually excludes significant cardiac disease, making an echocardiogram unnecessary and investigation for a non-cardiac cause of the patient's problems is likely to be more productive (see Box 15.2 for a summary of the use of BNP). BNP or N-terminal pro-B-type natriuretic peptide (NT-proBNP) may be measured, depending on local availability.

Box 15.2 BNP in the assessment of heart failure

- Previously untreated patients with BNP of <100pg/ml or NT-proBNP <400pg/ml are very unlikely to have heart failure
- Patients with BNP of 100–400 pg/ml or NT-proBNP of 400–2000pg/ml should be referred for further investigation (echocardiogram, specialist assessment)
- Patients with BNP of >400 pg/ml or NT-proBNP of >2000pg/ml should be assessed urgently

Limitations of the use of BNP or pro-BNP are:

- BNP is persistently elevated in some patients and so cannot be used to monitor treatment
- Levels may be lowered by ACE inhibitors, angiotensin-receptor blockers, beta-blockers, aldosterone antagonists, diuretics, and in obese patients
- Levels may be elevated in patients with tachycardia, liver cirrhosis, renal failure, (glomerular filtration rate <60ml/min), sepsis, diabetes, chronic obstructive pulmonary disease, right ventricular overload, left ventricular hypertrophy, cardiac ischaemia, and in some healthy people aged over 70 years

Case development

The patient's transthoracic Doppler two-dimensional echocardiogram showed:
- Left atrium diameter: 45mm
- Left ventricle systolic diameter: 32mm
- Left ventricle diastolic diameter: 48mm
- Left ventricle wall mass index: 150g/m^2
- Ejection fraction (EF): 65%
- Early mitral valve flow velocity (E)/early diastolic lengthening velocity (E')—(E/E'): >16 (normal <8)
- Aorta: normal ascending aortic root diameter, normal aortic and mitral valve appearance; right ventricle: normal size and function; right atrium: normal diameter and pressure.

This patient also had a heart MRI scan, which was unremarkable.

Questions continued

4. What do the echocardiographic findings indicate and what are the criteria for establishing the particular form of the syndrome illustrated by this patient?

5. What proportion of heart failure patients have preserved ejection fraction? How do these patients differ from those with compromised ejection fraction?

6. How would you manage this patient and what is the evidence to support your choice?

7. List the commoner conditions that may mimic heart failure with preserved ejection fraction.

8. List the most common non-cardiac conditions associated with heart failure in older people. How may some of these conditions affect management?

Answers continued

4 What do the echocardiographic findings indicate and what are the criteria for establishing the particular form of the syndrome illustrated by this patient?

The echocardiographic findings indicate that the patient has heart failure with preserved ejection fraction, as per the European Society of Cardiology guidelines (see also Table 15.2, Figs. 15.2–4):

- presence of signs and symptoms of congestive heart failure
- preserved LV ejection fraction of a non-dilated left ventricle
- evidence of diastolic dysfunction (impaired LV relaxation or increased LV diastolic stiffness) with elevated LV filling pressures.

Table 15.2 Criteria for heart failure with preserved ejection fraction

◆ Signs or symptoms of congestive heart failure
◆ Evidence of diastolic dysfunction on echocardiogram. The ratio of early mitral valve flow velocity (E) to early diastolic lengthening velocities (E) correlates with LV filling pressure. High ratio E/E, (Fig. 15.3) greater than 15 confirms diastolic left ventricle dysfunction. Values of <8 have high negative predictive value for the diagnosis of heart failure with preserved ejection fraction. E/E 8–15 is suggestive but not diagnostic of heart failure with preserved ejection fraction. If possible, such patients should have exercise echocardiography, where the level of exercise will depend on patients' individual circumstances, such as the presence of co-morbidities. Also, other measures may be necessary for the diagnosis: for example, a left ventricle wall mass index of >149g/m^2 in men or >122g/m^2 in women. There is evidence of increased LV filling pressure if E/A is high >2, with short deceleration time DT E <160ms (Fig. 15.4, the image from a different patient), with short isovolumic relaxation time (<60 ms) and with a low E
◆ Normal or only mildly abnormal left ventricular systolic function with an ejection fraction greater than 50% with a left ventricle end-diastolic volume index of <97 ml/m^2, LA volume index ≥34ml/m^2
E should always be interpreted in the context of LV and LA morphology, function, haemodynamics, and response to exercise of an individual patient

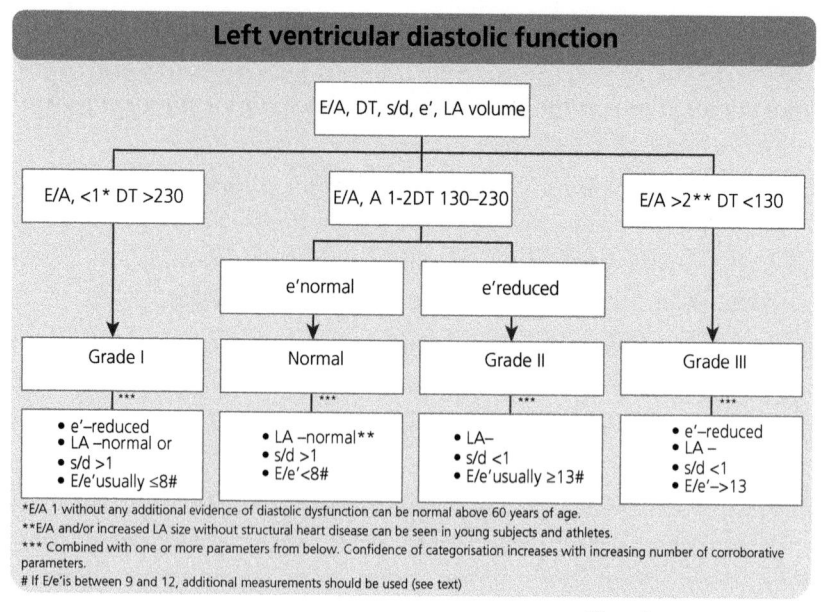

Left ventricular diastolic function

```
                    E/A, DT, s/d, e', LA volume
        ┌──────────────────┼──────────────────┐
   E/A, <1* DT >230    E/A, A 1-2 DT 130-230   E/A >2** DT <130
        │           ┌──────┴──────┐            │
        │        e'normal      e'reduced       │
        │           │              │           │
     Grade I      Normal        Grade II    Grade III
       ***         ***            ***          ***
```

- e'–reduced
- LA –normal or
- s/d >1
- E/e' usually ≤8#

- LA –normal**
- s/d >1
- E/e' <8#

- LA–
- s/d <1
- E/e' usually ≥13#

- e'–reduced
- LA –
- s/d <1
- E/e'–>13

*E/A 1 without any additional evidence of diastolic dysfunction can be normal above 60 years of age.
**E/A and/or increased LA size without structural heart disease can be seen in young subjects and athletes.
*** Combined with one or more parameters from below. Confidence of categorisation increases with increasing number of corroborative parameters.
# If E/e' is between 9 and 12, additional measurements should be used (see text)

Chamber Quantification

Fig. 15.2 Practical approach to assessment and grading of diastolic dysfunction:
* E/A <1 without any additional evidence of diastolic dysfunction can be normal above 60 years of age.
** E/A >2 and/or increased LA size without structural heart disease can be seen in young subjects and athletes.
*** Combined with one or more parameters already mentioned. Confidence of categorization increases with increasing number of corroborative parameters.
\# If E/e is between 9 and 12, additional measurements should be used.
In some diagnostically inconclusive cases, further investigations (e.g. cardiac MRI, radionuclide angiography, cardiac catheterization) may be considered where the results of echocardiography are inconclusive.
(Reprinted with permission of the British Society of Echocardiography)

CASE 15 | **163**

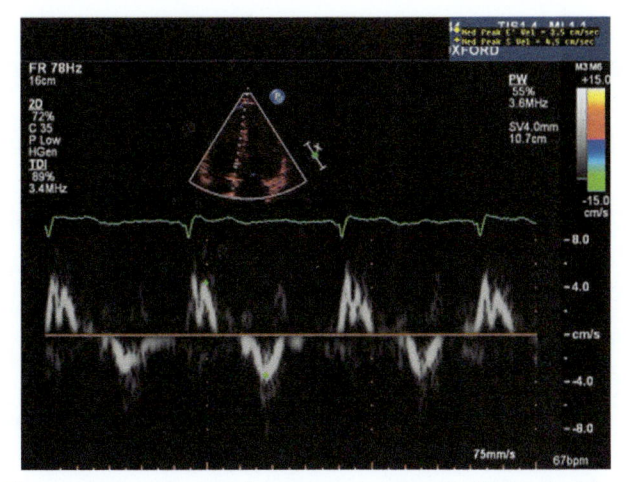

Fig. 15.3 Tissue Doppler of ventricular septum showing E' of 3.5cm/s giving an E/E' ratio of >30.

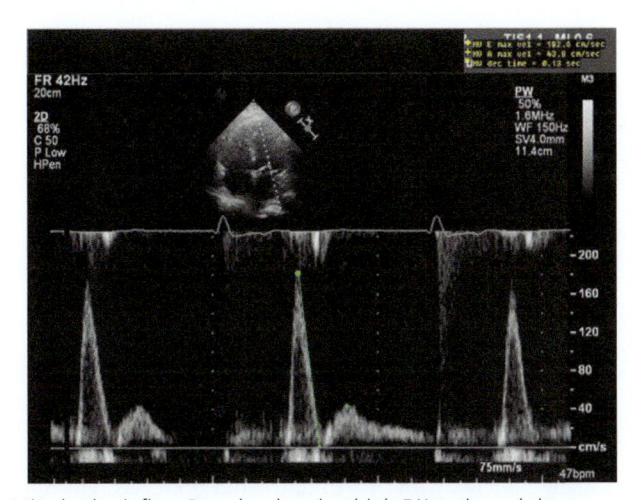

Fig. 15.4 Mitral valve inflow Doppler showing high E/A ratio and short deceleration time.

5 What proportion of heart failure patients have preserved ejection fraction? How do these patients differ from those with compromised ejection fraction?

Heart failure with preserved ejection fraction accounts for around 40–50% of all cases of heart failure and the prevalence increases with age.

Compared to those with reduced ejection fraction, patients with preserved ejection fraction are more likely to:

- have less severe symptoms
- be diagnosed as out-patients
- more likely to be hospitalized because of co-existing conditions
- have the following co-morbidities: diabetes mellitus (45% vs. 40%); anaemia; obesity; hypertension; and pulmonary disease
- have atrial fibrillation as in the current case
- have less elevated BNP levels
- be older (in one study 78 vs. 74 years)
- be female (the Framingham Heart Study had shown >2-fold increased risk)
- be obese
- survive hospital admission
- have obstructive sleep apnoea.

and are less likely to:

- have coronary artery disease (30% vs. 50%)
- have renal dysfunction (40% vs. 50%)
- have X-ray evidence of cardiomegaly
- be treated with ACE inhibitors and digoxin
- have a previous history of chronic heart failure
- require hospitalization
- have been previously hospitalized for heart failure.

Although many patients with heart failure and preserved ejection fraction have no underlying cardiac condition, common associated cardiac abnormalities include:

- chronic hypertension with left ventricular hypertrophy (as in the current case)
- constrictive pericarditis
- inherited or acquired restrictive cardiomyopathy (idiopathic or caused by infiltrative diseases, such as sarcoidosis, or amyloidosis)

- hypertrophic cardiomyopathy
- aortic stenosis with normal left ventricular ejection fraction.

6 How would you manage this patient and what is the evidence to support your choice?

This patient was given regular diuretics (furosemide and spironolactone) and angiotensin-converting enzyme inhibitor with clinical improvement. Warfarin and amlodipine were continued as before. He was also educated regarding restricting salt intake, checking his weight daily, and in recognizing the warning symptoms of worsening heart failure or overtreatment, e.g. postural hypotension.

There is a lack of data to guide the treatment of heart failure in older patients, particularly in heart failure with preserved ejection function. Overall, there is little evidence of mortality benefit for drugs proven to be effective for heart failure with reduced ejection fraction in those with preserved ejection function (e.g. the PEP-CHF study—perindopril versus placebo, CHARM-preserved trial-candesartan versus placebo, I-PRESERVE trial-irbesartan versus placebo, CHARM-Alternative trial-candesartan versus placebo). Also, there is no clear evidence to support statin therapy. Despite lack of evidence, targeting specific co-morbidities in patients with HFpEF may present an important part of the overall management.

In practice, treatment usually includes:

- Diuretics, to reduce fluid retention, and congestive symptoms
- Angiotensin-converting enzyme inhibitors or angiotensin-receptor blockers (hydralazine in combination with nitrate is an alternative)
- Beta-blockers licensed for heart failure, e.g. carvedilol, bisoprolol, nebivolol, which slow the heart rate, increase left ventricular filling time and coronary blood flow, and thus improve cardiac output.

Other therapies that may be considered include:

- aspirin (75–150mg/day) in coronary heart disease
- anticoagulation in patients with atrial fibrillation or for those in sinus rhythm, but with intracardiac thrombus, left ventricular aneurysm, or a history of thromboembolism
- digoxin for atrial fibrillation if beta-blockers are insufficient, or there is a contraindication
- calcium channel blockers for hypertension or angina, or AF rate control in certain cases
- influenza vaccine

- pneumococcal vaccine
- lifestyle modifications: diet; sodium restriction; weight loss in overweight patients; smoking cessation
- rehabilitation.

Elderly patients with heart failure benefit from multi-disciplinary team input and in the UK this is now recommended best practice. Such teams are led by a specialist (usually a consultant cardiologist). Specialist heart failure team management is particularly recommended for patients with:

- severe heart failure (NYHA Class IV; see Box 15.1)
- heart failure not responding to treatment
- heart failure that cannot be managed at home
- heart failure caused by valve disease
- heart failure with previous myocardial infarction.

Evidence of the benefit of cardiac rehabilitation in older patients with preserved ejection fraction is lacking, but small studies of exercise training in younger patients have shown improvements in exercise capacity and quality of life.

7 List the commoner conditions that may mimic heart failure with preserved ejection fraction.

Mimics of heart failure with preserved ejection fraction include:

- lung disease
- obesity
- myocardial ischaemia
- uncontrolled atrial fibrillation.

8 List the most common non-cardiac conditions associated with heart failure in older people. How may these conditions affect management?

The most common non-cardiac conditions associated with chronic heart failure (both with and without preserved ejection fraction) in older patients, are:

- Chronic renal impairment. This is an independent predictor of poor prognosis (~ 30% increase in mortality). Such patients are more likely to have lower blood pressure, higher plasma BNP levels, and to be older. Occasionally, renal impairment may be difficult to differentiate from heart failure, as pulmonary oedema, fluid overload, and elevated serum BNP may occur in both. A reduced glomerular filtration rate makes diuretics less effective and conversely, cardiac medications may worsen renal function. In addition, care is needed to reduce drug doses where necessary, e.g. digoxin, angiotensin-converting enzyme inhibitors, angiotensin-receptor blockers.

- Cognitive impairment. The prevalence of cognitive impairment varies between studies depending on the population and the method used to define impairment, but estimates range from 35% to 50% of older patients. Mechanisms include co-existent cerebrovascular disease, vascular risk factors, and the effects of brain hypoperfusion. Cognitive impairment is associated with functional deterioration and a five-fold increase in mortality. Recognition of cognitive impairment is important because of the need to ensure the patient is supported in taking their medication (e.g. use of a dosette box, supervision via carers).
- Depression is associated with heart failure and with renal impairment, morbidity, mortality, and hospitalization.
- Insomnia, anxiety, agitation.
- Obstructive sleep apnoea/hypopnoea and central sleep apnoea syndromes (see case 37, Sleep disorders). These conditions are twice as common in heart failure patients as in age-matched controls. Sleep-disordered breathing conditions are more severe and common in the older, male population. There are no data on the impact of such conditions on HFpEF outcomes.
- Diabetes mellitus. High rates of left ventricular diastolic dysfunction have been reported among normotensive patients with diabetes.
- Chronic anaemia.
- Obesity (body mass index (BMI) ≥35 kg/m^2 is associated with ~30% increase in cardiovascular hospitalization or death when compared to BMI 26.5–30.9 kg/m^2).
- Chronic obstructive pulmonary disease (see case 45) is present in around 30% of patients with heart failure, since both conditions are associated with smoking and ageing. It has higher prevalence in HFpEF patients. Symptoms and signs overlap, and patients often display poor echocardiogram windows, making it difficult to attribute symptoms correctly.
- Hypertension.
- Ischaemic heart disease.

- Postural hypotension and falls (see cases 11, 24, 27, 47).
- Nutritional disorders (see case 5).
- Incontinence (see case 7).
- Cerebrovascular disease (see cases 19, 26, 42).
- Musculoskeletal/joint problems requiring analgesia, such as arthritis (see case 41).
- Frailty (e.g. risk of falls, poor mobility see case 35).

Further reading

Betts T, Dwight J, Bull S (2010). Cardiology: Clinical cases uncovered. Chichester, UK: Wiley-Blackwell.

Cleland JGF, Tendera M, Adams J, et al. (2006). The perindopril in elderly people with chronic heart failure (PEP-CHF) study. *Eur Heart J*; **27**(19): 2338–2345.

Gure TR, Blaum CS, Giordani B, et al. (2012). Prevalence of cognitive impairment in older adults with heart failure. *J Am Geriatr Soc*; **60**(9): 1724–1729.

Hogg K, Swedberg K, McMurray J (2004). Heart failure with preserved left ventricular systolic function: epidemiology, clinical characteristics, and prognosis. *J Am Coll Cardiol*; **43**: 317–327.

Jong P, McKelvie R, Yusuf S (2010). Should treatment for heart failure with preserved ejection fraction differ from that for heart failure reduced ejection fraction? *BMJ*; 341: c4202.

Kotecha T, Fox K (2013). Investigating suspected heart failure. *BMJ*; **346**: f2442.

Lien CT, Gillespie ND, Struthers AD, McMurdo ME (2002). Heart failure in frail elderly patients: diagnostic difficulties, co-morbidities, polypharmacy and treatment dilemmas. *Eur J Heart Fail*; **4**: 91–98.

Mentz,RJ, Kelly, JP, von Lueder, TG, et al. (2014). Noncardiac comorbidities in heart failure with reduced versus preserved ejection fraction. *J Am Coll Cardiol*; **64**; 21:2281–2293.

Owan TE, Hodge DO, Herges RM, Jacobsen SJ, Roger VL, Redfield MM (2006). Trends in prevalence and outcome of heart failure with preserved ejection fraction. *N Engl J Med*; **355**(3): 251–259.

Paulus WJ, Tschope C, Sanderson JE, et al. (2007). How to diagnose diastolic heart failure: a consensus statement on the diagnosis of heart failure with normal left ventricular ejection fraction by the Heart Failure and Echocardiography Associations of the European Society of Cardiology. *Eur Heart J*; **28**; 2539–2550.

Penicka M, Vanderheyden M, Bartunek J (2014). Diagnosis of heart failure with preserved ejection fraction: role of clinical Doppler echocardiography. *Heart*; **100**: 68–76.

Case 16

An 82-year-old woman was admitted to hospital after a fall. No fractures were sustained, but she was unwell, and urine cultures grew coagulase negative staphylococci. She was treated successfully and received physiotherapy, but remained in hospital after three weeks. Her mobility improved, but she complained of tiredness. It was noted that her temperature increased every evening to between 38.3 and 38.8°C. She denied night sweats or headache, and did not have any rash. She was continent and had regular bowel opening.

There was no past medical history of note, but she described fatigue, loss of appetite, and weight loss of around 4kg over the preceding three months. Medications were paracetamol, calcium, and vitamin D. She was a non-smoker and drank only an occasional glass of wine.

She had been married for almost 60 years, but around 20 years ago had stopped being sexually active. There were no children. She had not travelled abroad for years, denied any allergies, and did not take over-the-counter medications.

On examination she was thin with a heart rate of 90bpm regular and blood pressure of 130/70 mmHg. External and rectal examination were unremarkable.

Investigations showed the following:

- Hb 12.7g/dl; WCC 11.05×10^9/L (7.24×10^9/L neutrophils, 4.0×10^9/L platelets, 0.2×10^9/L eosinophils)
- Na 135mmol/L; K 5.0mmol/L; adjusted calcium 2.38mmol/L; TFT, LFT—normal
- CRP 33mg/L; ESR 35mmh
- Serum electrophoresis: normal
- Urine dipstick, urine and blood cultures: negative
- CXR: normal
- Tuberculin skin test—negative; HIV—negative; HBsAg—not detected; Hepatitis C antibody—not detected; Lyme disease (*Borrelia burgdorferi*) antibody—negative.

- Echocardiogram: mild aortic sclerosis
- Ultrasound: no focal liver lesions or biliary dilatation; normal appearance of the spleen, kidneys, and pancreas; no free fluid.

Questions

1 What is the syndrome illustrated by this case?
2 What differential underlying diagnosis would you consider?
3 What are the most common causes of this syndrome in older patients?
4 How would you establish the underlying cause?

Answers

1 What is the syndrome illustrated by this case?

The syndrome is fever of unknown origin, which is defined as the presence of fever of 38.3°C or higher (measured rectally) on at least two occasions over at least three weeks, for which no cause can be identified after three days of investigations in hospital, after three or more out-patient visits, or after a week of intensive out-patient testing. Apart from history taking and thorough examination, tests should include C-reactive protein (CRP), erythrocyte sedimentation rate (ESR), full blood count, ferritin, renal function tests, electrolytes, liver function tests, lactate dehydrogenase, total protein, protein electrophoresis, creatine kinase, rheumatoid factor, antinuclear antibodies, tuberculin skin test, chest X-ray, abdominal ultrasound, urine microscopic analysis, urine, and three blood cultures. Fever of unknown origin is not:

- Fatal over a short period of time
- Caused by a condition diagnosed by common tests (e.g. urine or blood cultures, chest X-ray).
- Self-limiting—does not resolve over the period expected for self-limited infections.

The incidence and prevalence of fever of unknown origin is uncertain, but timely diagnosis and investigation is particularly important in older patients owing to increased likelihood of morbidity and mortality from delay in diagnosis and treatment, because of a reduced immune response, less physiologic reserve, etc.

There are four different types of fever of unknown origin:

- Classic fever of unknown origin. This was felt to be the most likely form in the current case since the patient had fever for weeks before admission to the hospital, and the cause was not found, despite routine investigation (excludes patients with known hypogammaglobulinaemia or patients who were taking prednisolone 10 mg (or equivalent) in preceding three months prior to the start of the fever).
- Neutropenic fever of unknown origin, associated with <500 neutrophils/µl, and at least two days of negative culture incubation.
- Nosocomial fever of unknown origin, in patients hospitalized for acute care who are appropriately investigated over three or more days without success, with at least two days of cultures without diagnosis.

- HIV-associated fever of unknown origin, in HIV patients investigated for at least three weeks as an out-patient, or for three days as an in-patient, and with cultures incubated for over two days without identification of the cause.

2 What underlying differential diagnosis would you consider?

The causes of fever of unknown origin can be divided into the following broad categories:

- noninfectious inflammatory disease (NIID) – include granulomatous disorders, autoimmune and rheumatic diseases, vasculitic syndromes.
- infectious
- malignant
- miscellaneous
- unknown.

The differential diagnosis of fever of unknown origin is similar in adults across the age spectrum, except that factitious and habitual fever is very rare in older patients, and common diseases presenting atypically are more often seen. Recent data suggest that infection as a cause of fever of unknown origin is diminishing in developed countries whereas NIID is becoming more important. Specific causes include:

- Neoplasm, found in around 10–20% of older patients, e.g. lymphomas, leukaemias, myeloproliferative disorders, solid tumours, of which colon cancer is the most common, renal carcinoma, breast, pancreas, liver, uterus, metastatic carcinoma.
- Infections, found in 20–50% of cases. Infections may cause abscesses, e.g. intra-abdominal, urinary tract infection, e.g. with *E coli*, endocarditis (see case 10), CMV infection, osteomyelitis and tuberculosis (more common in older patients), cat scratch disease, sinusitis, toxoplasmosis, trichinosis.
- Connective tissue disorders. Giant cell arteritis (see case 39) and polymyalgia rheumatica (see case 28) account for around 60%. Other conditions include systemic lupus erythematosus, rheumatoid arthritis, and polyarthritis nodosa (more common in older patients).
- Deep vein thrombosis, occult thrombophlebitis, and pulmonary emboli.
- Drug induced, suggested by correlation between initiation of the drug and the start of the fever, followed by resolution on stopping the medication. Commonly implicated drugs include antibiotics, often beta-lactam, isoniazid, alpha-methyldopa.

- Granulomatous disorders (e.g. sarcoidosis).
- Endocrine disorders (adrenal insufficiency, hyperthyroidism, subacute thyroiditis).
- Liver (alcoholic) cirrhosis, inflammatory bowel disease.
- Undiagnosed cases, estimated at around 10% in older patients compared to around 30% in younger adults, possibly because of spontaneous resolution in younger and fitter patients, or earlier appearance of disease specific symptom in older patients.

3 What are the most common causes of this syndrome in older patients?

In older patients, the most common underlying diseases causing fever of unknown origin are:

- Giant cell arteritis, polymyalgia rheumatica
- Deep vein thrombosis, occult thrombophlebitis, and pulmonary embolism.
- Tuberculosis (particularly miliary tuberculosis and extrapulmonary sites) usually from reactivation of old disease. Presentation is often non-specific with tiredness, confusion, and weight loss, while classic symptoms of night sweats or haemoptysis are much less common in older people.
- Abscess (abdominal and pelvis)
- Haematological malignancy (leukaemias, lymphomas)
- Colon cancer
- Drug related fever

4 How would you establish the underlying cause?

A thorough history should be taken asking systematically about specific symptoms, especially about any local or generalized pain, or discomfort. Patients may remember new and important details of the history, not previously mentioned, on further repeated questioning. It is important that an individual approach to each patient is adopted.

Potential diagnostic clues for further investigation and diagnosis may emerge from a history of night sweats, headache, weight loss, fatigue, contact with animals, travel history, occupational history, drugs (all drugs can cause fever, including over the counter or internet-purchased remedies and should be stopped, including antibiotics), sexual history (see case 30), animal contact, nutrition (ingestion of undercooked meats or unpasteurized dairy products), recreational habits, as well as previous history of, or exposure to, tuberculosis, cancer, or surgical procedures (see case 10), and indwelling joint prostheses, or pacemakers.

Clinical examination has to be scrupulous, as subtle abnormality in a particular system could reveal the cause. Particular attention should be paid to the presence of jaundice, pallor, and cachexia, and the examination must include: skin (e.g. rashes); mucous membranes; ears; nose; throat; eyes (including fundoscopy); lymph nodes; heart murmurs (new onset or changing character); temporal or occipital artery tenderness; neurological deficits; arthritis; abdominal tenderness; genitalia; liver; spleen; pelvic examination and examination of the feet. The whole body (including thyroid, spine, joints, and mouth) should be palpated for swellings and tenderness.

Daily physical examination should be performed, particularly searching for new lymphadenopathy. Fundoscopic examination and cryoglobulins should be performed early. If infective endocarditis is considered, echocardiography should be performed (see case 10). Other possible investigations may include thyroid function, synacthen tests, sputum and stool cultures, and bone marrow tests. Imaging should be guided by pain or discomfort, although a chest X-ray would be routine. In some cases, magnetic resonance imaging may also be warranted. Whole body imaging may be necessary and FDG-PET/CT (fluoro-2-deoxy-D-glucose positron emission computed tomography) is the preferred imaging technique. Computed tomography may be diagnostic as well as being able to identify abnormal tissue, but has lower diagnostic yield if compared to FDG-PET/CT. Labelled leucocyte scintigraphy or gallium scintigraphy has lower diagnostic yields when compared to FDG-PET/CT, but can be used as an alternative diagnostic test if FDG-PET/CT is unavailable. Invasive tests including endoscopy, bone marrow, or temporal artery biopsy may be required.

In this case, blood tests results did not indicate infection, and the examination findings did not indicate temporal arteritis or polymyalgia rheumatica.

Case continuation

On transfer to the rehabilitation ward, the patient was re-examined. Pelvic examination revealed a suprapubic mass and an enlarged supraclavicular lymph node.

CT scans of the chest, abdomen, and pelvis were performed (Figs 16.1, 16.2).

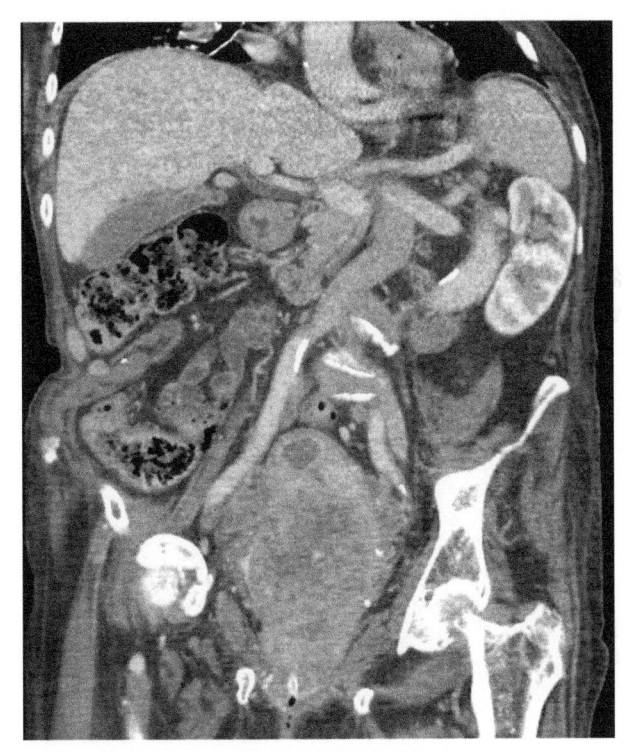

Fig. 16.1 CT of the abdomen/pelvis (coronal slice) with contrast.

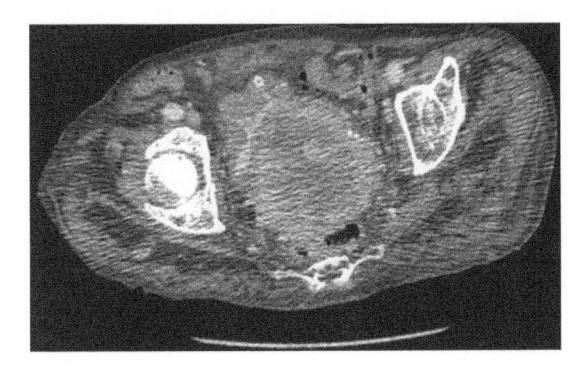

Fig. 16.2 CT of the abdomen/pelvis (axial slice) with contrast at the level of the bladder/uterus.

Questions continued

5 What do the abdominal and pelvic CT scans show? What is the most likely underlying diagnosis, and how would you confirm it?

6 How would you manage a fever of unknown origin in which the underlying cause is not established despite investigation?

Answers continued

5 **What do the abdominal and pelvic CT scans show? What is the most likely underlying diagnosis, and how would you confirm it?**

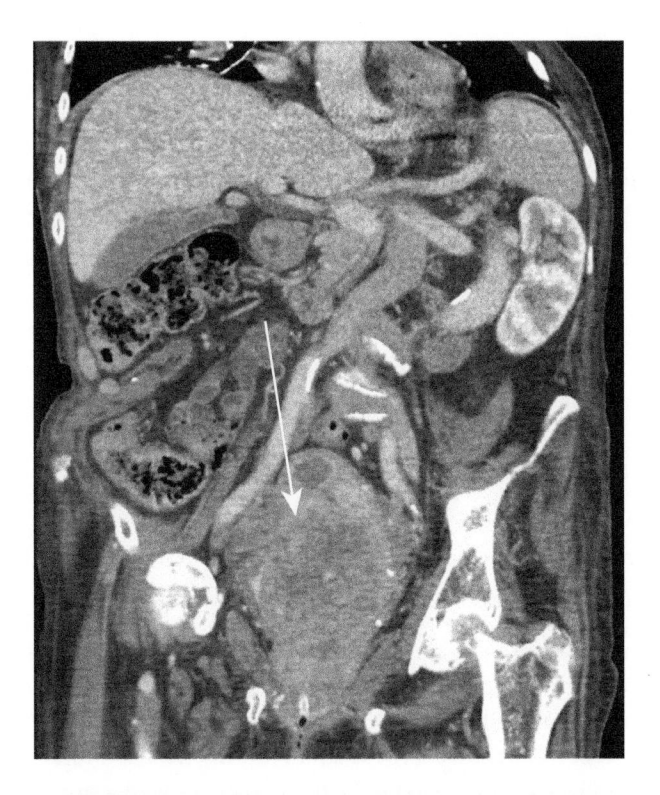

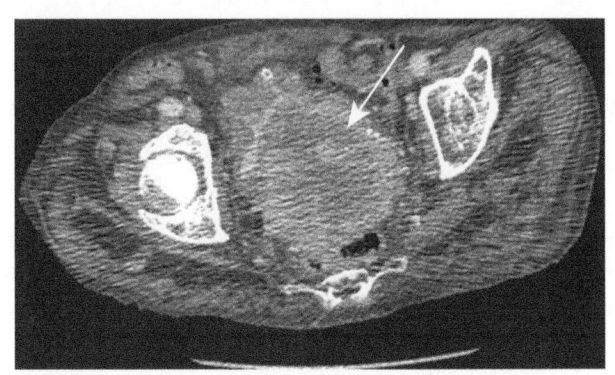

Figs 16.3 and 16.4 CT of the abdomen/pelvis shows an irregular mass (white arrow) arising from the pelvis, thought to be a uterine malignancy (carcinoma or sarcoma). The pelvic mass is inseparable from the catheterized bladder.

The CT scans show a large irregular pelvic mass and the most likely diagnosis is therefore fever caused by uterine malignancy. Fever of unknown origin may be the first or the most prominent symptom of malignancy.

Malignancy-related fever of unknown origin is most commonly seen with acute leukaemia, lymphoma, renal cell carcinoma, gastro-intestinal tract malignancies, and sarcoma. It is caused by tumour-related necrotic-inflammatory changes, as well as the endogenous pyrogens (cytokines).

To confirm the diagnosis, a biopsy of the uterus was suggested, but the patient refused any further investigation or intervention.

6 How would you manage a fever of unknown origin in which the underlying cause is not established despite investigation?

The management of fever of unknown origin in which investigations have failed to reveal a cause depends on the patient's clinical condition. In stable cases, simple observation is appropriate, and antipyretics in form of non-steroidal anti-inflammatory medications could be used. Patients who continue to deteriorate should have further investigations.

However, treatment should be considered if the following diagnoses are suspected:

- temporal arteritis (see case 39)
- disseminated tuberculosis
- culture-negative endocarditis (see case 10).

Neutropenic patients who are unwell should be given antibiotic treatment. In general, the empirical use of steroids in patients with fever of unknown origin is not recommended since this may delay diagnosis of haematological malignancy or worsen infection. Anakinra (the interleukin-1 receptor antagonist) could be tried for up to two weeks in patients with a suspected auto-inflammatory disorder. Clinically stable patients with fever of unknown origin, in whom investigations identify no cause, usually have a good outcome (spontaneous remission of fever in around 75% of patients). Overall prognosis in all patients will depend on the underlying condition.

Further reading

Efstathiou SP, Pefanis AV, Tsiakou AG, et al. (2010). Fever of unknown origin: discrimination between infections and non-infectious causes. *Eur J Intern Med*; **21**: 137–143.

Hot A, Jaisson I, Girard C, et al. (2009). Yield of bone marrow examination in diagnosing the source of fever of unknown origin. *Arch Intern Med*; **169**: 2018–2023.

Knockaert DC, Vanderschueren S, Blockman D (2003). Fever of unknown origin in adults: 40 years on. *J Intern Med*; **253**; 263–275.

Kouijzer IJ, Bleeker-Rovers CP, Owen WJ (2013). FDG-PET in fever of unknown origin. *Semin Nucl Med*; **43**: 333–339.

Mulders-Manders C, Simon A, Bleeker-Rovers C (2015). Fever of unknown origin. *Clin Med*; 15; **3**: 280–284.

Tal S, Guller V, Gurevich A (2007). Fever of unknown origin in older adults. *Clin Geriatr Med*; **23**: 649–668.

Turkulov V, Brkić S, Sević S, Marić D, Tomić S (2011). Fever of unknown origin in elderly patients. *Srp Arh Celok Lek*; **139**(1–2): 64–68.

Vanderschueren S, Eyckmans T, De Munter P, Knockaert D (2014). Mortality in patients presenting with fever of unknown origin. *Acta Clin Belg*; **69**: 12–16.

Case 17

A 68-year-old woman was admitted via the GP with a six-month history of worsening breathlessness and dry cough. She was now unable to manage the stairs without becoming short of breath, and also complained of occasional fleeting chest pains on exertion. She had no previous hospital admissions and had been in good health, working as a school dinner lady until one year earlier. She had no known allergies, and had recently been started on omeprazole for gastro-oesophageal reflux symptoms.

During the examination, she complained of swelling in her fingers, which caused the skin to 'feel tight', and that they often felt cold. Her facial appearance was a little unusual and her nose appeared 'pinched'. Blood pressure was 168/98mmHg, 72bpm regular with normal heart sounds, and the JVP was elevated at approximately 4cm. Respiratory rate was 18 breaths per minute with saturations of 92% on air, and she was noted to become slightly short of breath on getting up on to the couch. There were fine bi-basal inspiratory crepitations. There was mild pedal, but no sacral oedema. Telangiectasia were seen on the face and neck, and there was some thickening of the skin around the left elbow. The rest of the examination was normal.

Investigations revealed the following:

- Hb 8.2g/dl; MCV 84fL; WCC 8.2 × 10^9/L; neutrophils 5.3 × 10^9/L; platelets 270;
- sodium 136mmol/L; potassium 4.1mmol/L; urea 12mmol/L; creatinine 158μmol/L
- CRP: 20μmg/L
- Ferritin 350μg/L; iron 18μmol/L; folate 3μg/L; vitamin B_{12} 250ng/L; TIBC 54μmol/L
- CXR (see Fig. 17.1)
- ECG: right axis deviation and prominent p waves
- Urine dipstick: 2 + protein, nil else

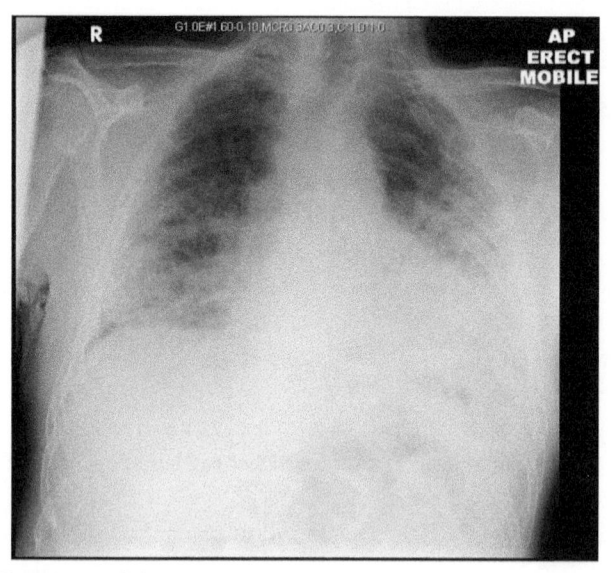

Fig. 17.1 Chest X-ray of the patient.

Questions

1. What is the most likely unifying underlying diagnosis that explains the clinical features in this case? What are the variants of this condition?
2. What is the most likely cause for this patient's shortness of breath given your answer for Question 1, and what initial investigations would you instigate?
3. How would you confirm the diagnosis in Question 1?
4. What is the prognosis, particularly in relation to the CXR abnormalities?
5. How does the underlying condition differ in older versus younger patients?
6. How does the immune system change with age?
7. Describe the pathophysiology of this type of anaemia.

Answers

1 What is the most likely unifying underlying diagnosis that explains the clinical features in this case? What are the variants of this condition?

The unifying diagnosis in this case is *diffuse systemic sclerosis*, leading to pulmonary fibrosis, anaemia of chronic disease, facial telangiectasia, and scleroderma, with sclerodactyly (swollen fingers with tight skin), and thickening of the skin around the left elbow. The term scleroderma is used to describe the presence of thickened, hardened skin (from the Greek 'scleros'). Scleroderma is the hallmark of a heterogeneous group of conditions in which only the skin and subjacent tissues may be affected or there may be systemic involvement (Box 17.1). The peak onset is between the ages of 30 and 50, and the disease is rare (<1:100,000) and more common in women, as observed for most other autoimmune diseases. This patient is therefore relatively elderly to be presenting *de novo*, although it is possible that epidemiological studies have been subject to bias being focused on selective younger populations. Also, the characteristic cutaneous features may be less obvious in older patients owing to age-related skin changes. Typical scleroderma may occur in patients with systemic lupus erythematosus, inflammatory arthritis, and inflammatory muscle diseases, termed so-called 'overlap syndrome'. In some cases, a diagnosis of mixed connective tissue disease is made inituially, but this often evolves over time into systemic sclerosis, systemic lupus erythematosus, or dermatomyositis.

Sclero-derma like skin changes may also occur as a result of toxin exposure, endocrine disorders (long-standing type 1 diabetes, hypothyroidism) renal failure, and amyloidosis.

Box 17.1 Classification of systemic sclerosis syndromes

Limited cutaneous scleroderma

- Raynaud phenomenon for years, occasionally decades.
- Skin involvement limited to hands, face, feet, and forearms (acral distribution).
- Nailfold capillary pattern typical of scleroderma—predominantly nailfold capillary loops with capillary dropout.
- A significant (10–15%) late incidence of pulmonary hypertension, with or without skin calcification, gastrointestinal disease, telangiectasias (CREST syndrome), or interstitial lung disease.

> **Box 17.1 Classification of systemic sclerosis syndromes** *(continued)*
>
> - Renal disease rarely occurs.
> - Anticentromere antibody (ACA) in 50–60%, but other patterns also occurring in 5–10% (especially anti-PM/Scl and anti-Scl-70).
>
> ### Diffuse cutaneous scleroderma
>
> - Raynaud phenomenon followed, within one year, by puffy or hidebound skin changes.
> - Truncal and acral skin involvement; tendon friction rubs.
> - Nailfold capillary pattern typical of scleroderma with dilatation (early), dilatation and dropout (active), and tortuosity with dropout (late).
> - Early and significant incidence of renal, interstitial lung, diffuse gastrointestinal, and myocardial disease.
> - Anti-Scl-70 (30%) and anti-RNA polymerase-I, II, or III (12–15%) antibodies.
>
> ### Scleroderma sine scleroderma
>
> - Presentation with pulmonary fibrosis or renal, cardiac, or gastrointestinal disease.
> - No skin involvement.
> - Raynaud phenomenon may be present.
> - Antinuclear antibodies may be present (anti-Scl-70, ACA, or anti-RNA polymerase-I, II, or III).
>
> ### Environmentally-induced scleroderma
>
> - Generally diffuse distribution of skin sclerosis and a history of exposure to an environmental agent suspected of causing scleroderma.
>
> ### Overlap syndromes
>
> - Features of systemic sclerosis that coexist with those of another autoimmune rheumatic disease, such as systemic lupus erythematosus, rheumatoid arthritis, dermatomyositis, vasculitis, or Sjögren's syndrome.
>
> ### Pre-scleroderma
>
> - Raynaud's phenomenon.

> **Box 17.1 Classification of systemic sclerosis syndromes** *(continued)*
>
> - Nailfold capillary changes (early or active pattern typical) and evidence of digital ischaemia.
> - Specific circulating autoantibodies—antitopoisomerase-I (Scl-70), anti-centromere (ACA), or anti-RNA polymerase-I, II, or III, or other hallmark scleroderma reactivity.
>
> ## CREST syndrome
>
> - Calcinosis, Raynaud's phenomenon, esophageal dysmotility, sclerodactyly, and telangiectasia syndrome, also called limited scleroderma or limited cutaneous form of systemic sclerosis; anti-PM/Scl: anti-polymyositis/scleroderma antinuclear antibodies, also called anti-exosome antibodies; anti-Scl-70: antinuclear autoantibody to the scleroderma 70 kD antigen fragment, also called the anti-topoisomerase I antibody; RNA: ribonucleic acid; ACA: anticentromere antibody.

When scleroderma is associated with internal organ involvement, the disease is termed systemic sclerosis (SSc). SSc is subcategorized further into diffuse cutaneous SSc (dcSSc) and limited cutaneous SSc (lcSSc) on the basis of the extent and distribution of skin involvement. lcSSc is commonly associated with the CREST syndrome. Systemic manifestations are diverse with abnormalities of the circulation (most notably Raynaud's phenomenon), and involvement of multiple organ systems, including the musculoskeletal, renal, pulmonary, cardiac, and gastrointestinal systems, with fibrotic and/or vascular complications (Table 17.1). Fatigue, arthralgia, and myalgia are frequent. Skin involvement is nearly universal, and is most obvious in the face and hands. Oedema may precede thickening and induration. Pruritus may occur together with digital ulcers.

Vascular dysfunction is a significant component of the pathogenesis of systemic sclerosis (SSc), the most characteristic manifestation being Raynaud's phenomenon. In lcSS, Raynaud's phenomenon may precede the development of other organ manifestations by many years whereas in dcSSc, it usually coincides with systemic disease.

This patient had recently been started on a proton pump inhibitor for gastro-oesophageal reflux symptoms, and blood and urine tests indicated renal impairment. Her blood pressure was elevated, a further indicator of renal damage. The patient mentioned that her hands frequently felt cold and

Table 17.1 Clinical features of the major systemic sclerosis subsets

Diffuse cutaneous	Early (< three years after onset)	Late (> three years after onset)
Constitutional	Fatigue and weight loss	Minimal, weight gain typical
Vascular	Raynaud's, often mild	Raynaud's, more severe, more telangiectasia
Cutaneous	Rapid progression involving arms, trunk, face	Stable or regression
Musculoskeletal	Prominent arthralgia, stiffness, myalgia, muscle weakness, tendon friction	Flexion contractures and deformities, joint/muscle symptoms less prominent
Gastrointestinal	Dysphagia, heartburn	More pronounced symptoms, midgut, and anorectal complications more common
Cardiopulmonary	Myocarditis, pericardial effusion, intersitital pulmonary fibrosis	Reduced risk of new disease, but progression of existing fibrosis
Renal	High risk	Renal crisis less frequent, uncommon after five years
Limited cutaneous	Early (<10 years after onset)	Late (>10 years after onset)
Constitutional	None	Only secondary to visceral complications
Vascular	Raynaud's often severe, telangiectasia	Raynaud's persists, often causing digital ulceration, or gangrene
Cutaneous	Mild sclerosis	Stable, calcinosis more prominent
Musculoskeletal	Occasional joint stiffness	Mild flexion contractures
Gastrointestinal	Dysphagia, heartburn	More pronounced symptoms, midgut, and anorectal complications
Cardiopulmonary	Usually no involvement	Lung fibrosis may develop but often slow. Anti-SCL-70 predicts increased risk of severe fibrosis. Pulmonary hypertension and right ventricular failure
Renal	No involvement	Rarely involved, anti-RNA polymerase predicts increased risk of renal involvement

on further questioning it transpired that she had recently developed Raynaud's phenomenon (see case 41, *Oxford Case Histories in Rheumatology* for further discussion of this syndrome).

2 What is the most likely cause for this patient's shortness of breath given your answer for Question 1, and what initial investigations would you instigate?

The CXR shows blunting of the costophrenic angles and patchy reticular nodular shadowing bilaterally in the lower zones (Fig. 17.2).

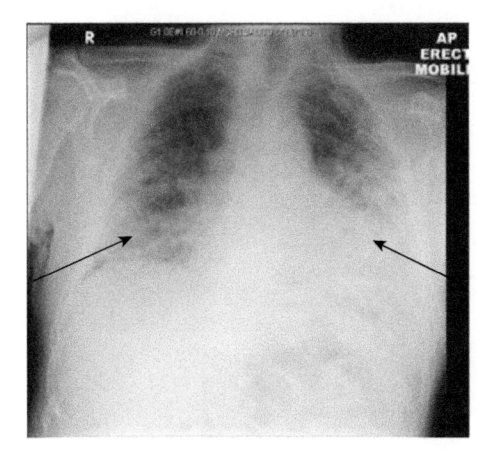

Fig. 17.2 Chest X-ray showing blunting of the costophrenic angles and patchy reticular nodular shadowing bilaterally in the lower zones (arrows).

The history of progressive breathlessness and dry cough coupled with the clinical findings of hypoxia, mild elevation of respiratory rate, bi-basal inspiratory crepitations, and the CXR findings are suggestive of interstitial pulmonary fibrosis. Lung disease is also suggested by the symptoms, consistent with right heart failure with elevated JVP, ankle swelling, and ECG showing right axis deviation with prominent p waves. The initial differential diagnosis includes left ventricular failure given the oedema and raised JVP, which may be difficult to distinguish radiologically from fibrosis when the latter is early, i.e. before the fibrotic changes are severe enough for the appearances to be characteristic. To investigate possible lung fibrosis further, a high resolution CT scan should be requested, which may show signs consistent with fibrotic change including ground glass appearance and honeycombing (see Fig. 17.3, from a different patient). Lung function tests should also be considered and in established pulmonary fibrosis, will demonstrate a restrictive pattern with impaired gas transfer.

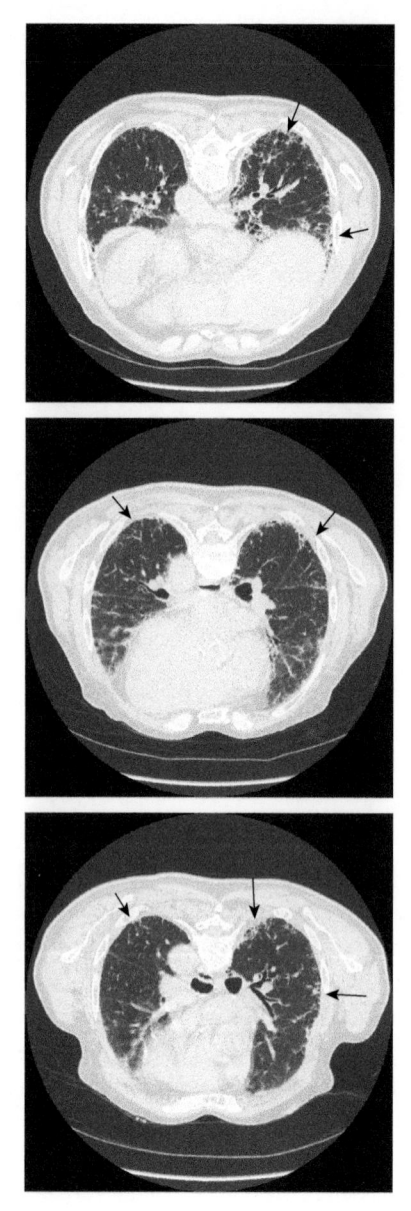

Fig. 17.3 Selective axial slices from a chest CT scan with lung windows. These demonstrate subpleural reticulation and honey-combing, most marked towards the lung bases, and are associated with traction bronchial dilatation consistent with usual interstitial pneumonia.

The patient has anaemia, which will contribute to the shortness of breath. Lower respiratory chest infection is unlikely given the history of breathlessness progressing over a six-month period, absence of fever, and little evidence for sepsis on the blood results. Although the patient complained of fleeting chest pains, there was no history of ischaemic heart disease, and clinical, ECG, and CXR findings did not convincingly support left ventricular failure.

3 How would you confirm the diagnosis in Question 1?

The diagnosis of SSc and related disorders is based primarily upon the presence of characteristic clinical findings and serum autoantibodies. Nailfold capilloroscopy, in which a drop of immersion oil is placed on the nailbeds to enable examination with a magnifying lens, may be considered to distinguish primary and secondary Raynaud's phenomenon in cases of diagnostic uncertainty. Secondary Raynaud's phenomenon (i.e. occurring in conjunction with underlying disease) is associated with discrete dilated capillary loops and loss of surrounding loop structures.

The extent of skin induration varies, but almost all patients have skin changes in the fingers (sclerodactyly), hands, and face. During the first few months, puffiness, arthralgia, and soft tissue swelling rather than skin induration may occur, and this may lead to erroneous diagnosis of rheumatoid arthritis, or another connective tissue disease. Calcinosis cutis, hyperpigmentation, and/or mucocutaneous telangiectasia point to SSc, but are often absent in early disease.

Thorough physical examination and investigation should be performed to look for extracutaneous disease if SSc is suspected. The combination of scleroderma plus the presence of one or more of the following clinical features supports the diagnosis of SSc:

- Heartburn and/or dysphagia of new onset (oesophageal dysmotility is the most frequent visceral complication of SSc).
- Hypertension and renal impairment.
- Dyspnea on exertion, interstitial pulmonary changes on CXR.
- Pulmonary hypertension.
- Diarrhoea with malabsorption (atonic bowel and bacterial overgrowth).
- Telangiectasia on the face, lips, oral cavity, or hands.
- Digital infarction and/or scars.
- Erectile dysfunction.

Serologic tests are helpful in confirming, but not in excluding, a diagnosis of SSc (i.e. sensitivity is not 100%). The antitopoisomerase-I, ACA, and anti-RNA polymerase III antibodies are highly specific (>99.5% in some studies) for SSc, but are only moderately sensitive (20–50%). Certain autoantibodies are associated with an increased likelihood of certain clinical manifestations and may also have prognostic implications.

A number of other autoantibodies may be present in patients with SSc; over 95% of SSc patients have at least one autoantibody.

4 What is the prognosis, particularly in relation to the CXR abnormalities?

In a systematic review of interstitial lung disease in systemic sclerosis, a variety of patient-specific, lung-specific, and SSc-specific variables predicted mortality and progression. However, most predictors were identified in only one study and most studies did not fully account for confounders. Older age, lower forced vital capacity, and lower diffusing capacity of carbon monoxide, predicted mortality in more than one study. Being of male gender, the extent of disease on high resolution CT (HRCT) scan, presence of honeycombing, and increased alveolar epithelial permeability were identified as predictors of both mortality and interstitial lung disease progression on unadjusted analysis. The extent of disease on HRCT scan was the only variable that independently predicted both mortality and interstitial lung disease progression. Further studies are required to better understand the predictors of outcome in older patients in whom the presence of additional co-morbidities and frailty will be important.

For overall mortality in SSc, one recent study reported a standardized mortality ratio of 1.34 (95% confidence interval (CI) 1.00–1.75) with slightly higher values in males (1.54 [95% CI 0.67–3.04] vs. 1.30 [95% CI 0.95–1.74]). The leading causes of death were infection, respiratory disease, and malignancy, while the most common cause of SSc-related mortality was pulmonary complications. Factors adversely affecting survival were older age at diagnosis, male gender, interstitial lung disease, and anti-RNA polymerase III antibody. Other studies have reported scleroderma renal crisis, pulmonary fibrosis, pulmonary arterial hypertension, cancer, and antitopoisomerase and anti-U1 antibodies, although there is heterogeneity in case mix and definitions across studies and types of cancer, and the strength of the associations are conflicting.

The current patient therefore has predictors for poor outcome including older age at presentation and presence of established interstitial lung disease with secondary cardiac changes.

5 How does the underlying condition differ in older versus younger patients?

Data comparing systemic sclerosis in older people aged >65 years versus younger age groups are relatively sparse partly because the age of onset appears to peak in middle age. However, available data suggest that older patients are at greater risk for pulmonary hypertension, renal impairment, cardiac disease, and muscle weakness, as seen to some extent in the current patient. Poor prognosis at older ages appears to be an independently associated with age (see earlier answer), but may also therefore be related to association with severe organ, particularly pulmonary, involvement.

In general, autoimmune disease in older versus younger patients is characterized by atypical features, insidious presentation, and lower expression of laboratory parameters. For example, in later onset rheumatoid arthritis, there is a lower incidence of rheumatoid factor positivity, insidious onset, and greater tendency for large joints to be involved, which may cause diagnostic confusion with polymyalgia rheumatica. There is also greater tendency for overlap between different disease phenotypes in older patients. At present, there are few studies focused on the clinical presentation of autoimmune disease in older people.

Secondly, some systemic vasculitis such as polyarteritis nodosa or Wegener's granulomatosis may show a similar clinical presentation in middle-aged and elderly patients, but are frequently associated with higher rates of morbidity and mortality in geriatric populations. Thirdly, the diagnosis of some autoimmune diseases in the elderly patients (inflammatory myopathies and antiphospholipid syndrome or APS) should lead to an active search for an underlying neoplasic disorder.

6 How does the immune system change with age?

Although most autoimmune diseases can occur at any age, some primarily occur in childhood and adolescence (e.g. type 1 diabetes), in the mid-adult years (e.g. myasthenia gravis, multiple sclerosis), or among older adults (e.g. rheumatoid arthritis, myositis, thyroiditis, Wegener granulomatosis and other primary systemic vasculitis) suggesting changes in immune function with age.

Ageing is accompanied by a progressive decline in the integrity of the immune system, a process known as immunosenescence (see Box 17.2). Although the quantity of antibodies produced in response to a stimulus remains much the same, older people produce fewer antibodies specific for the activating antigen and more nonspecific antibodies. It has been hypothesized that autoantibodies play a role in the ageing process through involvement in subclinical chronic tissue damage and also in age-related susceptibility to neoplasia.

Studies in the general population show that a large proportion of healthy older people have antibodies frequently associated with autoimmune disease. Such antibodies may be related to high exposure to exogenous factors

> **Box 17.2 Autoimmunity abnormalities in the elderly patients**
>
> **Cell-mediated immune disorders**
> Decrease of suppressive T cells
> Decrease of T helper cells
> Decrease of the expression of growth lymphocytic factors
> Decrease of the expression of specific lymphocytic receptors
>
> **Antibody-mediated immune disorders**
> Unaffected total number of B-cells
> Increase of the polyclonal response against diverse mitogens
> Decrease of specific-antigen response
> Intrinsic defects of the maturity of B-cells
>
> **Increased frequency of autoantibody synthesis and other immune system disorders**
> Effect of extrinsic factors (diet, drugs, exercise)
> Increase of CD95 expression with age
> Decrease of Th1 cytokines/increase of Th2 cytokines
> Disorders of polymorphonuclear apoptosis
> Increased serum levels of IgG, IgM, IgA
> Progressive thymus atrophy

such as viral infections or to medication use: certain medications are known to mimic autoimmune disease (e.g. drug-induced lupus-like syndrome; see case 9). Antibodies include rheumatoid factor (~20%), ANA (~15%), anticardiolipin (~30%), anti-mitochondrial (6%), anti-smooth muscle (5%) and anti-parietal cell antibodies (~4%) and ANCA (<2%). The extremely low rate of cANCA in the absence of pathology suggests that the presence of cANCA is almost always related to vasculitic disease (pANCA is much less specific). Similarly, anti-dsDNA and antibodies against the extractable nuclear antigens (anti-La/SSB, anti-Sm, and anti-RNP) are very infrequent in older people, and are closely associated with the presence of systemic autoimmune disorders.

The high prevalence of many autoantibodies in older people means that less significance may be attached to the presence of, e.g. rheumatoid factor in an older person and this, coupled with the increased likelihood of atypical symptoms, mean that there is frequent diagnostic uncertainty in older versus younger people with possible autoimmune disease. A better understanding of the underlying mechanisms of age-related changes in immunity may ultimately help prevent and treat illnesses associated with age. The development of biologic markers of immunosenescence may help identify subgroups at high risk of developing infections, neoplasia, and autoimmune disease.

7 Describe the pathophysiology of this type of anaemia.

This patient has a normal MCV, iron, reduced TIBC, and a raised ferritin, normal vitamin B_{12}, and folate consistent with a normocytic anaemia. A normocytic anaemia is unusual in systemic sclerosis unless there is concomitant renal failure since scleroderma rarely mounts an elevated CRP. The most common cause of normocytic anaemia is chronic disease. Other causes of normocytic anaemia include:

- renal failure
- bone marrow failure
- hypothyroidism
- haemolysis

In this case, although the renal function is impaired, it is not significant enough to cause the anaemia.

There are several factors which contribute to low haemoglobin levels in anaemia of chronic disease. Normal red blood cell life span is decreased from 120 days to 70–80 days, low levels of chronic inflammatory cytokines affect iron absorption and recirculation, and the effectiveness of erythropoietin is impaired. Pro-inflammatory cytokines such as IL-1, IL-6 and TNF-a are secreted in many chronic inflammatory conditions, and have a multifactorial role in the development of associated anaemias. Cytokines may cause the destruction of red blood cell precursor cells and a decrease in the number of erythropoietin receptors on progenitor cells. IL-6 also induces the secretion of heparin by the liver, which inhibits the expression of ferroportin-1, an iron transporter in the duodenum, and the release of iron from macrophages.

Further reading

Barnes J, Mayes MD (2012). Epidemiology of systemic sclerosis: incidence, prevalence, survival, risk factors, malignancy, and environmental triggers. *Curr Opin Rheumatol*; **24**(2): 165–170.

Cooper GS, Stroehla BC (2003). The epidemiology of autoimmune diseases. *Autoimmun Rev*; **2**(3): 119–125.

Deicher R, Hörl WH (2006). New insights into the regulation of iron homeostasis. *Eur J Clin Invest*; **36**: 301–309.

Howard WA, Gibson KL, Dunn-Walters DK (2006). Antibody quality in old age. *Rejuvenation Res*; **9**(1): 117–125.

Lindstrom TM, Robinson WH (2010). Rheumatoid arthritis: a role for immunosenescence? *J Am Geriatr Soc*; **58**(8): 1565–1575.

Manno RL, Wigley FM, Gelber AC, Hummers LK (2011). Late-age onset systemic sclerosis. *J Rheumatol*; **38**(7): 1317–1325.

Pérez-Bocanegra C, Solans-Laqué R, Simeón-Aznar CP, Campillo M, Fonollosa-Pla V, Vilardell-Tarrés M (2010). Age-related survival and clinical features in systemic sclerosis patients older or younger than 65 at diagnosis. *Rheumatology (Oxford)*; **49**(6): 1112–1117.

Ramos-Casals M, García-Carrasco M, Brito MP, López-Soto A, Font J (2003). Autoimmunity and geriatrics: clinical significance of autoimmune manifestations in the elderly. *Lupus*; **12**(5): 341–355.

Strickland G, Pauling J, Cavill C, Shaddick G, McHugh N (2013). Mortality in systemic sclerosis-a single centre study from the UK. *Clin Rheumatol*; **32**(10): 1533–1539.

Winstone TA, Assayag D, Wilcox PG, *et al.* (2014). Predictors of mortality and progression in scleroderma-associated interstitial lung disease: a systematic review. *Chest*; **146**(2): 422–436.

Case 18

Case 18.A

An 82-year-old man was referred to the geratology clinic by his GP with tiredness, loss of appetite, loss of weight, and 'general deterioration'. He was independent in all daily activities and lived alone in a ground floor flat following the death of his partner of 60 years. He described feelings of guilt and loneliness, and said that most of his friends had died.

He smoked 10 cigarettes per day, and had a pint of beer once or twice a week. Medication was paracetamol only for occasional knee pain.

On examination, he was unshaven and unkempt with dirty clothes and shoes. Temperature was 36.5°C, pulse 72bpm regular, and BP110/65mmHg. The general system examination was normal. He was alert and orientated with no focal neurological abnormality. MMSE was 25/30.

Investigations showed the following:

- FBC, LFTs, TFTs, CRP, calcium, PSA, urine dipstick: normal
- ESR, urea, and electrolytes, B_{12}, folate, serum and urine electrophoresis: normal
- ECG, sinus rhythm, heart rate 72bpm, regular
- CXR: normal

Case 18.B

A 72-year-old woman was referred to the out-patient clinic with poor memory, lethargy, and need for frequent rests during the day, as well as non-specific aches and pains. Her previous medical history included depression 10 years previously, diabetes mellitus type 2, and hypertension.

She was recently divorced and lived alone. Medications were metformin, amlodipine, ramipril, and bendroflumethiazide. She had never smoked and occasionally drank a small glass of sherry.

Examination was unremarkable except that her body mass index was 27. MMSE was 26/30.

Investigations showed the following:

- FBC, LFTs, TFTs, CRP, calcium, urine dipstick: normal
- ESR, urea, and electrolytes, B_{12}, folate, serum and urine electrophoresis: normal
- ECG, sinus, heart rate 68bpm, regular
- CXR: slightly enlarged heart
- Echocardiogram: normal, except for mild aortic sclerosis
- CT brain scan: periventricular patchy low-density areas consistent with small vessel disease.

Questions

1 What is the most likely unifying diagnosis in both cases, in view of the history and investigation results? What tools might you use to assist in further assessment?
2 How would you confirm your diagnosis?
3 List the most common reasons why this condition is often difficult to diagnose in older people.
4 List the risk factors for this condition in older patients.
5 Describe differences in this condition in older versus younger patients.
6 How would you manage this condition?
7 If patients do not respond to the usual treatment and are deteriorating, which further options could be considered and in what circumstances?

Answers

1 What is the most likely unifying diagnosis in both cases, in view of the history and investigation results? What tools might you use to assist in further assessment?

The most likely diagnosis is depression. Both patients have several risk factors for depression and all investigations were normal.

Depressive symptoms are found in around 15% of people in the community aged over 65 years, although reported prevalence rates vary between studies because of different diagnostic criteria and methodology. Rates are considerably higher among nursing home residents and hospitalized older patients. Depression is predicted to be the second largest cause of disability in the world in 2020 and may become the leading cause by 2030 in middle/higher income countries.

A high index of suspicion for depression is required in older people owing to atypical presentation in later life. It should be considered particularly where there is a history of depression, chronic illness, or recent traumatic life event with no organic basis for symptoms.

Both patients had a comprehensive medical history taken, revealing the previous depression in case B and presence of precipitating factors in both cases (bereavement, divorce). The diagnostic process was started with two short screening questions:

"During the past month, have you often been bothered by feeling down, depressed, or hopeless?" and

"During the past month, have you often been bothered by your finding little interest or pleasure in doing things?"

Both patients answered in the affirmative to both questions, as well as to the one-item screening question: 'Do you often feel sad or depressed?' However, these screening questions may not always be reliable and/or further assessment may be necessary. In both case A and case B, the Geriatric Depression Scale (GDS) was administered.

The GDS is validated in people aged over 60 years in acute general hospital settings and is accepted as a screening tool for depression in specific conditions, including Parkinson's disease. The full version consists of 30 items, but the shorter 15 item version is often used, in which a score of 0 to 5 is normal, above five suggests depression and ≥ 10 almost always indicates depression. It should be administered by experienced staff rather than being given to the patient to avoid inaccuracies and omissions.

Cognitive assessment should be considered, since depression is a frequent accompaniment of dementia/mild cognitive impairment and may also result in impaired cognitive scores. In both cases mentioned here, the cognitive scores were not completely normal, but further assessment did not indicate any impairment in daily functions as would be expected in dementia. In such cases, cognitive testing should be repeated after treatment of the accompanying mood disorder. The GDS is less reliable in patients with moderate/severe cognitive impairment (<15/30 on MMSE) in whom the Cornell Scale for Depression in Dementia may be preferable. Other validated screening instruments for depression in older patients, usable in most situations, include the Montgomery–Åsberg depression rating scale, the Hospital Anxiety and Depression Scale and the Evans Liverpool Depression Rating Scale (aimed at physically ill older people and focusing on the preceding four weeks). The Brief Assessment Schedule Depression Cards are useful for deaf patients.

GDS scores were 11/15 for case A and 8/15 for case B.

2 How would you confirm your diagnosis?

It is important to exclude organic disease mimicking or exacerbating depression (e.g. infection, medication, alcohol, or substance abuse). Specific investigations will be determined by the exact nature of the symptoms, but general investigations should include full blood count, fasting glucose, vitamin B_{12}, folate, calcium, renal, thyroid and liver function tests, urine analysis, and ECG (particularly since certain antidepressants may affect cardiac conduction). Computed tomography of the brain may be necessary in certain cases, e.g. to exclude space occupying lesions. In practice, the decision regarding how far to investigate may be difficult and should be considered on a case-by-case basis. A trial of antidepressants may be appropriate pending results of investigations.

Depression is a heterogeneous disease and its diagnosis should help clinicians to determine prognosis, treatment plans, and potential treatment outcomes for their patients, and can be helped by fulfilment of the criteria in the ICD-10 (The International Classification of Diseases and Related Health Problems 10th Edition) or the DSM-IV (Diagnostic and Statistical Manual of Mental Disorders of the American Psychiatric Association, 4th Edition). DSM-IV classifies depression as major depressive disorder (a heterogeneous symptom cluster that substantially overlaps with other syndromes e.g. anxiety disorders), subclinical or minor depression, and dysthymia. In cases of uncertain diagnosis, psychiatric review should be considered.

Both patients satisfied the DSM-IV criteria for major depression: either or both of depressed mood (1), and loss of interest or pleasure (2), and five or more of the other symptoms listed below for ≥ two weeks:

- depressed mood (for most of the day)
- loss of interest or pleasure in almost all activities
- change in appetite or weight
- sleep problems—insomnia (there may also be hypersomnia)
- loss of energy
- feeling of worthlessness (patients may also feel guilt)
- inability to concentrate
- thoughts of death or suicide
- psychomotor agitation or retardation

All older patients should be assessed for the impact of depression on their function. Risk of suicide must be assessed with direct questioning (e.g. intention, prior suicide attempts, family history of suicide). The suicide rate among older depressed patients is declining, but the highest rates of completed suicide are seen in >85-year-old white men: e.g. in the USA, it is more than five times the national age-adjusted suicide rate, or data from New Zealand show the highest average suicide rate among all was in men over the age of 85 years. Other risk factors for suicide in the older population include being unmarried or having a sleep disorder, bereavement, physical illness, untreated pain, history of alcohol and substance abuse, and evidence of planning, or previous suicide attempts. One small study had found that only around 40% of older people (the majority being women of Caucasian ethnicity) leave a suicide note, stating the reasons: health-related problems (physical health, inability to function independently); fear of institutionalisation reduced quality of life; stressful life events (e.g. legal, financial, and relationship related).

3 List common reasons why this condition is often difficult to diagnose in older people.

Depression may be difficult to diagnose in older patients because:
- The symptoms and signs of depression in older patients may be assumed to be a normal response to other medical conditions, life events, or part of ageing.

- Other diseases may mask or mimic depression. For example, the stooped posture, lack of facial expression, limited body movement, and speech changes (soft voice, use of monosyllabic words) of Parkinson's disease.
- Depression may present with symptoms of existing chronic medical conditions including pain, memory problems, loss of appetite and/or energy, fatigue, apathy, and weight loss.
- Depression may mimic dementia (a condition previously called pseudodementia) although recent evidence suggests that most such patients go on to develop true dementia.
- Depression may present with common non-specific complaints: not coping; irritability; insomnia; aches and pains; worrying.
- Depression may present with behavioural changes, e.g. new incontinence, screaming, biting, or aggressive behaviour, particularly in people with cognitive impairment dependent on carers.
- Depression may manifest only in reduced social relations.
- Older people commonly do not complain about their low mood and the 'stiff upper lip' generation of Britons was raised not to show their feelings.
- Loss of vision and hearing can make some patients withdraw from social interaction, for which depression can be a cause as well as a consequence.
- Different ethnic and social groups express distress or depression in different ways. Somatization is a common mechanism in which the location, form, and interpretation of symptoms have powerful cultural determinants.

4 List the risk factors for this disorder in older people.

The risk factors for depression in older people are:

- Loneliness (is independently associated with more severe depressive symptoms and is negatively associated with remission after two years).
- Insomnia. There is a complex relationship between sleep disorders (see case 37) and depression. Continuation of insomnia is associated with continuation of depression, but it is not clear whether insomnia is merely a symptom of depression or a co-morbid disorder in some older patients. In some cases, insomnia may lead to alcohol use as a hypnotic, causing worsening of depression and addiction.
- Stressful recent events, e.g. financial problems (including retirement) and especially bereavement (doubles the risk).
- Stressful past events, childhood trauma, or previous history of depression.

- Present and previous low socio-economic status and low level of education.
- Drugs (e.g. digitalis, benzodiazepines, beta-blockers, narcotics, calcium channel blockers, levodopa, diuretics, corticosteroids, antipsychotics).
- Low diastolic blood pressure according to some studies.
- Caring role—around 40% of informal carers suffer from depression.
- Female sex. Some authors claim that depression is up to twice as common in women as in men, although this gap narrows with increasing age, and lower reported rates in men may be secondary to their being less likely to admit to psychological symptoms.
- Physical co-morbidities especially pain, disability, multiple conditions, severe physical conditions of recent onset, and poor mobility/function. The prevalence of depression is reportedly around 30–50% in Parkinson's disease, 40% in chronic obstructive pulmonary disease, 25–75% in stroke, 45% in vascular dementia, and 30% in Alzheimer's dementia.
- Other psychiatric co-morbidity, especially anxiety disorder.

5 Describe differences in this condition in older versus younger patients.

Two groups of depressed patients aged over 60 years can be distinguished:

- New, late-onset depression, in which patients are less likely to have a family history of major mental health problems.
- Recurrent depression (in the majority of cases): a median of four episodes per lifetime is characteristic of recurrent depression, and over 10% will experience a chronic course.

In comparison with younger patients, older patients more often have the following symptoms:

- Hypochondriacal complaints, particularly preoccupation with cognitive and somatic symptoms.
- Loss of self-esteem.
- Poor insight and denial.
- Loss of interest in previously enjoyed activities.
- Depression causing functional impairment sufficient to cause malnutrition, poor muscle strength, poor mobility, and incontinence.
- A need for active rehabilitation to facilitate recovery.
- More frequent relapses of depression.
- Sleep disturbance.

- Psychotic symptoms. Auditory hallucinations are often of threats or accusations. Delusions may include irrational guilt, persecution, or that they are suffering from terminal illness. Such patients usually need input from mental health teams, and in many cases require hospitalization owing to a high risk of self-neglect and suicide.
- Suicidal thoughts.

Older patients with depression also show:

- A positive correlation between the presence and severity of white matter lesions in brain MRI and late-onset depression, consistent with the observed relationship between risks for cerebrovascular disease, history of transient ischaemic attacks, stroke, and so-called vascular depression. These patients often have a worse prognosis and poor response to the usual treatments for depression.
- Lower score on cognitive tests. Depression predicts decline in executive function, mild cognitive impairment, and dementia. Depressed patients also experience worse subjective cognitive symptoms in comparison with non-depressed contemporaries.
- Increased risk of falls (not caused by antidepressants).
- Increased risk for psychiatric re-admission for major depressive disorder.

In comparison with contemporaries without depression, characteristics of older depressed patients include:

- Lower educational level
- More likely to be a widow/widower or divorced.

6 How would you manage this condition?

Risk of self-harm and suicide should prompt urgent psychiatric referral. Patients should be asked about thoughts of self-harm, their attitude to suicide, plans, history of self-harm, severity of distress, hopelessness and helplessness, and impact of recent stressful events.

Treatment of depression comprises psychological interventions and/or drugs depending on the severity of the disease, patient's preference, and local availability of psychological interventions, e.g. cognitive behavioural therapy or a group physical activity. There is no convincing evidence for the superiority of any single treatment from a meta-analysis of 89 controlled studies, although early drug treatment is indicated if depression causes functional impairment. Older patients should be reassured that prescribed antidepressant drugs are not addictive. Physical exercises have been shown in systematic reviews to be beneficial for older patients. Outcomes appear better where patients are offered a choice of psychotherapy and drugs, and where there is care manager involvement.

Drugs should be initiated in low doses. Choice of drug depends on co-morbidities, other medication, and previous response. Drug monotherapy is preferred where possible. A Cochrane review of 32 randomized controlled trials of antidepressants in >55-year-old patients showed similar efficacy for selective serotonin reuptake inhibitors and tricyclic antidepressants, but the latter had more treatment withdrawals and side effects. However, selective serotonin receptor inhibitors are associated with high risk of falls, hyponatraemia (especially with older age, female sex, and low body weight), gastrointestinal bleeds, interaction with warfarin and heparin, as well as risk of serotonin syndrome (see case 36).

There is no evidence to guide length of drug therapy and drug cessation should be done slowly over several weeks. Patients should also be warned about discontinuation symptoms (e.g. for serotonin-specific reuptake inhibitors (SSRIs) these may include dizziness, electric shock-like sensations, or flu-like symptoms).

Full antidepressant response may take up to several weeks and around 20% of older patients need indefinite treatment. One study showed that the median duration of therapy was 18 months for a major depressive episode and that two thirds of patients needed around three years to recover, while another study (PRISM-E) showed that only 29% patients achieved complete remission after six months. Treatment should usually continue for 6–12 months after full remission in those with first episode of major depression. A psychiatric opinion should be sought for severe cases, or where there is persistent non-compliance, psychotic symptoms, lack of response, or deterioration despite therapy (assuming compliance with treatment), severe self-neglect and/or a complex psychosocial situation.

7 If patients do not respond to the usual treatment and are deteriorating, which further options could be considered and in what circumstances?

If patients do not respond to the monotherapy and continue to deteriorate, an alternative antidepressant should be tried. Combination therapy may be required in complex cases, but care must be taken regarding possible interactions, e.g. SSRIs and monoaminoxidase inhibitors causing serotonin syndrome (see case 36). Systematic evidence for the benefits and risks (e.g. impact on cognition) of electro-convulsive therapy in the treatment of depression in older people is lacking and practice is mainly based on case reports. Studies suggest that in the older patients suffering with major depression, but not dementia, short-term treatment outcome of electro-convulsive therapy treatment are not predicted by the baseline impairment of specific cognitive functions. At present, electro-convulsive therapy treatment may be recommended for older patients in cases of:

- Risk of suicide.
- Serious symptoms; for example in cases of severe self-neglect where the patient's physical condition is not compatible with antidepressant treatment and the associated four to six-week delay to maximal treatment effect.
- Depression with psychotic symptoms.
- Depression refractory to standard treatments.
- Intolerance to antidepressants.

Further reading

Arroll B, Khin N, Kerse N (2003). Screening for depression in primary care with two verbally asked questions: cross sectional study. *BMJ*; **327**: 1144–1146.

Bjølseth TM, Engedal K, Benth JŠ, Dybedal GS, Gaarden TL, Tanum L (2015). Baseline cognitive function does not predict the treatment outcome of electroconvulsive therapy (ECT) in late-life depression. *J Affect Disord*; **185**: 67–75.

Bruce ML, Ten Have TR, Reynolds CF 3rd, *et al.* (2004). Reducing suicidal ideation and depressive symptoms in depressed older primary care patients: a randomized controlled trial. *JAMA*; **291**: 1081–1091.

Cheung G, Merry S, Sundram F (2015). Late-life suicide: Insight on motives and contributors derived from suicide notes. *J Affect Disord*; **185**: 17–23.

Coupland C, Dhiman P, Morriss R, Arthur A, Barton G, Hippisley-Cox J (2011). Antidepressant use and risk of adverse outcomes in older people: population based cohort study. *BMJ*; **343**: d4551.

Fiske A, Wetherell JL, Gatz M (2009). Depression in older adults. *Annu Rev Clin Psychol*; **5**: 363–389.

Fried EI (2015). Problematic assumptions have slowed down depression research: why symptoms, not syndromes are the way forward. *Front Psychol*; **6**: 309.

Gardner BK, O'Connor DW (2008). A review of the cognitive effects of electroconvulsive therapy in older adults. *J ECT*; **24**(1): 68–80.

Holvast F, Burger H, de Waal MM, van Marwijk HW, Comijs HC, Verhaak PF (2015). Loneliness is associated with poor prognosis in late-life depression: Longitudinal analysis of the Netherlands study of depression in older persons. *J Affect Disord*; **185**: 1–7.

Kujala I, Rosenvinge B, Bekkelund S (2002). Clinical outcome and adverse effects of electroconvulsive therapy in elderly psychiatric patients. *J Geriatr Psychiatry Neurol*; **15**: 73–76.

Malik A, Junglee N (2015). A case of the serotonin syndrome secondary to phenelzine monotherapy at therapeutic dosing. *Case Rep Med*; **2015**: 931963.

Mitchell AJ, Subramaniam H (2005). Prognosis of depression in old age compared to middle age: a systematic review of comparative studies. *Am J Psychiatry*; **162**: 1588–1601.

Pinquart M, Duberstein PR, Lyness JM (2006). Treatments for later-life depressive conditions: a meta-analytic comparison of pharmacotherapy and psychotherapy. *Am J Psychiatry*; **163**: 1493–1501.

Rodda J, Walker Z, Carter J (2011). Depression in older adults. *BMJ*; **343**: d5219.

Suija K Rajala U, Jokelainen J (2012). Validation of the Whooley questions and the Beck Depression Inventory in older adults. *Scand J Prim Health Care*; **30**(4): 259–264.

Taylor D, Carol P, Kapur S (2012). The Maudsley Prescribing Guidelines, 11th Edition. Chichester, UK: Wiley-Blackwell.

Case 19

A 73-year-old woman was admitted to hospital having woken up with nausea and dizziness, accompanied by a couple of episodes of vomiting, and slight unsteadiness on standing and walking. She was previously fit and well, lived independently with her husband, and both were active members of a local bowling team. The patient had smoked socially while in her twenties, but had not smoked for over 45 years, and drank wine only on special occasions. She had no prescribed medication from her GP, but was self-medicating with 75mg of aspirin daily bought over the counter.

On examination, she was afebrile and in atrial fibrillation at 76bpm with blood pressure of 162/89mmHg. General systems were unremarkable. Cranial nerves appeared intact, but there was mild incoordination of upper and lower limbs bilaterally.

Blood tests showed the following:

- Hb: 12.2g/dl
- WCC: 6.6×10^9/L
- Urea: 10.2mmol/L
- Creatinine: 139μmol/L
- Sodium: 141mmol/L
- Potassium: 3.9mmol/L
- CRP: 12mg/L
- Cholesterol: 6.1mmol/L
- TSH: 2.34.

The admitting team organized a CT brain scan, which was reported as normal.

The following morning, nursing staff became concerned as the patient had become increasingly drowsy: the Glasgow Coma Scale (GCS) had decreased from 15/15 on admission to 10/15. After an assessment by the medical team, her GCS was found to have decreased further to 7/15, and a second CT scan was arranged (Fig. 19.1).

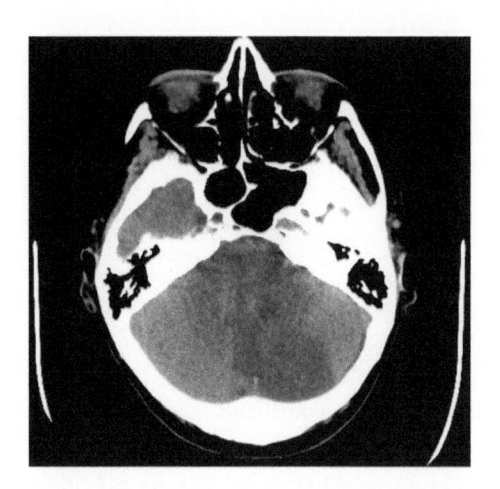

Fig. 19.1 Second CT brain scan from the patient, axial slice through cerebellum.

Questions

1 What was the likely diagnosis on admission? What other diagnoses would you have considered prior to the CT brain scan result?

2 What complication has occurred and what does the second scan demonstrate?

3 Discuss possible management strategies for this patient and what is the prognosis?

Answers

1 What was the likely diagnosis on admission? What other diagnoses would you have considered prior to the CT brain scan result?

The combination of nausea, vomiting, and unsteadiness in the context of atrial fibrillation and documented high blood pressure suggested a cerebellar stroke, which was confirmed on CT brain scan (see Fig. 19.2).

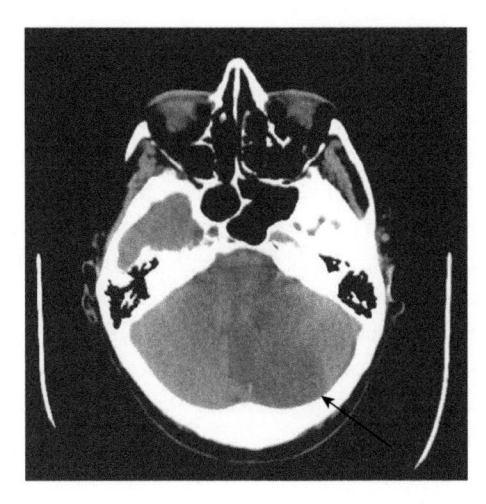

Fig. 19.2 The CT brain scan shows a large low attenuation area in the left medial cerebellar hemisphere with mass effect, consistent with a cerebellar infarct (arrow).

However, the initial differential diagnosis for the presenting symptoms and signs of acute unsteadiness, nausea, and vomiting, is wide and includes:

- *Labyrinthitis.* This is one of the most common differential diagnoses in patients with cerebellar stroke. There may be a viral prodromal illness.
- *Posterior fossa space-occupying lesion.* The relative likelihood of tumour is higher in older patients and may present with relatively sudden onset, particularly if there is haemorrhage into the tumour.
- *Brainstem encephalitis.* This is unlikely in comparison to vascular disease in older people, but should be considered in the presence of a normal CT brain scan. Cranial nerve abnormalities may occur, but are not always present.
- *Demyelinating disease.* In younger patients (in the sixth decade or below), the possibility of demyelinating disorders (e.g. MS) should always be considered in patients with symptoms of possible brainstem origin.

In cases of more subacute symptoms of unsteadiness and incoordination in older people, the differential diagnosis also includes:

- *Paraneoplastic disorder.* Cerebellar dysfunction may occur in association with certain tumours, particularly of the lung and ovaries.
- *Wernicke's encephalopathy.* Usually the ataxia is accompanied by eye movement disorder and confusion.
- *Thyroid disorders.* These may occasionally cause ataxia and unsteadiness.
- *Neurodegenerative syndromes.* Multi-system atrophy may present with cerebellar symptoms (see case 40).

This case illustrates the diagnostic difficulty that may arise in patients with cerebellar stroke in whom symptoms may be relatively mild and signs non-specific, even in large cerebellar hemispheric infarction (Figs 19.3 to 19.5). Although it is often stated that examination of the eye movements looking for vertical versus horizontal nystagmus enables discrimination of central versus peripheral (labyrinth) origin unsteadiness and vertigo, in practice it is very difficult. In older people, particularly those with vascular risk factors, the likelihood of stroke is high and scanning should be considered, particularly because of the possibility of later deterioration. It should also be noted that although strokes usually present with sudden onset maximal deficit, posterior circulation events may show a stuttering or even gradual onset, leading to diagnostic difficulty.

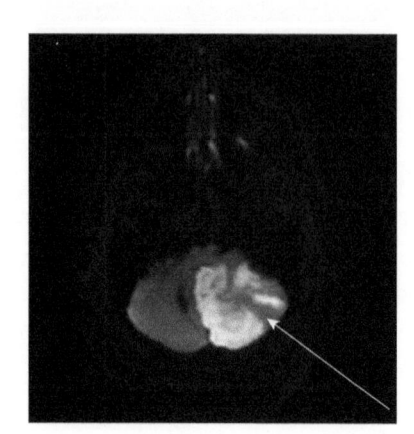

Fig. 19.3 This DWI MRI brain scan from another patient shows an acute cerebellar infarct.

2 What complication has occurred and what does the second scan demonstrate?

The complication of cerebellar oedema and brainstem compression (and possible obstructive hydrocephalus) has occurred and the second CT scan images demonstrate s a large cerebellar infarct and swelling around the infarcted tissue.

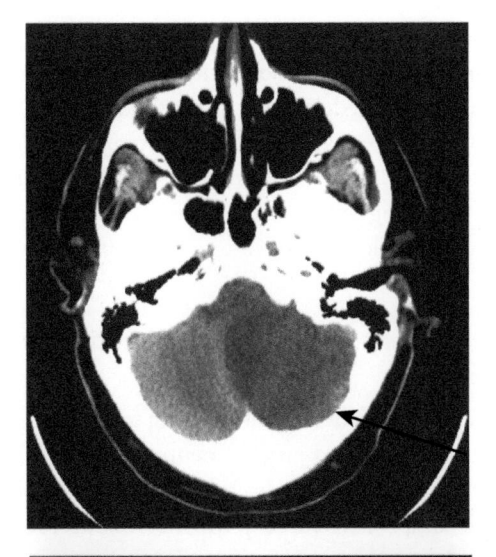

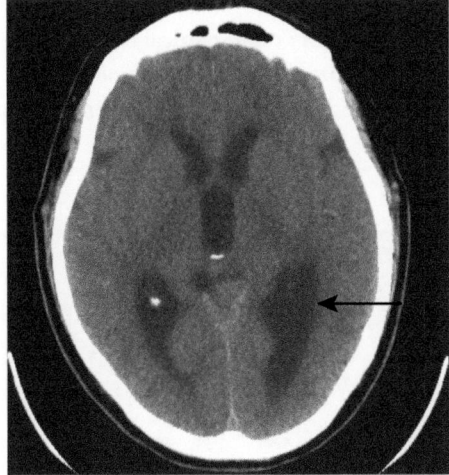

Figs 19.4 and 19.5 CT brain scan from the patient in Figure 19.3, now showing swelling of the cerebellar hemisphere (white arrow), and the development of acute hydrocephalus and ventricular enlargement (black arrow).

Cerebellar infarction is potentially life threatening, as seen in this patient. A large infarct causes cytotoxic and vasogenic oedema, and the resultant mass effect may compress the fourth ventricle and aqueduct of Sylvius, causing obstructive hydrocephalus (Figs 19.3–19.5). The midbrain and pons may also become compressed, and the cerebellar tonsils are ultimately forced downwards through the foramen magnum, while the superior cerebellar vermis herniates upwards through the tentorial notch. Obstructive hydrocephalus affects up to 20% of patients with cerebellar infarction. Reduced level of consciousness reflecting increasing oedema is most likely to occur two to four days after a cerebellar stroke, but may occur as late as nine days.

A significant cerebellar stroke may not be initially suspected in the presence of apparently minor symptoms (as seen in the current patient), leading to delay in CT scanning. Such a delay may result in lack of recognition of subsequent obstructive hydrocephalus. Even with prompt CT scanning, risk prediction of deterioration in individual patients is difficult although early signs of severity including stroke size, cranial nerve deficit, and oedema visible on the scan should prompt careful monitoring for change in GCS.

3 Discuss possible management strategies for this patient and what is the prognosis?

This patient's clinical condition has deteriorated owing to cerebellar oedema and brainstem compression, and urgent neurosurgical opinion is required. There is a lack of evidence to guide choice of surgical procedure, but ventriculostomy or decompressive surgery, with or without resection of infarcted brain tissue, or a combination of both may be considered (Figs 19.6 to 19.8). However, given the rapid clinical deterioration of this patient accompanied by severe obstructive hydrocephalus and tonsillar herniation, the outlook is poor, and neurosurgical intervention is unlikely to be of benefit.

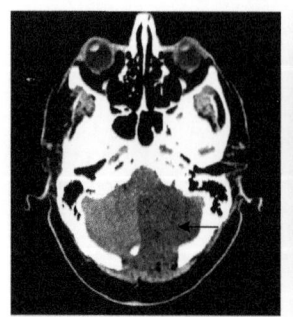

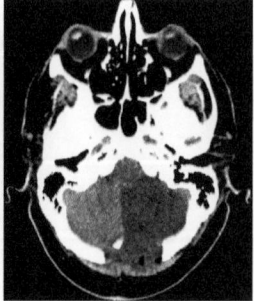

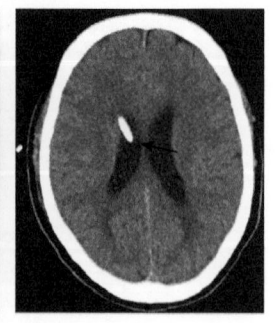

Figs 19.6, 19.7 and 19.8 (Scans taken from the patient in Fig. 19.3.) CT brain scan after postoperative decompression of the posterior fossa (arrow) and insertion of external ventricular drain (arrow).

Further questions

4 Generally speaking, is old age protective against 'malignant infarction' syndromes?
5 What is the most common cause of ischaemic stroke in middle aged versus older patients?
6 Is investigation more or less likely to find a cause for ischaemic stroke in older versus younger patients?

Answers continued

4 Generally speaking, is old age protective against 'malignant infarction' syndromes?

Malignant infarction syndromes comprise malignant middle cerebral artery (MCA) infarction and cerebellar infarction. In malignant MCA infarction, extensive tissue death in the MCA area is accompanied by oedema and hemispheric swelling, midline shift, and tonsillar herniation. Recently, trials have shown that hemicraniectomy is an effective treatment for such patients, resulting in reductions in the combined outcome of death and dependency. The proportion of large MCA infarcts that result in malignant space-occupying syndromes is substantially higher in younger patients partly because age-related cerebral atrophy is thought to be protective in older individuals. The proportion of posterior fossa strokes associated with the 'malignant infarction' syndrome shows less marked age differences because of the lack of available space to accommodate stroke expansion in the posterior fossa, even in the presence of age-related atrophy.

5 What is the most common cause of ischaemic stroke in middle aged versus older patients?

In middle age, lacunar stroke is the most common pathological type; the incidence of large artery stroke in this age group has reduced in line with decline in smoking and coronary heart disease. In older age groups, cardioembolic causes are most common, and are likely to become increasingly important with the ageing population and increasing prevalence of AF.

6 Is investigation more or less likely to find a cause for ischaemic stroke in older versus younger patients?

Investigation is much more likely to find a specific, underlying aetiology in older patients such as atrial fibrillation, carotid or intracranial stenosis, or malignancy. In younger patients, up to 50% of stroke is cryptogenic, and the cause remains unclear despite extensive investigation. Consequently, the tendency for clinicians to thoroughly investigate stroke in younger versus older individuals is not justified, particularly as the recurrence rate is also higher in older patients.

Further reading

Edlow JA, Newman-Toker DE, Savitz SI (2008). Diagnosis and initial management of cerebellar infarction. *Lancet Neurology*; 7: 951–964.

Jensen MB, St Louis EK (2005). Management of acute cerebellar stroke. *Arch Neurol*; **62**: 537–544.

Jüttler E, Schwab S, Schmiedek P, *et al.* (2007). Decompressive surgery for the treatment of malignant infarction of the middle cerebral artery (DESTINY). A randomised controlled trial. *Stroke*; **38**: 2518–2525.

Jüttler E, Schweickert S, Ringleb PA, Huttner HB, Köhrmann M, Aschoff A (2009). Long-term outcome after surgical treatment for space-occupying cerebellar infarction: experience in 56 patients. *Stroke*; **40**: 3060–3066.

Case 20

A 77-year-old man was referred to the rapid access clinic by his GP for an urgent assessment of acute confusion, thought to be caused by infection. The patient's wife had called the GP after she realized he was 'seeing things'. In the clinic he described 'different scenes, like on the television screen' of adults standing and talking, and of children running. He denied hearing any voices. On further questioning, he admitted that these symptoms had been present for weeks and were usually worse in the evenings, but he had not wanted to tell anybody for fear of being thought 'mentally ill'. The hallucinations were not frightening and he knew that they were not real, but he had become more worried after an episode two weeks earlier, when he saw people wearing hats running along beside the car in which he was a passenger. His GP had treated him empirically with antibiotics for a presumed urinary tract infection without effect.

He had had some symptoms of low mood over the past few weeks, but there was nil else of note. There was a past history of hypertension and macular degeneration, and he had had to stop driving about six months earlier as a result, but remained otherwise independent and self-caring. He was an ex-smoker and drank a glass of wine every night. Medication was nifedipine only.

Examination was normal and BP was 130/70mmHg. MMSE was 29/30 (copying the pentagons was incorrect) and CAM was negative.

Investigations showed the following:

- Blood tests (biochemistry and haematology results, including ESR): unremarkable
- Urine dipstick: normal
- Blood and urine cultures: normal
- ECG, CXR: normal
- CT head: mild small vessel disease; no focal atrophy.

Questions

1 Give a differential diagnosis.
2 How would you further assess this patient?
3 What do you think is the most likely diagnosis? What are the diagnostic criteria for this condition?
4 What is the pathophysiology of this syndrome?
5 How would you treat this patient?

Answers
1 Give a differential diagnosis.

This case illustrates the presence of complex visual hallucinations in the context of unremarkable investigation findings. Hallucinations are defined as gustatory, auditory, visual, tactile, or olfactory perceptions. Visual or auditory hallucinations may be complex (hearing music, seeing life-like scenes of people or animals), or simple (e.g. geometric shapes, circles, lines, colours, flashes of light).

The differential diagnosis in this case includes:

- *Charles Bonnet syndrome*: complex visual hallucinations occurring in the context of acquired (usually bilateral) visual impairment and intact cognition with retained insight. Investigations were normal.
- *Delirium (see case 1)*: acute confusion usually in the context of a physical illness. This was unlikely in the current case because MMSE was 29, CAM was negative, and investigations were normal.
- *Epilepsy (see cases 31, 44)*: visual hallucinations (simple or complex) develop in a characteristic fashion with rapid spread over a few seconds and are usually stereotypical. Patients may have déjà vu, somatosensory phenomena, motor activity, and postictal headache or confusion.
- *Alcohol or drug intoxication or withdrawal* (see case 27): visual hallucinations may be simple or complex. Patients usually lack insight and are confused. Auditory and/or tactile hallucinations are frequent accompaniments. The most commonly implicated drugs are opioids, antiepileptics, CNS stimulants (e.g. amphetamines), anti-parkinsonian drugs (e.g. dopamine agonists), sildenafil, and anticholinergics.
- *Dementia*: complex visual hallucinations are a characteristic feature of dementia with Lewy bodies (see case 25), occurring early in the course of the disease and may be the presenting feature. Alzheimer's disease (see case 46), vascular, and (rarely) frontotemporal dementia (see case 43,) may also be associated with visual hallucinations although this is usually a late feature.
- *Hemispheric lesions*: visual hallucinations may occur in stroke affecting the medial aspect of the occipital lobe, the parahippocampal gyrus, and hippocampus.
- *Sleep deprivation.*
- *Grief reaction or other intense emotional experience:* (e.g. post-bereavement). Complex hallucinations of the deceased may be reported by the bereaved.

- *Psychiatric illness:* hallucinations are usually complex and often disturbing. Visual hallucinations are rare in schizophrenia and affective disorders with auditory hallucinations being more common. Patients lack insight and may have other symptoms of psychiatric disorder, e.g. depression, anxiety, thought disorder, delusions.
- *Narcolepsy:* complex hallucinations may occur immediately before or after falling asleep. Patients usually have day-time sleepiness and may have poor insight.
- *Migraine with visual aura:* migrainous visual hallucinations are usually simple and rarely complex, and usually spread from near the centre to the periphery of the visual field. Onset is gradual over five minutes and symptoms last from five to 60 minutes. Characteristic abnormalities include zig-zag lines, localization to one hemi-field, and scotomata. Visual symptoms are nearly always followed by headache, nausea, and photophobia. The clinical features of the current case were not consistent with migraine.
- *Eye disease:* papilloedema may cause simple visual hallucinations; flashing lights, nausea, and vomiting may accompany elevated intraocular or intracranial pressure; scotomata, persistent or continuous blurred or distorted vision, or simple monocular hallucinations requireurgent ophthalmology review to exclude retinal injury.

2 How would you further assess this patient?

A detailed history was taken regarding the timing, repetition, length, and character (simple or complex) of the hallucinations, whether monocular or binocular, and presence of triggers such as bright lights and any accompanying symptoms. Medication was reviewed including use of over-the-counter therapies and any illicit drugs. In this patient MMSE was 29/30 and further history excluded any significant cognitive deficit (he was still managing the house finances, and remained an active member of his local political party).

This patient retained insight. The complex visual hallucinations usually lasted for several minutes and were of different character at different times, but always occurred in the evenings without obvious provocation. His low mood was secondary to his worry about the hallucinations and loss of ability to drive. He denied depression and his Geriatric Depression Scale (GDS) was 2/15. The patient's visual acuity was assessed as part of a complete eye examination and found to be low in both eyes.

3 What do you think is the most likely diagnosis? What are the diagnostic criteria for this condition?

This patient had recurrent complex, visual hallucinations with retained insight, and no evidence of psychiatric or neurologic disorder, except reduced vision from macular degeneration. Investigations were normal. The most likely diagnosis is thus Charles Bonnet syndrome, a diagnosis of exclusion.

The diagnostic criteria for Charles Bonnet syndrome are not yet established, but the following may be helpful:

1 Acquired visual impairment (e.g. due to diabetic eye disease, macular degeneration, cataract, glaucoma)
2 Persistent or recurrent complex visual hallucinations
3 No hallucinations affecting other sensory modalities
4 Retained insight
5 Grossly intact cognition and intellectual function
6 Absence of neurological or psychiatric disease.

Charles Bonnet syndrome affects older patients (mean age around 75 years), but its prevalence is unknown. Patients may be reluctant to seek help owing to fear of being labelled as mentally ill, as in the current case. Hallucinations are not usually stereotyped, and the frequency varies from a few times a year to several times a day. Episodes are usually short-lived, lasting seconds or minutes, but there are reports of longer duration. Patients usually have insight, although this may not be the case when hallucinations have recently developed or consist of shapes that fit the surroundings. Hallucinations are not usually disturbing, except in the minority of cases. Charles Bonnet syndrome has a worse outcome in patients who have one or more activities of daily living affected, and who have frequent and disturbing hallucinations, which may be attributed to serious mental illness.

4 What is the pathophysiology of this syndrome?

The mechanism underlying Charles Bonnet syndrome is unclear. There does not appear to be a correlation between severity of visual loss and likelihood of symptoms. Sensory deprivation, shyness, introversion, stress, and loneliness are contributing factors. Charles Bonnet syndrome has also been reported to occur in patients with non-ocular visual loss, e.g. after occipital infarction.

The deafferentation theory of hallucinations proposes that loss of sensory input to the visual cortex may result in spontaneous neuronal activity, resulting in regeneration of old visual images in a mechanism analogous to that of the 'phantom limb'. Neurons may also become more sensitive to residual visual stimuli in adapting to reduced visual input. It is notable that hallucinations appear to be most common immediately after loss of vision and become less prominent with time.

5 How would you treat this patient?

The patient was reassured and the lack of evidence to support an underlying psychiatric or other condition was summarized in lay terms. An explanation using the phantom limb analogy was given.

There is little evidence to guide treatment so management is based on sporadic case reports and on small observational studies. Many patients need only explanation as to the cause of the symptoms and do not need any intervention.

Treatment strategies include:

- Correction of vision (e.g. cataract operation), which may result in disappearance of the hallucinations.
- Changes in the environment (e.g. better lighting).
- Avoiding physical and social isolation.
- Joining support groups (e.g. The Macular Disease Society).
- Referral to a low vision specialist.
- Drugs: in distressing hallucinations where other measures are ineffective, drugs such as olanzapine, haloperidol, clonazepam, or gabapentin may be helpful. Selective serotonin reuptake inhibitor, or serotonin and norepinephrine reuptake inhibitor, may be considered where there is associated depression.
- Inform patients that hallucinations may cease as the vision stabilizes, or where there is progression to complete loss of vision.

Further reading

Cox TM, ffytche DH (2014). Negative outcome Charles Bonnet syndrome. *Br J Ophthalmol*; **98**(9): 1236–1239.

Eperjesi F, Akbarali N (2004). Rehabilitation in Charles Bonnet syndrome: a review of treatment options. *Clin Exp Optom*; **87**(3): 149–152.

Gold K, Rabins PV (1989). Isolated visual hallucinations and the Charles Bonnet syndrome: A review of the literature and presentation of six cases. *Compr Psychiatr*; **30**: 90–98.

Grimsby A (1993). Bereavement among elderly people: grief reactions, post-bereavement hallucinations and quality of life. *Acta Psychiatr Scand*; **87**(1): 72–80.

Kester EM (2009). Charles Bonnet syndrome: case presentation and literature review. *Optometry*; **80**(7): 360–366.

Menon GJ, Rahman I, Menon SJ, Dutton GN (2003). Complex visual hallucinations in the visually impaired: the Charles Bonnet syndrome. *Surv Ophtalmol*; **48**(1): 58–72.

Menon GJ (2005). Complex visual hallucinations in the visually impaired: a structured history-taking approach. *Arch Ophthalmol*; **123**(3): 349–355.

Santhouse AM, Howard RJ, Ffytche DH (2000). Visual hallucinatory syndromes and the anatomy of the visual brain. *Brain*; **123**: 2055–2064.

Case 21

A 74-year-old woman was brought into hospital by ambulance from her residential home after being found collapsed on the floor by a care worker. The care home staff had not witnessed the collapse, and had last seen her two hours earlier when she had appeared to be her usual self. The ambulance staff reported that when they arrived at the home, she had been incontinent of urine and had a Glasgow Coma Scale of 8/15 with oxygen saturation of 93% on air, heart rate of 74bpm regular, blood pressure 130/67mmHg, respiratory rate of 18 breaths per minute, temperature of 36.2°C, and BM of 2.9mmol/L. The ambulance team had given GlucoGel (formerly called Hypostop, containing carbohydrate) and intravenous fluid.

The patient had moved into the residential home 18 months previously following the death of her husband, who had been her carer. She had struggled to manage at home alone and had become more forgetful. She had settled well at the residential home, but over the preceding six months had had four episodes of mild drowsiness related to hypoglycaemia, which had improved each time after sugary drinks. She had a history of type 2 diabetes, which had required insulin for the past two years. As a result of the hypoglycaemic episodes, the GP had recently decreased the dose of insulin detemir (levemir) from 12 units to eight units and had asked the care home staff to keep a record of the blood glucose readings, which ranged from 2.2 to 11.4mmol/L. Other past medical history included a left fractured neck of femur, osteoporosis, hypertension, and a minor stroke three years previously, following which she had become incontinent of urine, and occasionally incontinent of faeces.

Medications were aspirin 75mg od, metformin 1g bd, gliclazide 160mg bd, amlodipine 5mg od, atenolol 50mg od, atorvastatin 10mg od, and bendroflumethiazide 2.5mg od, in addition to the levemir.

On examination in the emergency department, the BM was 5.6mmol/L, and GCS was 14/15, with AMTS of 6/10. There was mild dehydration and capillary refill of three seconds. General systems examination revealed a soft pansystolic murmur in the mitral region, the lung fields were clear, and the abdomen was soft and non-tender, with normal bowel sounds. There was decreased power in the left arm and leg, grade 4/5, consistent with previous examination findings following the stroke.

Investigations revealed the following:
- Hb: 10.3g/dL
- WCC: 6.2×10^9/L
- Neut: 3.6×10^9/L
- HCt: 0.42L/L
- MCV: 88fL
- Na: 134mmol/L
- K: 4.8mmol/L
- Urea: 10.3mmol/L
- Creat: 125µmol/L
- CRP: 4mg/L
- HBA1C: 5.6% (equivalent to <42mmol/mol IFCC-HbA1C)
- CXR: cardiomegaly; small left pleural effusion
- Urine dip: positive to protein; leucocytes; trace blood; no nitrites; urine culture negative
- ECG: 78bpm; AF; T wave inversion V 4–6; no change from previous ECGs.

Questions

1 What is the cause of this patient's collapse and why has this occurred? How would you manage this?
2 Why are older diabetic patients particularly at risk of this condition?
3 What are the potential complications of this condition?
4 What other alterations to this patient's medications would you consider?

Answer

1 What is the cause of this patient's collapse and how would you manage this?

This patient's collapse was caused by hypoglycaemia. Contributing factors include the drug regimen, and renal impairment.

There was no witness account available (see cases 11, 44), but the ambulance staff found a low BM on arrival. Further, there was a history of recurrent hypoglycaemia; the care home record showed episodes of low BM and the HbA$_{1c}$ demonstrated tight glucose control. The differential diagnosis would include syncope (see case 11) and seizure (see case 44, the risks of which are increased given the history of stroke and cognitive impairment (see cases 19 and 25)).

The patient's drug treatment included insulin in addition to the maximum doses of two oral anti-hyperglycaemic agents. Metformin, a biguanide, does not cause hypoglycaemia. It reduces gluconeogenesis and increases peripheral utilization of glucose, and is particularly useful in overweight patients in whom diet control has failed. The sulphonylureas, of which gliclazide is a short-acting example, promote islet beta-cell production of insulin and may all cause hypoglycaemia, which may persist for many hours, and usually therefore warrants hospital admission. Hypoglycaemia is more common with longer-acting sulphonylureas such as chlorpropamide and glibenclamide, which should be avoided in the older population (although are useful in younger patients with poor compliance). Older patients with impaired liver and renal function (as present in this case, Cr = 125) are especially prone to hypoglycaemia. Short-acting tolbutamide and gliclazide, which are principally metabolized in the liver, may be used in renal impairment, but careful monitoring is required. Insulin may be added in to oral therapy where the latter fails to control glucose adequately, and is usually commenced as a once daily long-acting form. Weight gain and hypoglycaemia are possible complications, but weight gain is less likely when the insulin is given at night, or in combination with metformin. Figure 21.1 shows a flow diagram illustrating the treatment of type 2 diabetes.

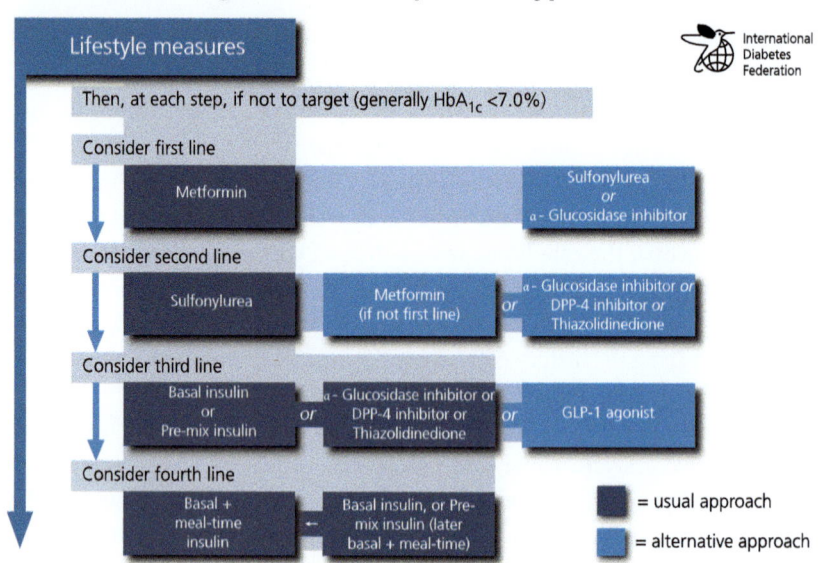

IDF Treatment Algorithm for People with Type 2 Diabetes

Fig. 21.1 Treatment algorithm for type 2 diabetes. (Reprinted by permission of the International Diabetes Federation.)

The United Kingdom Prospective Diabetes Study trial showed that tight glycaemic control using insulin and sulphonylureas in type 2 diabetics reduced the risk of microvascular complications, and that the use of metformin in overweight patients had a beneficial effect on the macrovascular risk. Measurement of glycosylated haemoglobin provides a good indication of glycaemic control over the previous two to three months. Ideally HbA1C should be maintained at 6.5–7.5% (48–59mmol/mol or less) with stricter control (<6.5%, <48mmol/mol) for those at risk of vascular disease. However, in older people, the benefit of tight glycaemic control (which is in any case less relevant in older patients with reduced life expectancy) has to be balanced against the adverse consequences of hypoglycaemia.

In the current case, there are several possible management strategies and the advice of the diabetic team should be sought early. The patient's food intake and weight should be reviewed to ensure that hypoglycaemia is not being exacerbated or precipitated by a lack of nutrition. Malnutrition and unintentional weight loss are prevalent in the care home population, and may be exacerbated by stays in hospital (see case 5). The care home should have a record of previous weights for comparison, and staff may need to be educated about the need for regular meals, and the risk of hypoglycaemia if meals are missed. Specific strategies in relation to the anti-diabetic regime include:

i. withholding the long-acting insulin. If the BMs remain within acceptable levels, i.e. 11–14mmol/L, then insulin should be discontinued. If hypoglycaemic episodes continue despite stopping insulin, then the gliclazide should be reduced. However, if withholding insulin causes the blood glucose to run too high, insulin could be reintroduced at a lower level.
ii. stopping the gliclazide, which will reduce the possibility of hypoglycaemia on insulin.
iii. stopping both the oral anti-diabetic medications and continuing with the insulin. In such cases, the insulin regime would usually be altered to a twice-daily intermediate acting insulin, with or without additional short-acting insulin before meals. The patient's renal impairment increases the risks of both sulphonylureas (see earlier) and metformin. Guidelines suggest reviewing the metformin dose in those with Cr above 130mmol/L, and discontinuing the drug in those with Cr >150. Metformin should also be used with caution in those (often older, frail patients) at risk of sudden deterioration in renal function.
iv. new anti-diabetic drugs could be considered although there is less experience with their use and there are some important side effects/contraindications. DPP-4 inhibitors (sitagliptin, vildagliptin) inhibit dipeptidylpeptidase-4 to increase insulin secretion and lower glucagon secretion. Thiazolidinediones (e.g. pioglitazone) reduce peripheral insulin resistance. Both groups of drugs are licensed for second line therapy in patients with inadequate control on metformin if there is failure to tolerate sulphonylureas, or in patients at risk from hypoglycaemia including older people, and those in dangerous jobs. These drugs may also be added to sulphonylureas in those intolerant of metformin, or as third-line additions to those already on metformin and sulphonylureas in whom insulin is undesirable. DPP-4 inhibitor therapy and thiazolidinediones should only be continued if there is a beneficial metabolic response (a reduction of at least 0.5% points in HbA_{1c} in six months).

Thiazolidinediones (pioglitazone) should be avoided in heart failure, or those at higher risk of fracture. Pioglitazone increases the risk of bladder cancer and should not be used in active cancer, or those with haematuria. The European licence for rosiglitazone has been suspended as the cardiovascular risk was felt to outweigh the benefits, and it should not be used.

A DPP-4 inhibitor (sitagliptin, vildagliptin) may be preferable to a thiazolidinedione (pioglitazone) if:

- further weight gain would be significantly problematic
- a thiazolidinedione is contraindicated

- there was a poor response to, or intolerance of, a thiazolidinedione.

A thiazolidinedione may be preferable to a DPP-4 inhibitor if:

- there is marked insulin insensitivity, or
- a DPP-4 inhibitor is contraindicated, or
- there was a poor response to, or intolerance of, a DPP-4 inhibitor.

Glucagon-like peptide-1 (GLP-1) mimetic (exenatide) binds to the GLP-1 receptor, increases insulin secretion, and suppresses glucagon secretion. It is given by subcutaneous injection, and is also licensed for third-line add-on therapy, particularly in obese patients. Acarbose may be considered if the patient does not tolerate other oral glucose-lowering medications.

Finally, this patient was reportedly forgetful, and admission AMTS was low. A cognitive assessment including collateral history should be undertaken and appropriate management instituted. The patient is in a care environment, where staff administer medication. However, cognitive impairment may cause particular difficulties in the management of diabetes for those living unsupported in the community, especially if they require insulin. Dosette boxes or other monitored dosage systems may be helpful to ensure safe administration of oral anti-diabetic medication, but carers may be required, and district nurse attendance may be necessary to administer insulin. In such cases, insulin regimes need to be simple (usually once daily long-acting insulin) to avoid the need for multiple costly home visits.

2 Why are older diabetic patients particularly at risk of this condition?

Older people are at increased risk of hypoglycaemia because of:

- reduced awareness of the symptoms of hypoglycaemia
- reduced intensity of symptoms
- inability to recognize or communicate symptoms because of cognitive impairment
- inability to take corrective action quickly, e.g. poor mobility
- presence of other medication blunting hypoglycaemic awareness (e.g. beta-blockers)
- presence of renal or hepatic impairment
- reduced or variable nutritional intake
- frequency of intercurrent illness.

There is an age-associated decrease in the autonomic response to hypoglycaemia, and symptoms such as sweating, tachycardia, and tremor are less pronounced. Physiological responses to hypoglycaemia, including secretion of glucagon, adrenaline, and growth hormone are also attenuated with age.

3 What are the potential complications of this condition?

The potential complications of hypoglycaemia include:

- *Hypoglycaemic coma.*
- *Episodic new or worsened confusion and/or other behaviour disturbance.* This may occasionally result in inappropriate treatment (e.g. antipsychotic medication).
- *Cognitive impairment.* Patients who have at least one episode of severe hypoglycaemia appear to be at increased risk of dementia and the cognitive trajectory may be adversely impacted in those with established cognitive impairment (see cases 25, 43, 46).
- *Falls* (see case 27).
- *Seizures* (see cases 31, 44). In the current patient, the history of cerebrovascular disease and likely cognitive impairment increase the risk.
- *Focal neurological symptoms.* Hypoglycaemia may cause focal as well as global nervous system deficits that may be mistaken for a further stroke. BM should always be checked in those with acute neurological deficit.

4 What other alterations to this patient's medications would you consider?

The patient is on three anti-hypertensive drugs including a beta-blocker, thiazide diuretic, and is in atrial fibrillation on aspirin.

Beta-blockers block the cardiac adrenoreceptors and also similar receptors in the lungs, peripheral vasculature, pancreas, and liver. They affect carbohydrate metabolism, may cause hypo- or hyperglycaemia, and attenuate the metabolic and autonomic response to hypoglycaemia. Beta-blockers should be avoided in diabetic patients with frequent hypoglycaemia and should not be used for the routine treatment of hypertension in diabetes or in those at high risk, especially not in combination with a thiazide diuretic, which may exacerbate diabetes. The atenolol should be stopped and the need for the bendroflumethiazide in addition to amlodipine should be assessed.

This patient is at high risk of a further stroke (see cases 19, 42), and yet is receiving aspirin and not warfarin. The risk versus benefit is usually in favour of warfarin, even in patients who have had a fall (see case 27). Adjustment of the medication to reduce the risk of hypoglycaemia would enable introduction of warfarin without undue concern regarding adverse outcomes, and her residence in a care home means that accurate INR monitoring and warfarin dosing will not be an issue, despite the likely cognitive impairment.

Further reading

Bo M, Gallo S, Zanocchi M, *et al.* (2014). Prevalence, clinical correlates, and use of glucose-lowering drugs among older patients with type 2 diabetes living in long-term care facilities. *J Diabetes Res*; Article ID 174316.

Chau D, Edelman SV (2001). Clinical management of diabetes in the elderly. *Clin Diabetes*; **19**(4): 172–175.

Meneilly GS, Cheung E, Tuokko H. Altered responses to hypoglycemia of healthy elderly people. *J Clin Endocrinol Metab*; **78**: 1341–1348.

Shashikiran U, Vidyasagar S, Prabhu MM (2004). Diabetes in the elderly. *Int J Geriatr Gerontol*; **1**: 2.

Whitmer RA, Karter AJ, Yaffe K, Quesenberry CP Jr, Selby JV (2009). Hypoglycemic episodes and the risk of dementia in older patients with type 2 diabetes mellitus. *JAMA*; **301**(15): 1565–1572.

Case 22

Case 22.A

A 66-year-old woman was admitted after a fall, having tripped while crossing the road. She sustained a fractured neck of femur and fractured right clavicle, and was eventually transferred to the rehabilitation ward.

There was a past history of hypothyroidism and diabetes mellitus, and medications included thyroxine and insulin. She had never smoked and did not take alcohol. During her admission, her brother and sister visited, and it was noticed that they were considerably taller and more strongly built. She commented that she had always been the smallest member of the family and a 'sickly child'.

On examination on the rehabilitation ward, she was thin and short, with a height of 156cm and BMI of 15. The rest of the examination was unremarkable.

Investigations showed the following:

- Hb 9g/dL; MCV 72fL; iron 5.0μmol/L; transferrin 3.0g/L; ferritin 9μg/L.
- PT 15 sec; APTT 26 sec.
- glc 6.4g/dl; alk phos 770 IU/L; bilirubin 14mmol/L; albumin 33g/L; AST 34 IU/L;CRP 7 mg/L; U&E; TFT normal; cholesterol 3.6mmol/L; ESR 14; folic acid 2.6mmol/L; B_{12} 200ng/L.
- Urine dipstick: negative for blood, nitrates, and leucocytes.
- Hepatitis A, B, and C serology: normal.
- Calcium 2.0mmol/L; vitamin D 22nmol/L (<30nmol/L indicates vitamin D deficiency); phosphate 0.94mmol/L.
- ECG: sinus rhythm; heart rate 72bpm regular.
- CXR: normal heart size; lungs clear.
- U/S abdomen: normal.
- Colonoscopy and flexible sigmoidoscopy: normal.
- Upper endoscopy: normal (histopathology results awaited).

Case 22.B

A 72-year-old man complained of a two-year history of tiredness, occasional abdominal pain, and increased flatulence. He also complained of a long-standing itch over his elbows and scalp. There was no loss of weight. He did not have any previous medical history, was teetotal, and never smoked.

Examination was unremarkable except that he was thin with a symmetrically distributed rash over the extensor surfaces of his elbows, knees, and buttocks (Fig. 22.1).

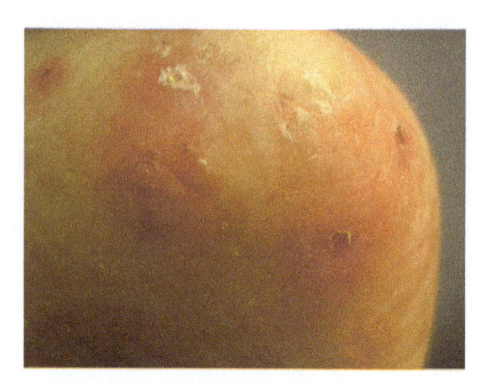

Fig. 22.1 Intact blister and excoriations/healing blisters on elbow of patient from case B.

Investigations showed the following:

- Hb 10.2g/dL; MCV 72f/L; iron 4.0μmol/L; transferrin 2.5g/L; ferritin 6μg/L.
- B_{12}, LFT, TFT, U&E, PT, APTT: normal.
- Folic acid: 3mmol/L.
- Calcium 2.0mmol/L; vitamin D 20nmol/L.
- Parathyroid hormone: 12pmol/l (normal range <0.8–8.7pmol/L).
- CXR: normal heart size; lungs clear.
- U/S abdomen: no abnormalities seen.
- Colonoscopy and flexible sigmoidoscopy: normal.
- Upper endoscopy: normal, but histopathology results showed inflammatory cells, with intraepithelial lymphocytes, and shortened intestinal villi.

Questions

1 What is the diagnosis applicable to both cases?
2 Define this condition and its prevalence in the older population.
3 What are the criteria for confirming the diagnosis?
4 Describe the clinical presentation of this condition in older people.
5 What is the differential diagnosis for this condition, and what complications and associated problems may occur particularly in older patients?
6 How would you manage the condition in older people?

Answers

1 What is the diagnosis applicable to both cases?

The diagnosis is coeliac disease, which in case A is most likely to have been present from childhood given the patient's short stature in comparison to her siblings. There is an association of coeliac disease with type 1 diabetes mellitus and hypothyroidism. In case B, the disease is more likely to have been of recent onset. It was previously assumed that coeliac disease developed in childhood, but it may arise *de novo* in older people.

2 Define this condition and its prevalence in the older population.

Coeliac disease is a multifactorial, chronic autoimmune disorder, caused by intolerance to gluten (a protein in barley, rye, and wheat) in genetically predisposed individuals, causing maldigestion, and malabsorption of nutrients. Human leukocyte antigen (HLA)-DQ2, HLA-DQ8, as well as some non-LA genes, have been identified as genetic risk factors for coeliac disease, which mainly affects populations of Northern European origin with highest prevalence in North America, Australia, Ireland, and Finland. Populations of African, Chinese, or Japanese descent, in which the prevalence of these genes is very low, have a correspondingly low incidence of coeliac disease.

Coeliac disease affects all age groups and its likelihood increases with age. The UK prevalence is 1.2% in adults and 1% in children. The prevalence in first-degree relatives is about 10%. Between 4–30% of cases of coeliac disease are diagnosed in patients >60 years, and there is a female preponderance. Despite significant associated morbidity and mortality, diagnosis may be delayed owing to atypical or non-specific symptoms, and failure to consider the diagnosis in older people in whom investigations may be directed towards malignant disease. There may be a previous diagnosis of irritable bowel syndrome or multiple hospitalizations before the diagnosis of coeliac disease is reached.

3 What are the criteria for confirming the diagnosis?

The definitive test for coeliac disease is small bowel biopsy (at least four biopsy samples should be taken because of patchy mucosal changes) showing typical small-intestinal villous atrophy, lymphocyte infiltrate, and crypt hyperplasia (modified Marsh classification), as seen in case B. Endomysial antibodies have a sensitivity of >90%, but may be absent in partial and milder degrees of atrophy. Anti-tissue transglutaminase autoantibodies have a sensitivity of ~90% and specificity ~95%, and are the test of choice for screening. In cases of low total serum IgA, IgG isotopes of test antibodies should be requested. The diagnosis is supported by disappearance of antibodies on a gluten-free diet. Antigliadin antibodies are no longer used, owing to poor sensitivity, and specificity.

Duodenal biopsy should be performed if there is a strong suspicion of coeliac disease even if serological tests are negative, but a high-gluten diet must be taken for at least two weeks prior to the endoscopy and biopsy for this to be reliable. Duodenal biopsy allows follow-up evaluation of the response to treatment, and excludes other conditions that may mimic the symptoms and laboratory findings of coeliac disease. It is important to note that patients with a negative duodenal biopsy may subsequently develop the disease, and thus investigations may need to be repeated.

In uncertain cases, HLA typing may help in excluding the diagnosis. HLA-DQ2 is present in 90–95% of patients with coeliac disease and its absence, if associated with an absence also of HLA-DQ8, provides a negative predictive value of almost 100%.

4 Describe the clinical presentation of this condition in older people.

The mean age of diagnosis of coeliac disease in the >65 years population is 71.7 ± 4.4 years, with a predominance of female patients at 1.3:1 (compared with 3.8:1 at ages 18–30 years). In older people, it may be asymptomatic, and there are conflicting reports about the pattern of symptoms in later life. It has been thought that older patients have more non-specific symptoms such as flatulence, abdominal discomfort or bloating, and even constipation, while younger patients have diarrhoea, abdominal pain, and weight loss. However, recent reports suggest that diarrhoea and weight loss occur with similar frequency in older and younger patients. Coeliac disease is a common cause of steatorrhoea in older patients.

Clinical features include: fatigue; weakness (due to poor nutrition, anaemia, hypokalaemia, hypocalcaemia); arthritis; arthralgia; osteopaenia; osteoporosis; neurological symptoms (peripheral neuropathy, ataxia); ascites in severe hypoproteinaemia; bleeding diathesis due to malabsorption of vitamin K; low levels of magnesium and cholesterol; dental enamel hypoplasia; cheilosis; glossitis; and Chvostek's sign (see case 23). Micronutrient deficiencies are common and may be the only indicator of the disease. Anaemia is present in up to 80% (usually from iron deficiency), but low folate and occasionally low vitamin B_{12} (indicating ileal involvement) may co-exist, producing a dimorphic blood picture. Low calcium and vitamin D can lead to metabolic bone disorder. In some cases, deranged liver function tests indicate so-called 'coeliac hepatitis': silent coeliac disease may be the underlying diagnosis in up to 10% of patients with otherwise unexplained elevated transaminase levels.

Skin disorders are common and around 15% of patients (with a male predominance) have dermatitis herpetiformis, which is characterized by a papulovesicular rash affecting buttocks, elbows, scalp, and knees, as seen in Figure 22.1 from case B.

5 What is the differential diagnosis for this condition, and what complications and associated problems may occur?

The differential diagnosis includes:

- Small bowel ischaemia
- Small intestine bacterial overgrowth
- Exocrine pancreatic insufficiency
- Bowel malignancy
- Irritable bowel syndrome
- Lactose intolerance
- Intestinal injury from drugs (e.g. non-steroid anti-inflammatory drugs) causing microscopic colitis.

Complications and associated problems of coeliac disease in older people include:

- *Gastro-intestinal adenocarcinoma* (mouth, pharynx, oesophagus, jejunum).
- *Lymphoma.* This is more common in older patients, particularly if coeliac disease was diagnosed between 50 and 80 years of age. T-cell lymphomas are most frequent (Fig. 22.2) and carry a high risk of bowel perforation.
- *Neurological disorders.* Neuropathy (motor or sensory) may occur and there is an increased incidence of seizures, the aetiology of which is unclear.
- *Splenic atrophy and hyposplenism,* usually in untreated disease.
- *Disorders of bone metabolism* (osteopenia, osteoporosis) as seen in case A. There is malabsorption of vitamin D, calcium, and hypoalbuminaemia.
- *Chronic hepatitis.*
- *Ulcerative jejuno-ileitis* with ulcerations, strictures, or both.
- *Short stature.* If the disease starts in childhood patients may be of short stature, as nutrient malabsorption causes failure to thrive and stunted growth as in patient A.
- *Cognitive impairment.* There are reports of so-called 'accelerated dementia', which may not respond to a gluten-free diet.

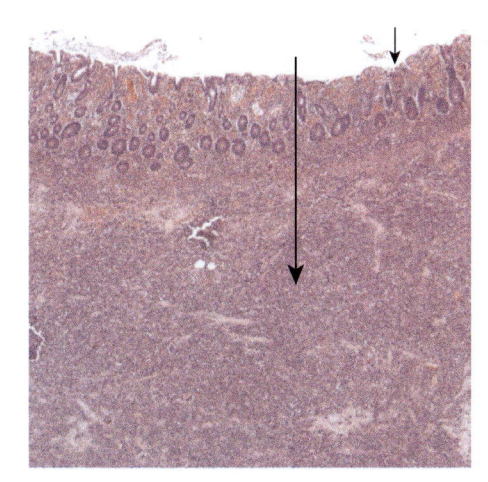

Fig. 22.2 A photomicrograph showing the infiltration of the duodenum by an enteropathy-associated T-cell lymphoma in an older patient (not the described case) with a long history of poorly controlled coeliac disease. The intestinal wall is infiltrated (long arrow) and the residual mucosa shows ulcerations (short arrow).

- One study reported increased cataract risk in patients compared with age- and sex-matched controls.
- Autoimmune disorders are 3 to 10 times more prevalent than in people without coeliac disease, and include type 1 diabetes mellitus and abnormalities of thyroid function as in patient A. Hypothyroidism in particular is more common among older patients. Rheumatoid arthritis, polymyalgia rheumatica, pernicious anaemia, and Sjögren's disease are also more common in older people with coeliac disease.

6 How would you manage the condition in older people?

Referral to a gastroenterologist and dietitian is required. Patients should be advised to omit gluten from the diet and be warned that some pills, capsules, preservatives, and food stabilizers may contain gluten. Gluten-free diets may be problematic for older people owing to reduced financial resources, limited mobility, and thus access to gluten-free food. Care home residence, impaired vision, and inability to read ingredients lists, together with a lifetime's dietary habits add to the difficulties. Education and the continued involvement of the dietitian, with careful monitoring of symptoms as well as supplementation of calcium, iron and vitamins, are essential.

About 5% of all patients develop refractory coeliac disease characterized by persistence of symptoms and villous atrophy, despite a gluten-free diet. The majority of such patients are older. The early recognition of refractory coeliac disease is important, since it is associated with an increased risk of developing T-cell lymphoma, the principal cause of death in such patients, and ulcerative jejunitis.

Further reading

Collin P, Kaukinen K, Vogelsang H, *et al.* (2005). Antiendomysial and antihuman recombinant tissue transglutaminase antibodies in the diagnosis of coeliac disease: a biopsy-proven European multicentre study. *Eur J Gastroenterol Hepatol*; **17**(1): 85–91.

Gasbarini G, Ciccocioppo R, De Vitis I, Corazza GR, Club del Tenue Study Group (2001). Coeliac disease in the elderly: a multicentric Italian study. *Gerontology*; **47**: 306–310.

Green PH, Cellier C (2007). Celiac disease. *N Engl J Med*; **357**(17): 1731–1743.

Green PH, Jabri B (2003). Coeliac disease. *Lancet*; **362**(9381): 383–391.

Tack GJ, Verbeek WH, Schreurs MW, Mulder CJ (2010). The spectrum of celiac disease: epidemiology, clinical aspects and treatment. *Nat Rev Gastroenterol Hepatol*; **7**(4): 204–213.

Jones R, Sleet S (2009). Coeliac disease. *BMJ*; **338**: 539–540.

Ludvigsson JF, Bai JC, Biagi F, *et al.* (2014). Diagnosis and management of adult coeliac disease: guidelines from the British Society of Gastroenterology. *Gut*; **63**: 8 1210-1228.

Mukherjee R, Egbuna I, Brar P, *et al.* (2010). Celiac disease: similar presentations in the elderly and young adults. *Dig Dis Sci*; **55**(11): 3147–3153.

Patel D, Kalkat P, Baisch D, Zipser R (2005). Celiac disease in the elderly. *Gerontology*; **51**: 213–214.

Rashtak S, Murray JA (2009). Celiac disease in the elderly. *Gastroenterol Clin North Am*; **38**(3): 433–446.

Rubio-Tapia A, Kyle RA, Kaplan EL, *et al.* (2009). Increased prevalence and mortality in undiagnosed celiac disease. *Gastroenterology*; **137**(1): 88–93.

Case 23

A 77-year-old woman was referred to the acute medical team by her GP following a home visit. She complained of fatigue, muscle cramps and constipation, and had been seen three weeks previously for lethargy and anaemia with Hb of 9.3g/dL, and MCV of 111fL. A diagnosis of pernicious anaemia had been made on the basis of low vitamin B_{12} and positive intrinsic factor antibodies. She had subsequently received intramuscular hydroxocobalamin on alternate days over the 10 days preceding admission. The past medical history included hypertension and osteoarthritis, and medications were amlodipine, aspirin, and paracetamol with occasional tramodol. She was still driving and independent, and lived with her husband.

On arrival in the medical assessment unit, temperature was 35.9°C, respiratory rate was 16 breaths per minute, heart rate was 58bpm regular and oxygen saturations were 98% on air. On auscultation, the lung fields were clear, and heart sounds were normal. The abdomen was soft and there were no palpable masses. Cranial nerves were intact, and power was grade 4/5 in upper and lower limbs. Sensation and coordination were normal, and the reflexes were found to be slow relaxing.

Investigations revealed the following:

- Hb: 9.4g/dL
- MCV: 107fL
- WCC: 8.2×10^9/L
- Neut: 4.3×10^9/L
- Na: 138mmol/L
- K: 2.7mmol/L
- Urea: 8.9mmol/L
- Creat: 116μmol/L
- ALT: 16IU/L
- Bili: 7μmol/L
- Alp: 326U/L
- CRP: 6mg/L

- Urine dip: NAD
- CXR: NAD
- ECG: sinus rhythm; heart rate 60bpm; no acute changes.

Questions

1 What is the most likely cause for this patient's hypokalaemia? What is the aetiological mechanism?
2 How would you manage this patient?
3 What is the time course of response to vitamin B_{12} therapy?
4 Discuss the prevalence and causes of vitamin B_{12} deficiency.

Answers

1 What is the most likely cause for this patient's hypokalaemia? What is the aetiological mechanism?

The most likely cause for the hypokalaemia is the hydroxycobalamin injections. During initial treatment of vitamin B_{12} deficiency, reticulocytosis occurs, which causes rapid consumption of potassium leading to hypokalaemia.

2 How would you manage this patient?

This patient requires:

- potassium replacement
- vitamin B_{12} injections should continue once the hypokalaemia has been corrected
- investigation of the underlying cause of the bradycardia, hypothermia, and constipation.

Hypokalaemia cannot completely explain the patient's symptoms. The bradycardia, hypothermia, constipation, and slow relaxing reflexes are suggestive of concomitant hypothyroidism, the incidence of which is increased (along with other autoimmune disorders) in patients with B_{12} deficiency. In this patient, thyroid stimulating hormone was elevated, levothyroxine treatment was initiated, and the patient's symptoms improved.

3 What is the time course of response to vitamin B_{12} therapy?

Patients often feel better before any improvement in anaemia. Bone marrow erythropoiesis changes from megaloblastic to normoblastic within one to two days and elevated serum iron, bilirubin, and lactate dehydrogenase fall rapidly. Reticulocytosis occurs in three to four days and peaks at one week, followed by a rise in haemoglobin and a fall in red blood cell mean corpuscular volume. Hypersegmented neutrophils disappear at 10–14 days and the haemoglobin concentration usually returns to normal within eight weeks. A delayed or incomplete response suggests the presence of an additional abnormality or an incorrect diagnosis (e.g. concomitant iron deficiency, infection, hypothyroidism as seen in the current case, or malignancy).

Neurological abnormalities, if present, improve over the ensuing three months, with maximum improvement attained at 6–12 months. The degree of improvement is inversely related to the extent and duration of disease.

4 Discuss the prevalence and causes of vitamin B$_{12}$ deficiency.

Causes of vitamin B$_{12}$ deficiency include:

Gastric abnormalities

- Pernicious anaemia
- Gastrectomy/bariatric surgery
- Gastritis
- Autoimmune metaplastic atrophic gastritis.

Small bowel disease

- Malabsorption syndromes
- Ileal resection or bypass
- Crohn's disease
- Blind loops
- *Diphyllobothrium latum* (fish tapeworm) infestation.

Pancreatitis

- Pancreatic insufficiency

Diet

- Strict vegans
- Vegetarian diet in pregnancy.

Agents that block or inhibit absorption

- Neomycin
- Biguanides (e.g. metformin)
- Proton pump inhibitors
- Histamine 2 receptor antagonists (e.g. cimetidine).

Inherited transcobalamin II deficiency

Vitamin B$_{12}$ deficiency has a prevalence of around 12% in community dwelling older patients, but is higher in older people who are unwell, and those in care home settings. Dietary insufficiency is rarely a cause of vitamin B$_{12}$ deficiency except among vegans. The average western diet contains 5–30µg of vitamin B$_{12}$ per day, of which 2–3µg is absorbed. Vitamin B$_{12}$ is mostly stored in the liver and it can take around two years for the stores to become deplete. A more common cause of B_{12} deficiency is pernicious anaemia, which is an autoimmune condition affecting 1 in 8,000 over 60-year-olds in the UK. In pernicious anaemia, autoimmune destruction directed against hydrogen-potassium ATPase in the gastric parietal cells of the gastric mucosa leads to failure of production of intrinsic factor and malabsorption of vitamin B_{12}. The presence of intrinsic factor antibodies strongly suggests the diagnosis of pernicious anaemia, since specificity approaches 100%, sensitivity being 50 to 70%. In patients without intrinsic factor antibodies, elevated serum gastrin levels, low pepsinogen I levels, and a low ratio of pepsinogen I to pepsinogen II are highly sensitive for the diagnosis of pernicious anaemia (90 to 92%), although these tests lack specificity.

Other causes of atrophic gastritis include chronic *helicobacter pylori infection*. Malabsorption secondary to pancreatic insufficiency, small bowel bacterial overgrowth, Crohn's disease, and ileal resection can also lead to vitamin B_{12} deficiency. Observational studies suggest that metformin may affect vitamin B_{12} absorption, but the mechanism is not understood.

Further reading

Hermann LS, Nilsson BO, Wettre S (2004). Vitamin B_{12} status of patients treated with metformin. *BJDVD*; **4**(6): 401–406.

Case 24

An 82-year-old female retired teacher was admitted with decreased mobility, left hip and lower back pain, tiredness, loss of appetite, recent weight loss, and pyrexia. Six weeks before admission, she had sustained a fall while overseas after tripping on an uneven pavement. That fall had led to two admissions to hospital with the aforementioned symptoms and she had been diagnosed with the condition shown in Figure 24.1. During the first admission, it had been noted that the inflammatory markers were moderately elevated, but chest X-ray, urine dipstick, and cultures were unremarkable. On the second admission, however, blood cultures had grown multi-drug resistant extended-spectrum β-lactamase-producing *Escherichia coli*, presumed to originate from a urinary tract infection. She had been prescribed a course of intravenous antibiotics and discharged home. However, the pain and fever continued, and she was readmitted to the medical ward a week later.

There was a history of osteoarthritis and right hip replacement four years previously. She lived with her husband in a cottage in the countryside, and prior to the fall she had been independent in all daily activities, including driving twice a week to a nearby town to help a friend run a charity shop. She was a non-smoker and moderate drinker. Medications were paracetamol, codeine phosphate, lactulose, and senna.

On examination, she was pyrexial at 37.8°C, with a pulse of 90bpm and blood pressure of 120/65mmHg. General systems and neurological examinations were normal, except for a decreased range of left hip movement, and pain and tenderness over the parasymphyseal, and sacral areas on the left side. AMTS was 10/10.

Investigations showed the following:

- Hb 11.5g/dL; WCC 13.8 × 10^9/L; (80% neutrophils); plt 350 × 10^9/L
- U&E, TFT, LFT: normal, except for alkaline phosphatase 600IU/L
- CRP 120mg/L; ESR 80mm/h
- Urine dipstick: no protein; blood, leucocytes, and nitrate positive
- Urine culture: negative
- Blood culture: awaited

- CXR: normal heart; clear lungs
- ECG: sinus rhythm; heart rate 90bpm; occasional ventricular ectopics
- Pelvic X-ray: see Figure 24.1.

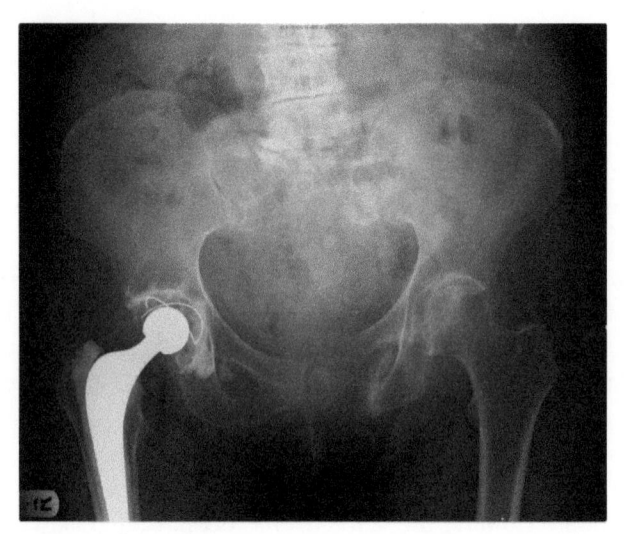

Fig. 24.1 Plain X-ray of the pelvis.

Questions

1. What does Figure 24.1 show? What is the incidence and prognosis of this condition?
2. How should patients with this condition be managed?
3. This patient's symptoms and signs cannot be explained solely by the condition shown in Figure 24.1. What complications or accompanying conditions might have occurred and what specific points in the history and examination should be looked for?

Answers

1 What does the X-ray in Figure 24.1 show? What is the incidence and prognosis of this condition?

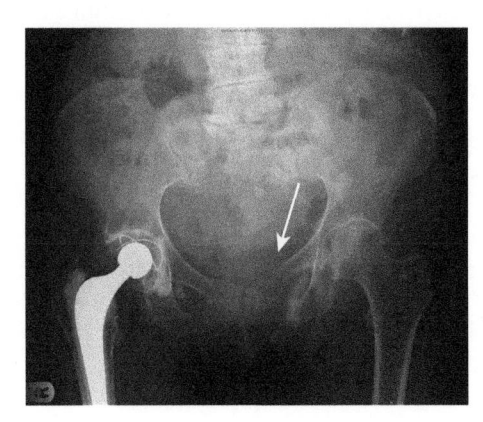

Fig. 24.2 Plain X-ray of the pelvis with arrow showing fractures of the left superior and inferior pubic rami.

The X-ray shows fractures of the left superior and inferior pubic rami (arrow, Fig. 24.2). Such fractures are the most common form of pelvic fracture, usually occurring after falling from a standing position. The incidence of pubic rami fractures in people older than 60 years is 26/100,000 per year, and it will affect 0.5% of males and 2% of Caucasian females by 85 years of age. Mean age of presentation is 77 years and 63 years for women and men respectively, with around a quarter of all patients having a diagnosis of dementia prior to the injury. A high resting heart rate, older age, history of pelvic irradiation, or corticosteroid treatment, conditions related to propensity to falls, and the presence of indicators for frailty (e.g. functional loss with dependence for activities of daily living, or recent loss of weight), and osteoporosis confer an increased risk.

Historically, it has been assumed that pubic rami fractures are benign, but if admission to hospital is required, the mean time spent in a geriatric orthopaedic unit is around 40 days. The complication rate is 20%, mostly related to infection, and in-patient fatality is around 14%. Post-mortem examinations of patients with pubic rami fractures show estimated blood loss in the soft tissue surrounding the fracture of around 1L.

When compared with age- and sex-matched controls, either in-patient or general population, post-discharge mortality rates of in-patients with pubic rami fractures are much higher, reaching 25% at one year. Most excess deaths are in the 60–69 year age group, and age by itself does not determine mortality. By five years, mortality rates have fallen to levels matching the general population, indicating that the excess mortality reflects the immediate effects of the fracture and its complications.

The factors predictive of poorer prognosis in patients with pubic rami fractures are:

- immobilization and increased risk of falls
- dependency
- poor mental and physical health, particularly dementia
- fractures closer to the acetabulum.

Fewer than 50% of patients will reach pre-admission mobility levels by the time of discharge and the rate of re-fracture is high at around 25% (compared with a 10% risk for re-fracture in patients >50 years with any fracture). Although up to 60% will return to independent living overall, this falls to only 30% in the over 80s.

2 How should patients with this condition be managed?

Immobilizing pain in the pelvic region is the main symptom of pelvic fractures, together with groin, or lower back pain. The priority of management is therefore pain control, early mobilization, and prevention of thromboembolic complications, as well as early treatment of underlying osteoporosis. Treatment is mostly on an out-patient basis with pain relief and early mobilization at home.

A minority of patients will require surgical intervention depending on fracture type (bone displacement is usually minimal) and associated complications, e.g. concomitant genito-urinary injury or presence of hypovolaemic shock. Patients with inadequate pain control and difficulty mobilizing may require admission to hospital, preferably to a specialist geriatric medical ward, and patients on anticoagulants may also warrant hospital admission for observation.

Geriatric input improves outcomes for frail older patients with hip fracture and is likely to do so for other fractures. Patients should have comprehensive geriatric evaluation including: multidisciplinary team input; osteoporosis evaluation; falls risk assessment; drugs review; and cognitive and continence assessments. GP liaison and careful discharge planning by the multidisciplinary team including the social worker, occupational therapist, and physiotherapist is required.

3 This patient's symptoms and signs cannot be explained solely by the condition shown in Figure 24.1. What complications or accompanying conditions might have occurred and what specific points in the history and examination should be looked for?

The clinical findings and symptoms suggest the possibility of one or more of the following:

i. **Sacral fracture.** This patient was slow to mobilize with difficult-to-control pelvic pain, lower back pain, and new onset of sacral tenderness on the same side as the pubic rami fractures.

Magnetic resonance imaging (MRI) and bone scintigraphy are highly sensitive, but occasionally the latter may confuse fractures with malignancy or infection. In inconclusive cases, or when MRI is not available, CT imaging may be used (Fig. 24.3).

Small studies have shown that sacral fractures are associated with pubic rami fractures in the majority of low-impact pelvic ramus fractures of older patients. These fractures can affect the ipsilateral or bilateral wings of the sacrum, and are often missed or diagnosed late, owing to insensitivity of routine pelvic X-rays, and poor awareness among clinicians. Such accompanying sacral fractures are often associated with generalized osteoporosis. Sacral fractures are a significant injury, not least because they are a cause of chronic pain and if non-displaced, treatment with sarcoplasty may be considered, although its validity is yet to be determined. Surgical intervention with stabilization is recommended for the displaced fractures, thus allowing earlier mobilization, and significant pain reduction. There are recent reports of successful treatment with a combination of sarcoplasty and surgical intervention.

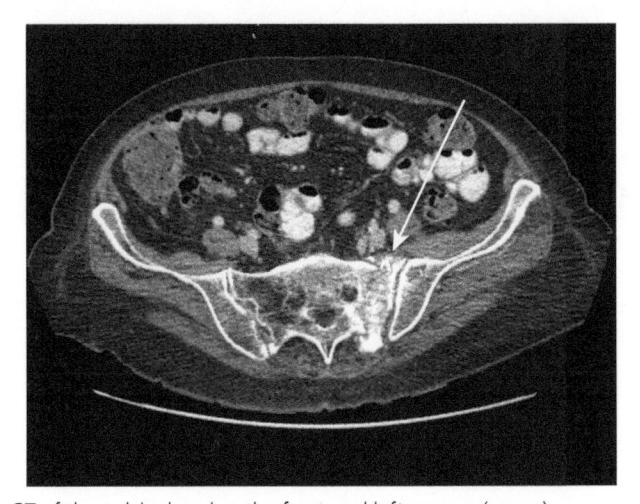

Fig. 24.3 CT of the pelvis showing the fractured left sacrum (arrow).

ii. **Bladder injury.** This may result from direct injury by bone fragments in pelvic fractures. Bladder injury is associated with pelvic or suprapubic pain, an inflammatory response and often, urinary infection.
iii. **Urethral injury.** This was less likely in this patient, as urethral injury usually presents with overt haematuria, or inability to void. It is more common in men, who may also rarely display a high-riding prostate on rectal examination.
iv. **Infection.** Infection in this case was suggested by difficult-to-control pain, pyrexia, and raised inflammatory markers, persisting for weeks after the original injury in a patient who had been previously well. The multiple hospital admissions were also a risk factor for hospital-acquired infection. Pelvic abscess, osteomyelitis, and peritonitis (from a bladder leak or pelvic haematoma) should be considered.
v. **Sacral nerve injuries,** which are unlikely in this case given the lack of neurological abnormality on examination. The neurological examination should include sphincter function testing.
vi. **Haemorrhage** was also unlikely, since it is usually associated with anticoagulant treatment. Significant haemorrhage is associated with hypovolaemic shock and swelling, bruising, and pain in the abdomen (particularly in the suprapubic or periumbilical regions), groin, or perineum (see Figs 24.4 and 24.5).

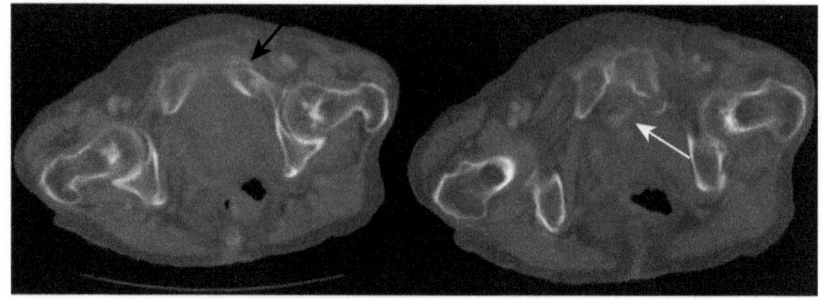

Fig. 24.4 CT pelvis post intravenous contrast on bony windows from a different patient. This demonstrates fracture of the left pubic ramus (black arrow), with active bleeding into the pelvis (white arrow).

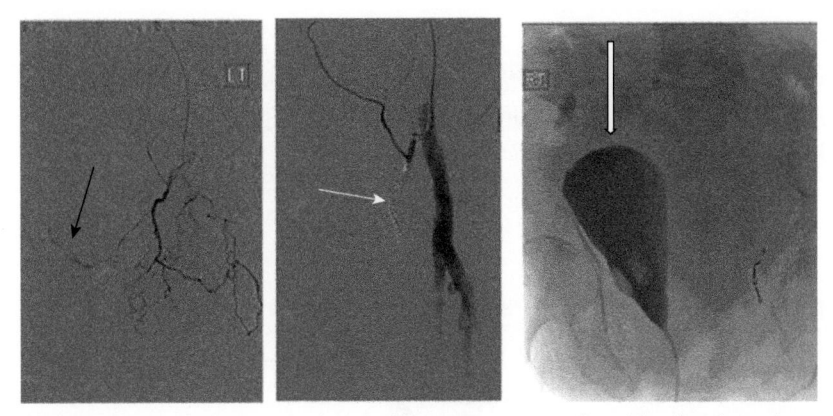

Fig. 24.5 Selective angiography from a different patient confirms bleeding from the corona mortis artery (left, black arrow), which was embolised with multiple coils (middle, white arrow). There is large haematoma post procedure displacing the bladder to the right (right, thick arrow).

Case development

After admission to hospital, the patient continued to feel unwell with poor appetite. Blood culture was positive for multi-drug resistant extended-spectrum β-lactamase-producing *Escherichia coli*.

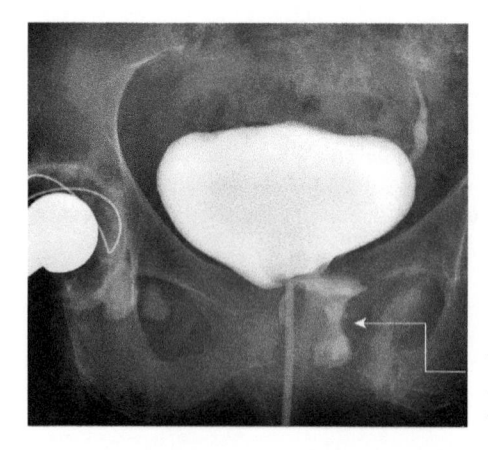

Fig. 24.6 Cystogram from the patient with relevant abnormality, indicated by the arrow.

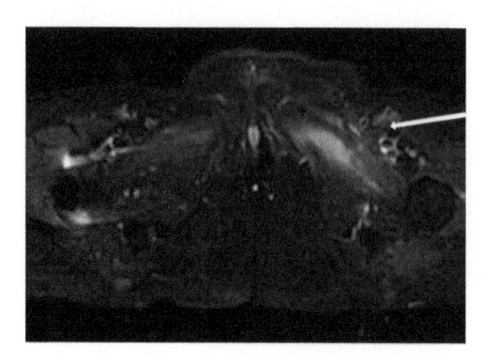

Fig. 24.7 MRI of the pelvis with arrow indicating abnormalities in the left pectineus muscle.

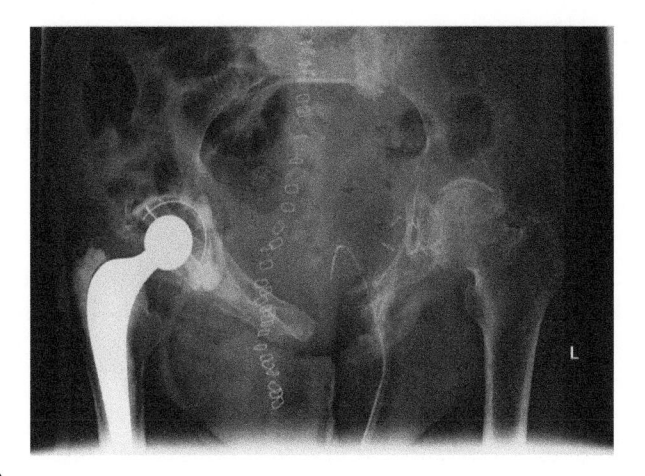

Fig. 24.8

Questions continued

4 What is the implication of recurrent positive blood cultures with multi-drug resistant extended-spectrum β-lactamase-producing *Escherichia coli* in this patient?
5 How would you proceed further? What is the role of comprehensive geriatric assessment in this case?
6 Review the patient's subsequent images (Figs 24.6 and 24.7). What is the most likely diagnosis based on these?
7 Describe Figure 24.8. What do you think has now happened to the patient?

Answers continued

4 What is the implication of recurrent positive blood cultures with multi-drug resistant extended-spectrum β-lactamase-producing *Escherichia coli* in this patient?

Extended-spectrum β-lactamase-producing *Escherichia coli* are resistant to penicillin, cephalosporin, fluoroquinolone, trimethoprim, and cefoxitin, and are usually associated with indwelling devices (e.g. urinary catheters, central venous lines, and PEG tubes), decubitus ulcers (see case 14), recent surgery, and/or poor nutritional state (see case 5). Recent studies report increasing rates of community-acquired infections with extended-spectrum β-lactamase-producing *Escherichia coli* in patients with urinary tract infections, and in some cases, bacteraemia. Such patients are usually older and may have diabetes mellitus, a history of prior hospital admissions, and/or prior quinolone use.

In this patient urgent investigation to locate the source of the underlying infection was required. Possible sources for infection included:

- bladder leak and intra-abdominal infection
- pelvic abscess from an infected haematoma
- osteomyelitis/discitis/joint space infection
- endocarditis (unlikely to be present in isolation given the pelvic pain and urinary dipstick findings).

5 How would you proceed further? What is the role of comprehensive geriatric assessment in this case?

This patient needed further:

- assessment (to establish the underlying diagnosis)
- treatment of the inter-current illness
- achievement of homeostasis
- prevention of complications.

Further assessment included a cystogram, MRI pelvis, and cystoscopy. Antibiotic prescription was guided by blood and urine culture sensitivities, and she received pain control, nutritional intervention, thromboembolic prophylaxis, and osteoporosis treatment.

Comprehensive geriatric assessment (CGA) was performed at the point of admission, where medical, psychological, and functional capabilities were assessed and coordinated (systematic assessment of an older patient), and an integrated plan for the treatment was devised (management of an older patient). There is no standardized protocol for CGA; however, it encompasses the following:

i. history of complaints (e.g. present and past complaints). Symptoms may be non-specific or atypical.
ii. history of all conditions/admissions/interventions (e.g. previous disease, the presence of multi-morbidities) and in this case, the possibility of osteoporosis requiring treatment.
iii. functional assessment—the assessment of physical activity, is done either by interview and/or by the use of assessment instruments for activities of daily living including the Barthel Activities of Daily Living, and the Nottingham Extended Activities of Daily Living Scale.
iv. assessment of continence (urinary symptoms, bowel opening, see cases 7, 32).
v. drug history (e.g. polypharmacy, drug allergies).
vi. social history.
vii. habits (e.g. use of alcohol, smoking, illicit drugs).
viii. cognitive function and mood assessment for delirium, depression, or dementia using the appropriate tests guided by the clinical picture (see cases 1, 18, 25).
ix. nutritional assessment (see case 5) (e.g. Malnutrition Universal Screening Tool (MUST); BMI (Body Mass Index)). It should be noted that obesity does not imply adequate nutrition or the absence of sarcopenia: 'sarcopaenic obesity' describes obesity with loss of muscle strength/mass, see case 5.
x. environmental assessment (e.g. house condition, presence of stairs, heating).

CGA takes a holistic approach to the patient and may be delivered:

- at a dedicated acute geratology ward
- by mobile interdisciplinary geriatric teams (such teams give recommendations to the non-specialist physicians).

In this patient, there was history of a fall and subsequent loss of mobility, loss of appetite, and of feeling unwell. Her symptoms were relatively non-specific and the systemic response to infection was relatively muted. She was assessed for activities of daily living and the Barthel Activities of Daily Living score was reduced compared to the estimated pre-morbid level. There was no polypharmacy, but nutritional assessment revealed recent loss of weight associated with her illness. Living arrangements were adequate as she lived in a bungalow, which did not need much adjustment prior to her discharge. Osteoporosis with 'low trauma fracture' was diagnosed and treatment started. The fall was felt to be mechanical.

There is evidence that CGA improves patient survival, function, and quality of life, reduces length of stay in hospital, prevents deterioration and institutionalization, and re-admission to hospital.

6 Review the patient's subsequent images (Figs 24.6 and 24.7). What is the most likely diagnosis based on these?

Figure 24.6 shows a cystogram with a leak from the left base of the bladder anteriorly (arrow), thought to be caused by a fragment of the fractured pubic ramus. This was confirmed on cystoscopy where a bone fragment was seen protruding into the bladder. Figure 24.7 is an MRI of the pelvis showing an intramuscular abscess in the left pectineus. Other images also revealed osteomyelitis in the pubic bones.

Her fall was thus assumed to have caused fractures of pubic rami, symphysis and sacrum with a bladder injury from a bone fragment complicated by osteomyelitis of the pubic bones and an intramuscular abscess.

7 Describe Figure 24.8. What do you think has now happened to the patient?

The patient had surgery with removal of the osteomyelitic pubic rami, muscle abscess excision, and a successful bladder repair. Figure 24.8 shows the pelvis after surgical intervention and removal of fractured bone fragments (bilateral pubic rami, arrow). She was given a further course of antibiotics and recovered well. She returned home continent, continuing with physiotherapy in the community. Six months later she was independently mobile with a stick.

Further reading

Cosker TDA, Ghandour A, Gupta SK, Tayton KJJ (2005). Pelvic ramus fractures in the elderly: 50 patients studied with MRI. *Acta Orthop*; **76**(4): 513–516.

Dijk WA, Poeze M, Helden SH, Brink PRG, Verbruggen JPAM (2010). Ten-year mortality among hospitalised patients with fractures of the pubic rami. *Injury*; **41**(4): 411–414.

Ellis G, Whitehead MA, Robinson D, O'Neill D, Langhorne P (2011). Comprehensive geriatric assessment for older adults admitted to hospital: meta-analysis of randomised controlled trials. *BMJ*; **343**: d6553.

Hill RMF, Robinson CM, Keating JF (2001). Fractures of the pubic rami. Epidemiology and five-year survival. *J Bone Joint Surg (Br)*; **83**-B: 1141–1144.

Kelsey JL, Prill MM, Keegan THM, Quesenberry CP Jr, Sidney S (2005). Risk factors for pelvis fracture in older persons. *Am J Epidemiol*; **162**: 879–886.

Macdonald DJM, Tollan CJ, Robertson I, Rana BS (2006). Massive haemorrhage after a low-energy pubic ramus fracture in a 71-year-old woman. *Postgrad Med J*; **82**(972): e25.

Paterson DL, Bonomo RA (2005). Extended-spectrum beta-lactamases: a clinical update. *Clin Microbiol Rev*; **18**: 657–686.

Rommens PM, Wagner D, Hofmann A (2012). Surgical management of osteoporotic pelvic fractures: a new challenge. *Eur J Trauma Surg*; **38**: 499–509.

Case 25

A 76-year-old man was admitted via the emergency department after his wife, who reported that he had fallen three times in the previous week, found him on the floor. He was unable to recall the circumstances of the falls, found it difficult to stay awake and answer questions, although he was easily roused from the sleepy episodes. His wife said he had first fallen a year earlier, but had fallen more frequently over the past six months. He had also developed memory difficulties over the past year. She was also concerned that he had been talking to an imaginary cat that sat in the corner of the room, and spoke of seeing a little girl from time to time on the stairs.

His past medical history included osteoarthritis, pancreatitis, cholecystectomy, and diverticulitis. Medication included paracetamol, lactulose, and omeprazole. He was a retired mechanical engineer and was a non-smoker. Alcohol intake was 10 units a week.

On examination, observations were stable, but supine blood pressure was 158/72mmHg and standing blood pressure was 132/68mmHg. General systems were unremarkable but neurological examination demonstrated bilateral increased rigidity of the upper limbs, with decreased plantar responses.

Mini Mental State Examination (MMSE) score was 26/30 with points lost on copying the intersecting pentagons, recall, and the date.

Investigations showed the following:

- Hb: 13.6g/dL
- WCC: 4.6×10^9/L
- Neut: 2.2×10^9/L
- HCt: 0.37L/L
- Na: 135mmol/L
- K: 4.6mmol/L
- Urea: 6.9mmol/L
- Creat: 97µmol/L
- Calcium: 2.4mmol/L
- Magnesium: 0.85mmol/L

- ALT: 34IU/L
- Bili: 22μmol/L
- Alp: 220U/L
- Albumin: 42g/L
- CRP: 2mg/L
- Urine dipstick test: negative
- Chest X-ray: normal
- ECG: unremarkable
- CT brain: minor small vessel disease with no focal atrophy.

Questions

1 What is the most likely diagnosis? List other possible diagnoses. What other bedside test might you consider?
2 What other investigations should be considered?
3 What are the next steps in the management of this patient?
4 What is the prognosis in this condition?

Answers

1 What is the most likely diagnosis? List other possible diagnoses. What other bedside test might you consider?

The most likely diagnosis is dementia with Lewy bodies (DLB). A MoCA or other cognitive test including visuoexecutive function should be considered.

DLB comprises approximately 20–30% of all dementia, with Alzheimer's disease and vascular dementia making up the majority of remaining dementia in older people. DLB is a neurodegenerative disorder of unknown cause that is characterized by cognitive decline, fluctuation, parkinsonism and visual hallucinations, autonomic dysfunction, sleep disorder, and neuroleptic sensitivity. DLB affects males more than females with a ratio of 2:1 and the mean age at presentation is 75 years, with death occurring around 6.5 years after diagnosis. Early incontinence and swallowing problems, more severe parkinsonian, and/or psychiatric features are associated with increased mortality.

The neuropathology is characterized by the presence of round, intracytoplasmic neuronal inclusions, containing ubiquitin and alpha-synuclein (Lewy bodies). Lewy bodies are seen in the deep cortical layers throughout the brain, especially in the anterior frontal and temporal lobes, the cingulate gyrus, the insula, and also in the pigmented neurons of the substantia nigra, locus ceruleus, raphe nuclei, nucleus basalis of Meynert, and other brainstem nuclei. The pathologies of DLB and Parkinson disease dementia are similar, and Lewy bodies eventually develop in the cortex in patients with Parkinson's disease as cognitive impairment develops. There is also some overlap with Alzheimer's disease: most patients with DLB have amyloid plaques, although the burden appears overall less than in patients with pure Alzheimer's disease, in whom amyloid PET imaging shows marked amyloid marker retention (Fig. 25.1). The consensus criteria for DLB are shown in Table 25.1

Fig. 25.1 Serial planes showing the topography of amyloid deposition as evidenced by ^{11}C-PIB compound retention in the brain of a control individual and a patient with AD. The axial (top two rows) and sagittal (bottom two rows) standardized uptake values (SUV) of PIB images are shown. Images from the control individual are shown in rows one and three, and the corresponding data from the patient with AD are shown in rows two and four. The scale bar indicates the relative levels of PIB SUV values.
(Reproduced with permission from WE Klunk, H Engler, A Nordberg, et al. Imaging brain amyloid in Alzheimer's disease with Pittsburgh Compound-B. *Ann Neurol*; 55: (2004), pp. 306–319, Wiley-Liss Inc.)

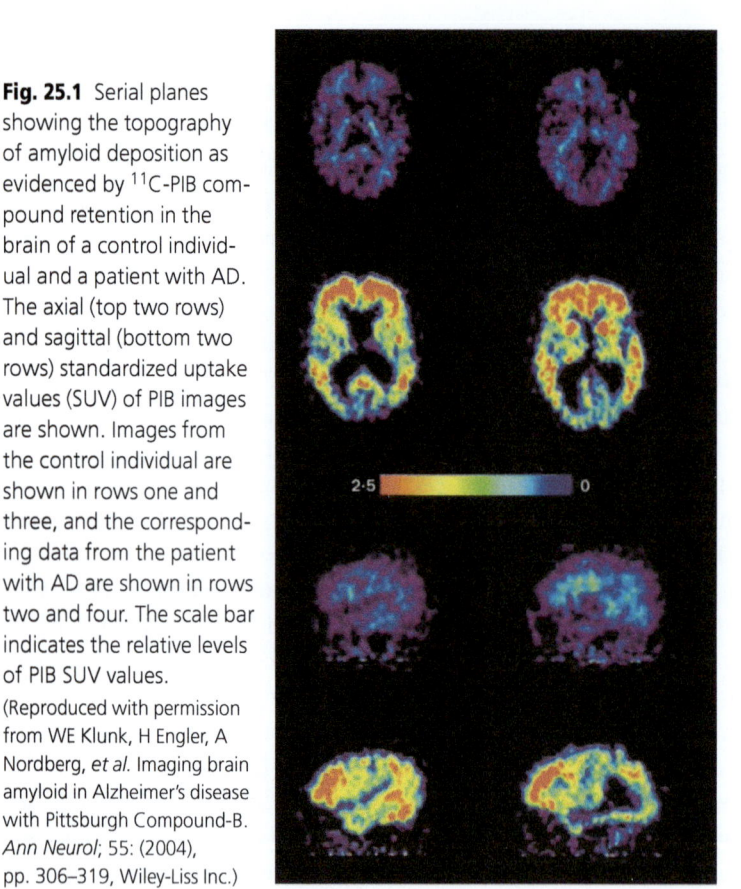

Table 25.1 Consensus criteria for DLB

	Frequency in DLB (%)
Central feature (essential for the diagnosis)*	
Progressive cognitive decline, dementia	100
Core features (two features essential for diagnosis of probable DLB, one for possible DLB)*	
Fluctuating cognition	60–80
Recurrent well-formed, detailed visual hallucinations	50–75
Spontaneous features of parkinsonism	80–90

Table 25.1 (continued) Consensus criteria for DLB

	Frequency in DLB (%)
Suggestive features (one suggestive feature with one core feature may diagnose probable DLB, one or more suggestive features may diagnose possible DLB)*	
REM sleep disorder	85
Severe neuroleptic sensitivity	30–50
Low dopamine transporter uptake in basal ganglia on SPECT or PET	
Supportive features (common features with undetermined diagnostic specificity)*	
Repeated falls	33
Syncope or transient loss of consciousness	
Severe autonomic dysfunction	
Hallucinations in other modalities	20
Systematized delusions	55–75
Depression	30–40
Relative preservation of medial temporal lobe on MRI or CT	
Generalized low uptake on SPECT or PET perfusion imaging with reduced occipital activity	
Abnormal (low uptake) MIBG myocardial scintigraphy	
Prominent slow wave activity and temporal lobe transient sharp waves on EEG	
Conflicting features (features which make DLB less likely)*	
Cerebrovascular disease evidenced by focal neurological signs or neuroimaging	
Other physical illness or brain disorder, which is consistent with some or all of clinical features	
First appearance of parkinsonism at late stage (severe) dementia	
Temporal sequence (features which distinguishes DLB from Parkinson disease dementia)*	
Dementia should occur before or concurrently with onset of parkinsonism	

* Consensus criteria of the third report of the DLB consortium. McKeith IG, Dickson DW, Lowe J, et al. (2005). Diagnosis and management of dementia with Lewy bodies: third report of the DLB Consortium. *Neurology*; 65: 1863.

The differential diagnosis includes:
- Alzheimer's disease
- Delirium (see case 1)
- Parkinson's disease (see case 40)
- Parkinson's plus syndrome (see case 40)
- Normal pressure hydrocephalus (see case 6)
- Vascular dementia (see case 46)
- Charles Bonnet syndrome (see case 20).

The patient in this case has at least two core features of DLB (visual hallucinations and parkinsonism), and some supportive features (falls, postural hypotension, preserved temporal lobes on CT brain scan). The sleepiness is also characteristic (fluctuating conscious level), and fluctuations in cognition and levels of alertness may occur early in the course of the disease. Severity, duration, and type of symptoms vary even within a given patient. There may be subtle brief decline in ability, or more overt somnolence, bizarre behaviour, or speech or motor arrest. Episodes may last hours to days and be interspersed with relatively normal function. The aetiology is unclear, but seems to involve an impairment of alerting/attentional processes. Although patients with other types of dementia may show variable cognitive function, this is usually non-specific and related to external stressors, rather than occurring abruptly and spontaneously.

The visual hallucinations in DLB are complex as seen here (also see case 20) and often take the form of humans or animals, but typically are not distressing. Hallucinations may precede the onset of other symptoms by years, and conversely, early visuospatial dysfunction predicts risk of future hallucinations. Parkinsonian features including rigidity, cogwheeling, bradykinesia, and shuffling gait often occur within 12 months of onset, but resting tremor is not typical. The extrapyramidal features tend to respond less well to levodopa treatment than in idiopathic Parkinson's disease and such medications may exacerbate cognitive symptoms. The distinction between DLB and Parkinson's disease dementia is made somewhat arbitrarily based on the time of onset of cognitive impairment, relative to the parkinsonism. Onset of cognitive problems before or within one year of parkinsonism indicates DLB.

The pattern of cognitive deficits in DLB is subcortical with prominent impairment in attention and executive function (planning and sequencing) and visuospatial memory, in contrast to Alzheimer's disease in which there is usually an initial prominent deficit in short-term memory with relative preservation of other domains. Cognitive tests should therefore include tests of executive function, e.g. MoCA, ACE III, and CLOX test. The MMSE is relatively insensitive to visuoexecutive dysfunction being weighted towards memory and language, and this patient's relatively good score of 26/30 is unsurprising.

Vascular cognitive impairment may be associated with parkinsonism, including shuffling gait, but the increased tone is generally largely confined to the lower limbs. Hallucinations would not be expected, and there may be focal neurological signs and focal vascular lesions on brain imaging.

The CT brain scan was not consistent with normal pressure hydrocephalus (see case 6) and there were no specific clinical features to suggest Parkinson's plus syndrome (see case 40). Delirium (see case 1) is often part of the differential in patients with DLB when they first present, and so collateral history to determine the time course of symptoms is key. Even then, the typical fluctuating cognition and hallucinations may make it difficult on first assessment to exclude delirium. In the current case, there was little on investigation to support a diagnosis of systemic illness (although delirium may occur in the absence of an overt precipitant). In such cases, it is prudent to recheck the patient's drug history not only with GP records, but with family and carers to make sure that the patient is actually taking the medication as prescribed, and to check for any additional over the counter medications or supplements, which may contribute to symptoms.

Although the different dementia sub-types are classically described as having distinct clinical features, it should be noted that the majority of older people (age >75 years) dying with dementia show a mixed neuropathology with Alzheimer's (amyloid plaques and neurofibrillary tangles), with or without Lewy bodies together with vascular pathology. Unsurprisingly therefore, many older patients with dementia have overlapping clinical features, e.g. typical AD with added hallucinations. Also, drugs may cause parkinsonism in patients with non-DLB dementia and result in diagnostic confusion.

2 What other investigations should be considered?

Investigations must exclude reversible or exacerbating factors for cognitive impairment. In this case, as with all cases of cognitive impairment, screening for reversible or contributing causes should include:

- thyroid function tests
- vitamin B_{12} and folate
- septic screen to exclude underlying infection.

Brain imaging should be performed to exclude treatable or unexpected cerebral pathology (the sleepiness and history of fall means that subdural haemorrhage must be considered). There are no diagnostic features of DLB on CT or MRI brain scans, but hippocampal atrophy is generally less marked than in Alzheimer's disease. SPECT or fluoro-deoxy-glucose PET imaging may be useful to look for typical patterns of reduced cerebral perfusion or metabolism in atypical cases where the clinical features overlap. Occipital hypoperfusion/metabolism is thought to indicate DLB, whereas temporoparietal reductions are more suggestive of Alzheimer's disease (Fig. 25.2). Using specific ligands for dopamine transporter, SPECT and PET studies have demonstrated low dopaminergic activity in the striatum in DLB (Fig. 25.3). This is also seen in Parkinson's disease, multiple system atrophy (see case 40, MSA) and progressive supranuclear palsy, but not in AD. Sensitivity of around 80% and specificity of 90% of ioflupane I-123 dopamine transporter SPECT imaging (DaTscan) has been reported for the diagnosis of DLB, and positive DaT scan is considered a suggestive feature in the diagnosis of probable or possible DLB (Table 25.1).

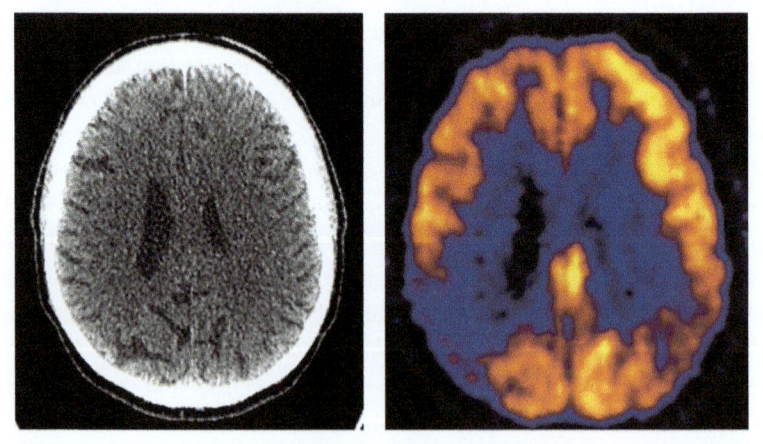

Fig. 25.2 Axial CT scan (left) and fluoro-deoxy-glucose PET axial scan image (right) from a patient with Alzheimer's disease showing markedly reduced parietal metabolism.

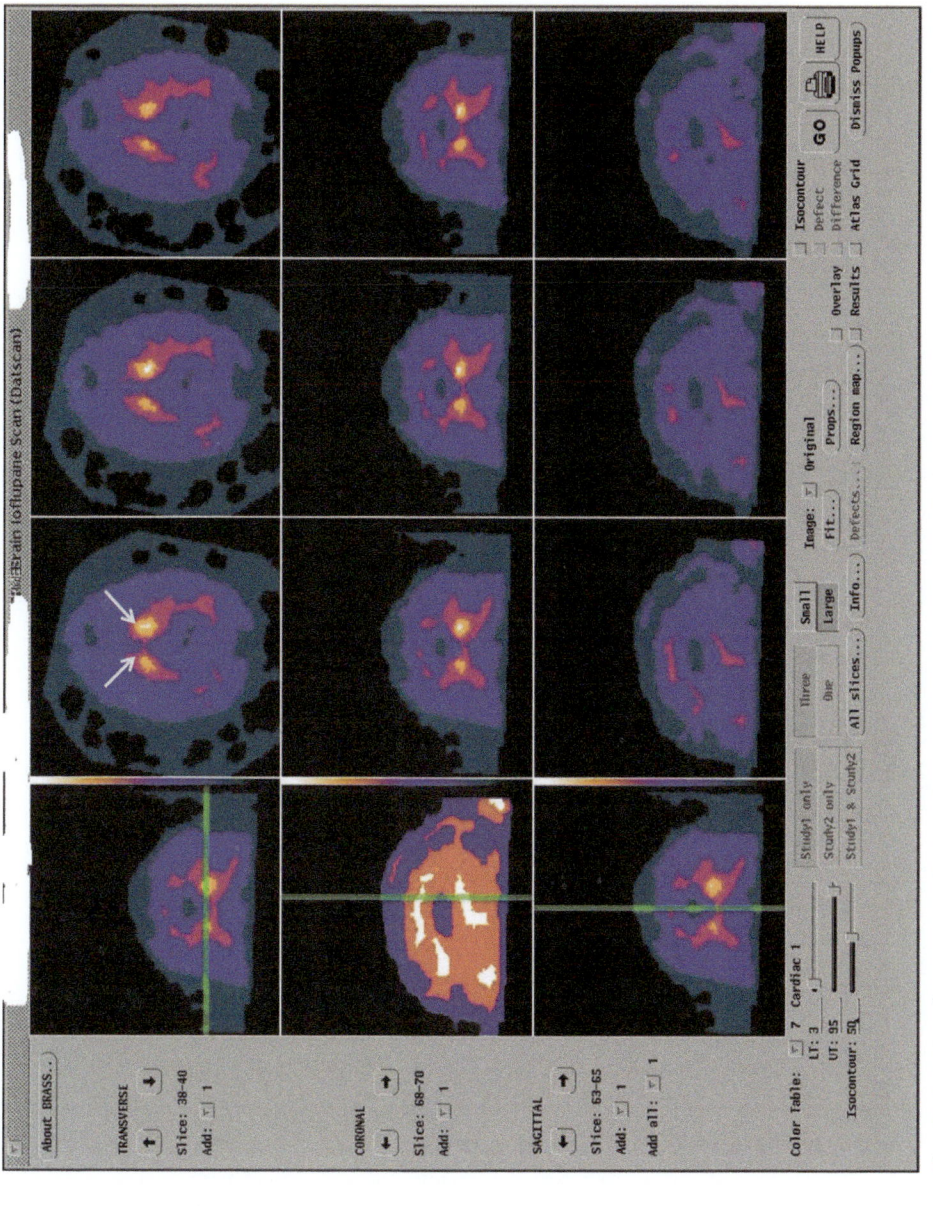

Fig. 25.3 Brain ioflupane scan (Datscan) shows reduced uptake in both basal ganglia.

3 What are the next steps in the management of this patient?

This patient's management can be divided into two components: non-pharmacological and pharmacological.

Non-pharmacological interventions

The diagnosis and its implications need to be communicated sensitively to the patient and his family. It is important to discuss driving, and power of attorney, and to make sure that there is a robust handover to the community team including the GP on discharge. Carer support in the form of advice on local services should be given. The patient should undergo a multidisciplinary team assessment including a falls risk assessment, and a further history regarding the falls should be taken with the help of the patient's wife. The physiotherapist may be able to offer advice and/or walking aids to reduce the risk of falls, and input from an occupational therapist and social services may also be required to help the patient, and his wife, to cope at home.

Pharmacological interventions

As with all dementias, there are no treatments with disease-modifying effects. Treatment is targeted at specific symptoms and may include behavioural management strategies in the context of challenging behaviour. Fludrocortisone or sodium chloride may be considered for orthostatic hypotension, and might help reduce the frequency of falls.

There is limited evidence for the use of cholinesterase inhibitors in DLB, but there are multiple reports from case series and limited trials of benefit not only on cognition, but also for fluctuations, psychotic symptoms, and parkinsonism. The effect size is thought to be larger than in patients with AD, consistent with the greater cholinergic deficit in DLB.

Agitation and hallucinations may respond particularly well to cholinesterase inhibitors. This patient was started on rivastigmine with improvement in his cognitive function and hallucinations.

4 What is the prognosis in this condition?

The extrapyramidal features of DLB tend not to respond well to levodopa treatment, which in some cases can worsen confusion and increase the likelihood of falls. Depression is a common feature of DLB. Screening for depression should be performed and treatment considered if necessary.

REM sleep disorder often responds to low doses of clonazepam or melatonin given at bedtime. Melatonin may be preferred in the setting of cognitive impairment and quetiapine may also be considered, but has potentially serious side effects.

Neuroleptics such as haloperidol, or the phenothiazines chlorpromazine and prochlorperazine should generally be avoided, as they may precipitate catastrophic parkinsonism, autonomic dysfunction, and stupor. Severe psychotic symptoms should be treated with cholinesterase inhibitors as first line treatment, with reduction in anti-parkinsonian treatment if relevant. If antipsychotic therapy is required despite these measures, atypical neuroleptics such as olanzapine or quetiapine should be used at low doses, and patients and caregivers should be warned about the possibility of severe side effects. Antipsychotic drugs are associated with an increased risk of death when used in older patients with dementia and trials suggest limited efficacy in dementia in general, and in DLB in particular.

Further reading

Goldman JG, Williams-Gray C, Barker RA, Duda JE, Galvin JE (2014). The spectrum of cognitive impairment in Lewy body diseases. *Mov Disord*; 15; **29**(5): 608–621.

McKeith IG, Dickson DW, Lowe J, *et al.* (2005). Consensus criteria of the third report of the DLB consortium. Diagnosis and management of dementia with Lewy bodies: third report of the DLB Consortium. *Neurology*; **65**: 1863.

Molano JR (2013). Dementia with Lewy bodies. *Semin Neurol*; **33**(4): 330–335.

NICE guidelines: Dementia: Supporting people with dementia and their carers in health and social care (2006): http://www.nice.org.uk/guidance/cg42

Rolinski M, Fox C, Maidment I, McShane R (2012). Cholinesterase inhibitors for dementia with Lewy bodies, Parkinson's disease dementia and cognitive impairment in Parkinson's disease. *Cochrane Database Syst Rev*; **14**: 3.

Savica R, Grossardt BR, Bower JH, Boeve BF, Ahlskog JE, Rocca WA (2013). Incidence of dementia with Lewy bodies and Parkinson disease dementia. *JAMA Neurol*; **70**(11): 1396–1402.

Case 26

A 79-year-old man was admitted with slurred speech on a background of recurrent episodes of left arm weakness, confusion, and worsening mobility over a period of a month. He had no significant past medical history and was not taking any medication. He lived with his wife and had previously been independent and driving. He had never smoked and drank around 10 units of alcohol per week.

General systems examination revealed no abnormalities and in particular, blood pressure was around 110/65mmHg. AMTS was 7/10. There was mild slurring of speech, and some word-finding difficulties, which improved over several hours. There was no other neurological abnormality.

A presumptive diagnosis of stroke was made. Blood, urine analysis, chest X-ray, ECG, carotid ultrasound, and echocardiogram were unremarkable. CT brain scan showed an infarct in the right frontal region (Fig. 26.1).

The patient made a complete recovery, AMTS on repeat was 9/10, and he was discharged home after a week on aspirin and a statin.

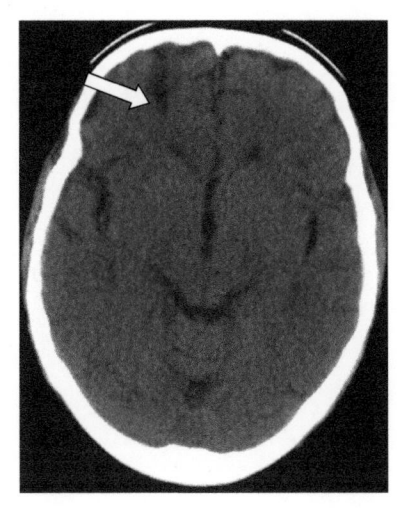

Fig. 26.1 CT brain scan (axial slice) showing infarct in the right frontal region (arrow).

Questions

1 What are the prognostic implications of confusion associated with acute stroke?
2 Which clinical features are associated with confusion in patients with stroke?

Answers

1 What are the prognostic implications of confusion associated with acute stroke?

Confusion in acute stroke often fulfils the criteria for delirium (see case 1), but less overt changes in global (as opposed to focal) changes in cognition may occur. Even mild cerebrovascular events may impact on cognition acutely, although this may only be apparent on formal cognitive testing. Confusion in acute stroke (as for delirium in general) is associated with poor outcomes including:

- longer length of hospital stay
- increased risk of institutionalization
- greater risk of post-stroke dementia
- higher mortality.

2 Which clinical features are associated with confusion in patients with stroke?

Stroke-related confusion is associated with:

- age >65
- pre-stroke dementia/cognitive impairment, which may have been previously unrecognized
- unsafe swallow
- poor vision
- intracerebral haemorrhage
- seizures
- multifocal strokes in embolic conditions
- total anterior circulation infarction
- lesions of the caudate nucleus, thalamus, or basal forebrain
- concurrent systemic illness, particularly infection, or presence of other delirium risk factors (see case 1).

Case progression

A week later, he was readmitted with recurrent episodes of transient confusion, bilateral hand weakness, and mild expressive dysphasia. Clinical examination revealed brisk reflexes in the right arm, left visual neglect, and a left extensor plantar response. Another CT brain scan was performed, which showed no new lesion. Blood and urine tests were normal and the ECG confirmed sinus rhythm. An EEG showed slow wave activity over both cerebral hemispheres, more pronounced on the right, consistent with diffuse cerebral dysfunction compatible (but not specific for) cerebrovascular disease. Over the following 24 hours, he once again recovered completely and was keen to go home, refusing further investigations. Dipyridamole was added to his medication.

Questions continued

3 Give a differential diagnosis.

Answers continued
3 Give a differential diagnosis.
This patient has recurrent, multiple stroke, or stroke-like episodes accompanied by fluctuating confusion. The differential diagnosis is wide and includes vascular, neoplastic, inflammatory, infectious, and metabolic disorders, as follows (see also *Neurological Case Histories* and *Case Histories in TIA and Stroke* for examples of many of these conditions):

- *Cardioembolic strokes,* e.g. associated with atrial fibrillation, structural heart disease, cardiomyopathy, infective endocarditis (see case 10).
- *Cerebral vasculitis.*
- *Neoplastic conditions,* including space occupying lesion (CT scan did not suggest this diagnosis in the current case, but intravenous contrast was not given), paraneoplastic disorders and intravascular large B-cell lymphoma (IVLBCL). IVBCL is high on the list of differential diagnoses, since it is associated with multiple strokes and confusion/encephalopathy.
- *Hashimoto's encephalopathy,* associated with elevated thyroid antibodies and characterized by stroke-like episodes and encephalopathy.
- *Creutzfeldt-Jakob disease.* This is a cause of rapid cognitive decline, but stroke-like episodes would not be expected and myoclonus was not seen in the current case.
- *Cerebral infection* (e.g. tuberculosis, cryptococcus, Whipple's disease).
- *Seizure* with postictal state and Todd's paralysis, non-convulsive status epilepticus.
- *Metabolic, toxic, and endocrine encephalopathies* (e.g. hypoglycaemia, renal/hepatic failure, hyponatraemia, hypercalcaemia, hyper/hypothyroidism).
- *Demyelination* (unlikely given the age of the patient and the presence of a moderate-sized lesion on CT brain scan compatible with his initial symptoms).
- *Subdural haematoma* may cause stroke-like episodes and fluctuating confusion, but the CT brain was not compatible with this diagnosis.
- *Migraine* may cause recurrent focal neurological symptoms, but was unlikely in the current case given the lack of a previous history.
- *Cerebral autosomal dominant arteriopathy, subcortical infarcts, and leukoencephalopathy.* This is an inherited condition characterized by recurrent stroke in middle age, migraine, and dementia. There were no clinical features in this case to support this diagnosis.

- *Cerebral amyloid angiopathy (see case 42).* This condition is not associated with systemic amyloidosis, but is caused by the deposition of β-amyloid in small and mid-sized arteries (and rarely veins) of the cerebral cortex, and the leptomeningae. It can cause recurrent transient neurological events (e.g. focal weakness, seizures), confusion, and headache.
- *Conversion disorder.* This may be a cause of neurological symptoms, including focal neurological abnormality, but was unlikely here given the patient's age, and presence of a lesion on CT brain scan.

Further developments

Over the following weeks, the patient continued to have recurrent episodes of transient expressive dysphasia and weakness in both arms and left leg, and was eventually readmitted. He had developed intermittent tremor in the hands and occasional jerky movements in the left arm. His mobility had deteriorated and he was unsteady on his feet.

On examination, he remained cardiovascularly stable, and in sinus rhythm. Neurological system review showed focal myoclonic jerks in the left arm and leg. Tone was increased and power was reduced in the left leg. Reflexes were brisk bilaterally, but more so on the left. Coordination was impaired bilaterally, but sensation was preserved. He remained variably confused with MMSE between 1–18/30.

MRI brain scan was obtained (Figs 26.2 and 26.3) followed by a cerebral angiogram (Fig. 26.4).

Other investigations showed the following:

- Hb 14.9g/dL; WCC 6.6 × 10^9/L (neutrophils 6.51 × 10^9/L; lymphocytes 1.91 × 10^9/L); platelets 234 × 10^9/L; ESR 32mm/h
- CRP, U&E, LFT, TFT, B_{12}, folate, Ca, PO_4: all normal
- Chol 5.5mmol/L; glucose 4.5mmol/L; lactate dehydrogenase 1200 (60 to 160 IU/L)
- Serum/urine electrophoresis, immunoglobulins, ANA, ANCA, lupus anticoagulant, complement, antiphospholipid antibody, cryoglobulins: negative
- Urine dipstick and microscopy: no protein, blood, or casts seen
- ECG, 24-hour ECG, transoesophageal echocardiogram, CXR: normal
- LP: opening pressure 14cm H_2O; protein 0.65g/L; cell count 8/mm^3 (8 lymphocytes); glucose 4.0mmol/L (blood glucose 4.5mmol/L); oligoclonal bands negative. No malignant cells were seen and subsequent cultures were negative.

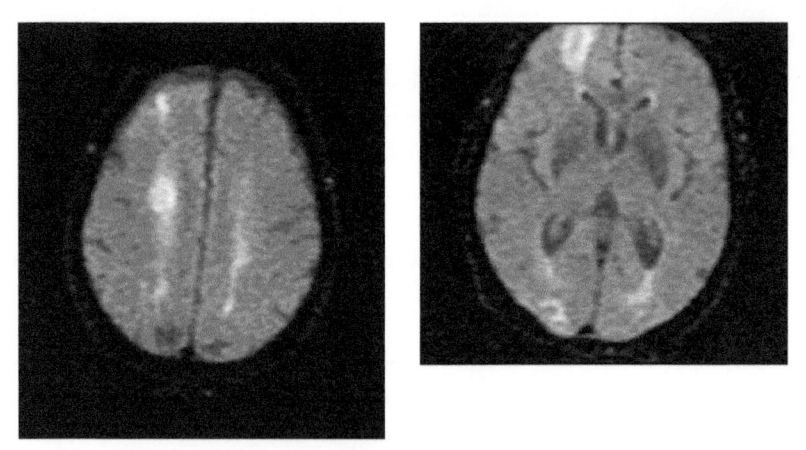

Figs 26.2 and 26.3 MRI brain (DWI sequence, axial slices).

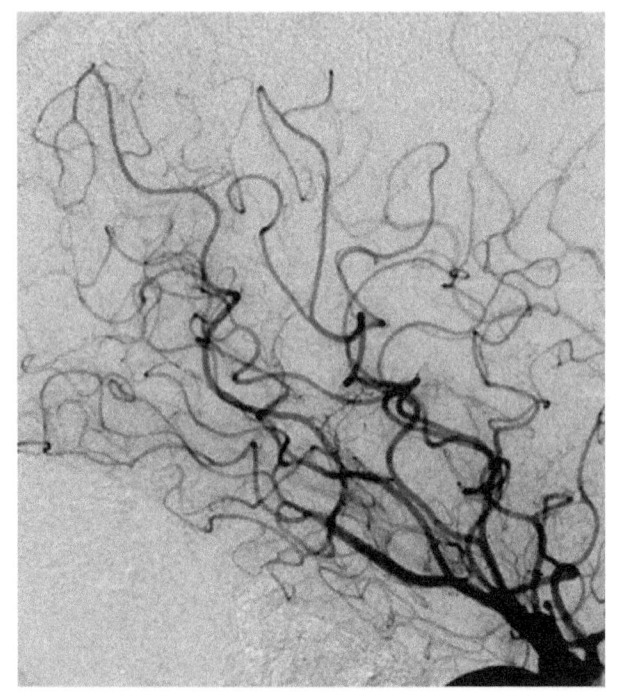

Fig. 26.4 Cerebral intra-arterial angiogram lateral view.

Questions continued

4 Describe the findings on the MRI scan.
5 What abnormality does the cerebral angiogram indicate?
6 What is the most likely diagnosis and why?
7 How would you confirm the diagnosis?

282 | CASE HISTORIES IN GERIATRIC MEDICINE

Answers continued

4 Describe the findings on the MRI scan.

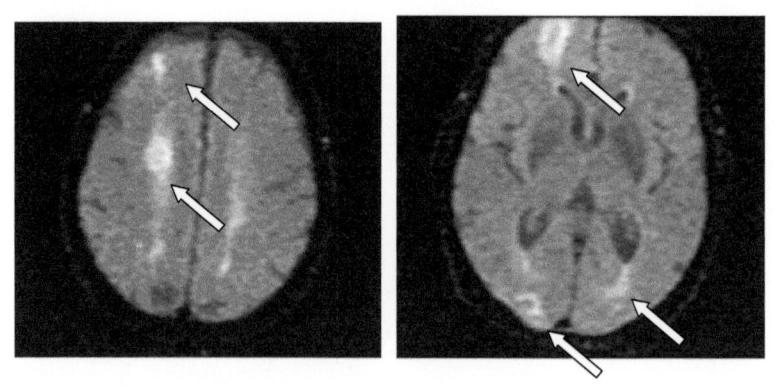

Fig. 26.5 MRI brain (DWI sequence, axial slices) with arrows showing multiple acute infarcts in the anterior and posterior circulation territories.

The MRI (DWI sequence) brain scan shows multifocal subcortical areas of hyperintense signal change, indicating multiple acute infarcts in the anterior and posterior circulation territories (arrows on Fig. 26.5).

5 What abnormality the cerebral angiogram indicate?

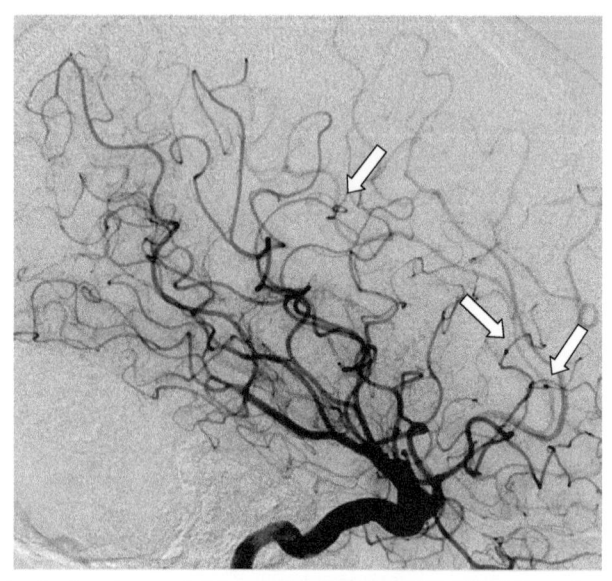

Fig. 26.6 Cerebral angiogram with arrows indicating the multiple irregular stenoses and aneurysms of small and medium sized arteries, consistent with vasculitis.

The cerebral angiogram shows multiple irregular stenoses and aneurysms of small and medium sized arteries, consistent with vasculitis (Fig. 26.6, arrows).

6 What is the most likely diagnosis and why?

Intravascular large B-cell lymphoma is the most likely diagnosis as suggested by progressive multifocal neurological deficits, diffuse encephalopathy, angiographic appearances resembling vasculitis, high serum LDH, high CSF protein, and rapid decline, together with the older age of the patient, and lack of evidence for cardiac embolism, or vasculitis.

Intravascular large B-cell lymphoma is an unusual, aggressive sub-type of non-Hodgkin lymphoma, which affects predominantly elderly patients with a median age of 70 years, without a gender bias. Neoplastic cell growth is almost exclusively limited to small and medium sized blood vessels, causing thrombosis, and ischaemic damage. The large arteries and veins are exempt and there is a characteristic absence of tumour cells from the parenchymal tissue of affected organs. Tumour cells express mainly B-cell antigens and only rarely T-cell antigens, with usually positive CD_{20} and CD_5 on immunohistochemical staining.

The most common presenting symptom in intravascular large B-cell lymphoma is fever of unknown origin (see case 16) with general fatigue. Other common, non-specific symptoms are loss of appetite, weight loss, and functional decline. Specific clinical manifestations relate to the particular organ involvement and degree of vessel obstruction. Organ involvement may be disseminated or isolated, and almost any organ may be affected: central nervous system (CNS); gastrointestinal tract; endocrine glands (adrenals, hypopituary gland); eyes; lungs; heart; kidney; prostate; testis; skin; uterus.

Intravascular large B-cell lymphoma shows regional characteristic differences with Western and Asian variants. In the Western variant, the CNS, and skin are most commonly affected. The CNS symptoms may include: cognitive and gait impairment; hemiparesis; speech disorders; incontinence; altered sensation; ataxia; seizures; dysarthria; vertigo; transient visual loss; myoclonus; cauda equina syndrome; and neuropathy. Patients usually present with more than one neurological symptom and may commonly be misdiagnosed with stroke, vasculitis, multiple sclerosis, encephalomyelitis, and Creutzfeldt-Jakob disease. Magnetic resonance brain imaging may suggest vasculitis, small vessel ischaemia, and/or demyelination. Skin abnormalities take the form of tumours, plaques, maculopapular eruptions, ulcers, palpable purpura, nodules, haemangioma, and senile angiomas. The Asian IVBCL variant has dominant haemophagocytosis, with the majority of patients presenting with thrombocytopenia, spleen, liver, and bone marrow infiltrations, without skin involvement and neurological impairment. It is linked to endemic helmentic infections.

7 How would you confirm the diagnosis?

Definitive diagnosis of intravascular large B-cell lymphoma requires biopsy of the affected organ. There are no diagnostic clues such as lymphadenopathy, or specific blood abnormalities (a minority of patients may have elevated LDH, which is non-specific) to suggest a lympho-proliferative disorder. The lack of diagnostic algorithms and laboratory or imaging results specific to the disease contribute to the diagnosis being delayed, or acquired post-mortem. Rates of antemortem diagnosis have improved recently owing to increased awareness of the disease and the use of skin biopsies (random sample of skin with or without evident lesions). Further studies are needed to assess random skin biopsies as a useful diagnostic procedure although skin biopsies may be negative in both IVBCL variants.

Final developments in the case

The patient and his wife refused brain biopsy, and he was empirically treated for cerebral vasculitis. However, he continued to deteriorate, and died six weeks later. Figures 26.7 to 26.9 show histopathological biopsy samples from his brain obtained post-mortem.

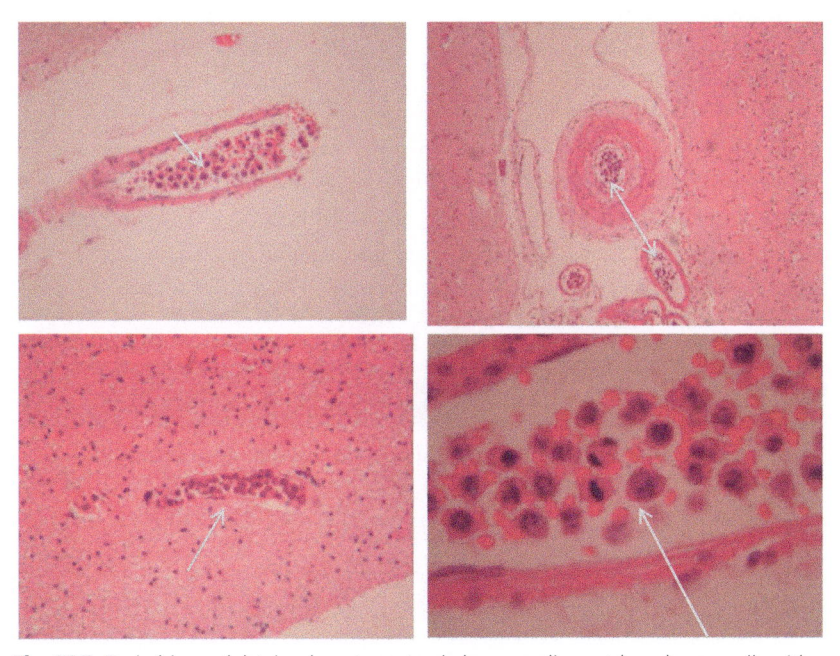

Fig. 26.7 Brain biopsy (obtained post-mortem) shows malignant lymphoma cells within the small arteries, causing occlusion and brain infarcts.

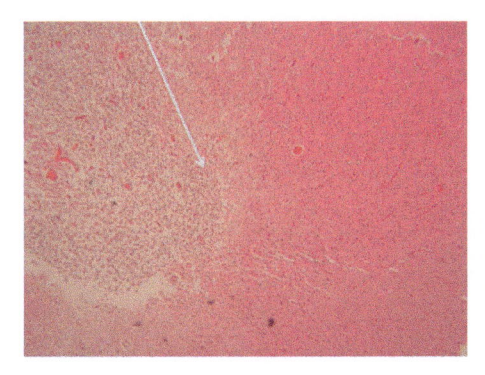

Fig. 26.8 Brain biopsy showing the edge of a subacute cortical infarct (on left of figure) in the frontal lobe.

Fig. 26.9 Brain biopsy shows brown stain for a B-cell epitope staining B-cells blocking a small leptomeningeal artery close to the infarct. This section is counterstained with haematoxylin, which shows the cell nuclei, and one cell is seen in mitosis.

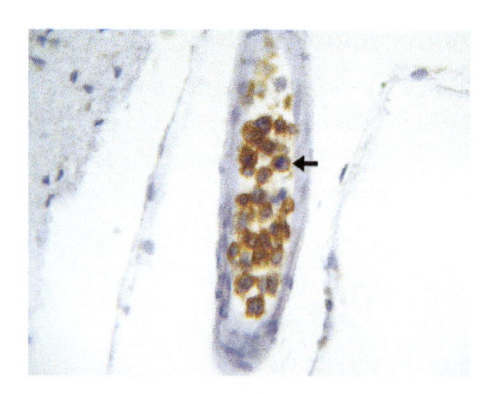

The samples from the post-mortem brain biopsy showed malignant lymphoma cells within the small arteries causing occlusion and brain infarcts. Immunostaining revealed these cells to be B-lymphocytes, and the diagnosis was confirmed to be intravascular large B-cell lymphoma.

Questions continued

8 What is the prognosis of IVBCL and how has this changed recently?

Answers continued

8 What is the prognosis of IVBCL, and how has this changed recently?

Median survival in untreated patients from the date of clinical presentation varies between two and eight months, but may be up to two years in patients treated with rituximab (anti-CD_{20} B-cell antigen monoclonal antibody) and chemotherapy (CHOP-cyclophosphamide, doxorubicin, oncovin-vincristine, prednisolone). The use of rituximab has significantly improved the outcome of the disease and in patients with CNS involvement, the additional use of high dose methotrexate is recommended. Treatment options may include autologous stem cell transplantation in some cases. Favourable prognostic factors include the skin variant of the disease and younger age. The presence of cognitive impairment and age >60 years are associated with poorer prognosis.

Further reading

Ferreri AJM, Campo E, Seymour JF, *et al.* (2004). Intravascular lymphoma: clinical presentation, natural history, management and prognostic factors in a series of 38 cases, with special emphasis on the 'cutaneous variant'. *Br J Haematol*; **27**: 173–183.

Ferro JM, Caeiro L, Verdelho A (2002). Delirium in acute stroke. *Curr Opin Neurol*; **15**: 51–55.

Gill S, Melosky B, Haley I, ChanYan C (2003). Use of random skin biopsy to diagnose intravascular lymphoma presenting as fever of unknown origin. *Am J Med*; **114**: 56–58.

Murase FT, Yamaguchi M, Suzuki R, *et al.* (2007). Intravascular large B-cell lymphoma (IVLBCL): a clinicopathologic study of 96 cases with special reference to the immunophenotypic heterogeneity of CD-5. *Blood*; **109**: 478–485.

Pendlebury ST, Wadling S, Silver LE, Mehta Z, Rothwell PM (2011). Transient cognitive impairment in TIA and minor stroke. *Stroke*; **42**(11): 3116–3121.

Ponzoni M, Ferreri AJM (2006). Intravascular lymphoma: a neoplasm of 'homeless' lymphocytes? *Hematol Oncol*; **24**: 105–112.

Satti S, Castillo R (2005). Intravascular B-cell lymphoma. *Comm Oncol*; **2**: 55–60.

Sheng AZ, Shen Q, Cordato D, Zhang YY, Yin Chan DK (2006). Delirium within three days of stroke in a cohort of elderly patients. *J Am Geriatr Soc*; **54**(8): 1192–1198.

Shimada K, Kinoshita T, Naoe T, Nakamura S (2009). Presentation and management of intravascular large B-cell lymphoma. *Lancet Oncol*; **10**: 895–902.

Shimada K, Matsue K, Yamamoto K, *et al.* (2008). Retrospective analysis of intravascular large B-cell lymphoma treated with rituximab-containing chemotherapy as reported by the IVL study group in Japan. *J Clin Oncol*; **26**: 3189–3195.

Zuckerman D, Seliem R, Hochberg E (2006). Intravascular lymphoma: the oncologist's 'great imitator'. *Oncologist*; **11**: 496–502.

Case 27

An 87-year-old woman was brought to the emergency department after being found on the floor at 9am by her carers. She was disorientated and complaining of pain in her back. It emerged that she had been helped to bed the previous evening by her carer, but was unable to remember events afterwards. There was a past medical history of COPD, TIA, gastro-oesophageal reflux disease, and diabetes. Medication included amlodipine 5mg od, aspirin 75mg od, omeprazole 20mg, simvastatin 40mg, gliclazide 80mg bd, seretide and salbutamol inhalers. The social history was somewhat unclear as she was unwilling/unable to give much information and there was no informant present, but she was known to live alone, her husband having died two years previously, and was an ex-smoker who enjoyed a gin every evening. She was usually mobile indoors with a stick, but rarely ventured outside alone.

On examination, she smelt of urine. Temperature was normal, and heart rate was mildly elevated at 100bpm regular, with respiratory rate of 18 breaths per minute. Oxygen saturations were 89% on air. She had difficulty sitting forwards because of the back pain. Examination revealed tenderness over the lumbar spine and scattered crepitations at the right base. There were no focal neurological signs. AMTS was 7 and CAM was negative.

Investigations revealed the following:

- Hb: 10.1g/dL
- WCC: 14.2×10^9/L
- MCV: 108×10^{-15}/L
- Neut: 8.0×10^9/L
- Plat: 88
- Na: 133mmol/L
- K: 3.3mmol/L
- Urea: 10.3mmol/L
- Creat: 188μmol/L
- Calcium: 2.6mmol/L
- ALT: 66IU/L

- Bili: 58μmol/L
- Alk phosp: 654U/L
- Albumin: 24g/L
- CRP: 88mg/L
- CXR: patchy shadowing right base
- Urine dip: positive for protein and leukocytes; nitrite negative
- Lumbar spine X-ray: see Figure 27.1.

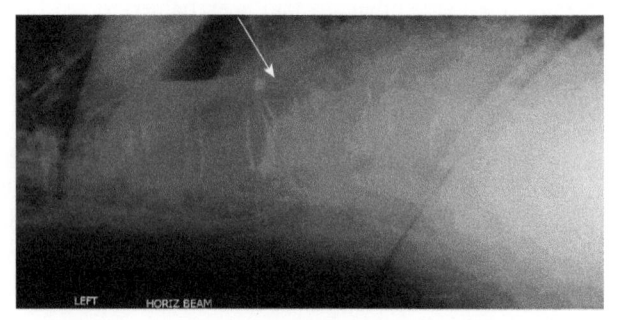

Fig. 27.1 Plain X-ray of the lumbar spine with abnormality demonstrated by arrow.

Questions

1. What does the lumbar spine X-ray demonstrate?
2. Discuss the initial management plan for this patient.

Answers

1 What does the lumbar spine X-ray demonstrate?

The X-ray shows lumbar spine vertebral wedge fracture. There are no features to suggest any additional pathology other than osteoporosis, although bony metastasis must be included in the differential as a cause for a vertebral fracture as this may easily be missed on a plain X-ray. If there is a suspicion of other pathology, such as malignancy, or infection, then further investigations such as MRI scanning should be arranged (Fig. 27.2).

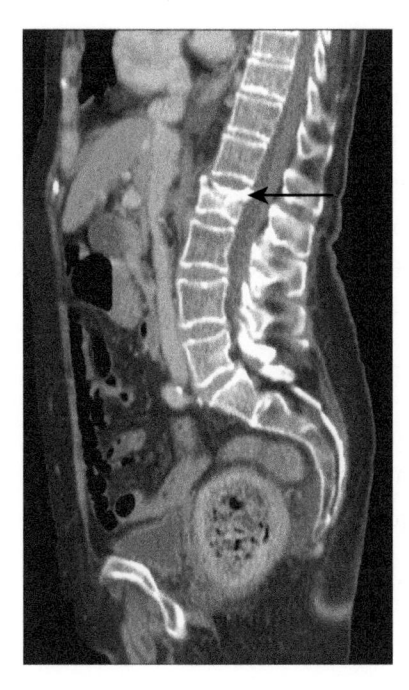

Fig. 27.2 CT scan lumbo-/sacral spine from the same patient: there is depression of the L2 upper end plate with mild retropulsion of the superior endplate (arrow).

Vertebral wedge fractures are a common incidental finding on spinal imaging. It is necessary to seek further history to establish whether these have occurred acutely. There may be local tenderness on palpation of the spine, and it is often useful to compare with previous X-ray imaging, or look for characteristic changes on MRI. Alkaline phosphatase is also often raised following an acute fracture and may take several weeks to settle. As in this case, there may also be a history of a recent fall.

The clinical presentation of vertebral fractures varies. Many vertebral fractures can be asymptomatic, or present with minor pain and discomfort. Some cause pain, which may be severe for only a few days, while other patients will have prolonged periods of pain that can render them immobile for weeks to months. Patients with severe pain require regular analgesia and the side effects of these can also contribute to illness and disability. Vertebral fractures also cause kyphosis, which can lead to restricted lung capacity and exacerbation of underlying respiratory disease. A vertebral fracture also signals an increased likelihood of other fragility fractures within the next year and particularly if this is a hip fracture, the consequences may be serious (see case 47 for further discussion of fragility fractures). The thoracolumbar junction is particularly vulnerable to osteoporotic vertebral fractures, as the change in structure of the vertebral facets provides less resistance to anteroposterior displacement.

2 Discuss the initial management plan for this patient.

The initial management plan for this patient includes:

a. Further investigations:

   Blood cultures; urine cultures

   BM; haematinics; B_{12}; folate; thyroid function; clotting screen

   ECG; postural blood pressure

   Liver ultrasound

   CT brain scan should be considered (subdural haemorrhage is a possibility)

b. Treatment of respiratory and possible urine infection
c. Rehydration and potassium replacement
d. Analgesia
e. Monitoring of inflammatory markers and electrolytes
f. Monitoring for delirium (see case 1) and further cognitive assessment
g. Collateral history
h. Bone protection.

The blood glucose level should be checked, as in any patient with confusion, or reduced conscious level. The raised white cell count, CRP, and CXR suggest lower respiratory tract infection, although it is possible that the oxygen saturations of 89% on air may be near normal for her given the COPD history. Blood cultures should be taken and a mid-stream urine sample should be sent for analysis. Although the bedside urine test was not positive for nitrites, infections caused by enterococci and staphylococcus do not reduce dietary nitrates to nitrites, so may be missed on bedside screening tests. The anaemia requires further work-up, the high MCV raises the possibility of vitamin B_{12} or folate deficiency (both of which are associated with cognitive impairment), but thyroid dysfunction or alcohol excess are other causes. The liver function is abnormal with an obstructive picture, and the macrocytosis and low platelets could be consistent with alcohol excess.

The possibility of infective discitis should always be considered in any patient with back pain and signs of infection, or if there are abnormalities in two neighbouring vertebrae. Discitis affects the lumbar spine in 50%, the thoracic spine in 30%, and the cervical spine in 20% of cases. It is less likely in this case given the history of a fall and the wedge fracture shown on the X-ray. Other causes should also be considered if the pain persists, or there are features to suggest other conditions, e.g. myeloma or spinal metastasis. As stated, elevated alkaline phosphatase levels point towards an acute fracture, and are therefore not typically raised in cases of myeloma. However, alkaline phosphatase maybe elevated if the myeloma has caused the pathological wedge fracture.

Treatment of infection

Antibiotics should be prescribed according to local guidelines. The patient was taking regular inhaler therapy, but may benefit from a short course of nebulized treatment.

Analgesia

Pain relief should be given promptly to provide comfort and reduce complications secondary to reduced mobility. Respiratory infection will be exacerbated by poorly controlled back or thoracic pain, which inhibits deep breathing and coughing, making patients more susceptible to further atelectasis and infection.

Pain from vertebral wedge fractures can often be managed with simple oral analgesics and usually improves within six weeks. Oral opiates including morphine with liquid morphine for breakthrough pain may be required if simple analgesia is insufficient (see case 41 for further discussion of pain relief). Excess analgesia predisposes to delirium and falls (see cases 1 and 47), but pain is also a potent cause of delirium and complications as described.

In severe cases where pain is persistent and limiting despite analgesia, vertebroplasty may be considered, although this remains a somewhat controversial procedure owing to a lack of definitive evidence of benefit. In vertebroplasty, bone cement is injected under fluoroscopic guidance into the damaged vertebral body with a view to easing pain and stabilizing the fracture. The procedure is reportedly generally well tolerated and complications are rare, but include migration of cement, damage to neural structures during the injection, and cement pulmonary embolism. In the longer term, there may be acceleration of local bone resorption caused by the cement, and an increased risk of fracture in the treated or adjacent vertebrae, owing to changes in surrounding mechanical forces.

Collateral history and cognitive screening

Collateral history is required to establish whether the confusion is acute or chronic. The patient is at high risk of delirium (infection, low admission cognitive score, advanced age, severe illness—raised heart rate, CRP, elevated respiratory rate) and should be closely monitored. A multicomponent intervention for delirium prevention should be put in place (see case 1). A CT brain scan should be considered to exclude a subdural haematoma or intraparenchymal haemorrhage, particularly if there is deterioration in cognitive state since the patient has had a fall, has reduced platelet count (although the count is above the level usually associated with significant bleeding problems), and has possible acute change in mental state.

ECG and postural BP

Exclusion of overt cardiac arrhythmia is required in patients with fall or unwitnessed collapse. However routine requests for 24-hour tapes in asymptomatic patients often provide a poor yield. It is worth repeating the ECG at regular intervals throughout the admission, particularly if the patient complains of dizziness or palpitations, or following a further fall. Lying and standing blood pressures should be carried out alongside a review of medications to ensure that they are not a contributing factor to her fall (she is on amlodipine).

Case continuation

The patient was commenced on antibiotics, fluids and analgesia, and initially began to improve. However, on the second afternoon after her admission, she became more confused, and the nursing staff reported that she was having visual hallucinations. On examination, heart rate was 102bpm, oxygen saturations were 92% on air and temperature was 37.4°C. She was shaky and agitated so it was only possible to perform a limited examination, but the respiratory signs had improved, and the abdomen was soft and non-tender.

Questions continued

3 What is the most likely cause of her deterioration?
4 How would you manage this condition?

Answers continued

3 What is the most likely cause of her deterioration?

The most likely cause for this patient's deterioration is acute alcohol withdrawal.

The admission bloods show a low platelet count, raised MCV, low albumin, and deranged liver function tests consistent with long-term alcohol use. Alcohol dependence among older patients is often not recognized owing to a lack of awareness in clinical and nursing staff, and therefore may be missed as an underlying cause of delirium. In the current case, further enquiry revealed that a neighbour visited frequently and helped with the shopping, which included several bottles of gin a week.

4 How would you manage this condition?

This patient needs a withdrawal regimen of long acting benzodiazepines together with high dose thiamine to prevent Wernicke–Korsakoff syndrome from vitamin B_1 deficiency caused by alcoholism. Wernicke encephalopathy is characterized by acute confusion, eye movement disorders and ataxia, and may progress to coma and death. Korsakoff's syndrome results from untreated Wernicke encephalopathy and is associated with profound inability to form new memories, which may be associated with confabulation. Patients with suspected Wernicke encephalopathy require close monitoring for seizures and electrolyte/glucose abnormalities. Once stabilized, a full neurological examination should be performed, looking particularly for cognitive impairment, cerebellar signs, and/or peripheral neuropathy, together with general systems examination looking particularly for signs of chronic liver disease. A liver ultrasound should be performed to look for cirrhosis and evidence of portal hypertension. Patients must also be counselled about cutting down significantly on alcohol.

Further reading

Crome I (2013). Substance misuse in the older person: setting higher standards. *Clin Med*; 13(6): s46–s49.

Esses SI, McGuire R, Jenkins J, *et al.* (2011). The treatment of symptomatic osteoporotic spinal compression fractures. *J Am Orthop Surg*; 1(3): 176–182.

Longo UG, Loppini M, Denaro L, Maffulli N, Denaro V (2012). Osteoporotic vertebral Fractures: current concepts of conservative care. *Br Med Bull*; 102(1): 171–189.

O'Connell H, Chin AV, Cunningham C, Lawlor B (2003). Alcohol use disorders in elderly people-redefining an age old problem in old age. *BMJ*; 327: 664.

Case 28

An 84-year-old retired business woman was referred to the geratology rapid access clinic with a four-week history of tiredness, poor appetite, decreased mobility caused by hip pain, new onset anaemia, and low mood. She had been well previously and lived independently, spending half the year abroad in Italy. Since her return to the UK around 10 days before, the neck and hip pain had worsened, and she had felt feverish on occasion, although when her temperature was checked it was normal. The symptoms were worse on waking, with marked stiffness in the neck, shoulders, and hips, which improved during the day.

The past medical history included a left hip replacement three years earlier. She was an ex-moderate smoker having given up more than 20 years before. Alcohol intake was between two and four units of alcohol per week. There were no known drug allergies.

Examination was unremarkable, except for pain on palpation of the shoulders, which became more acute on lifting the arms. Blood pressure was 130/70mmHg, without postural drop. AMTS was 10/10. During the clinical consultation, she expressed concern that the other hip might need to be replaced.

The GP had checked the urine dipstick, which was negative. Other tests revealed:

- Hb 9g/dL; MCV 86fL; ESR 100mm/h (Westergren method)
- CRP 77mg/L; the rest of biochemistry results were normal, including creatine kinase
- Hepatitis serology: negative
- CXR: normal
- X-ray hips: left-sided prosthesis in situ. There was a minor loss of joint space on the right side, consistent with age-associated osteoarthritis
- ECG: sinus rhythm; occasional ventricular extrasystoles; heart rate 72bpm.

Questions

1. What is the most likely diagnosis in this case and why? Describe this condition and its aetiology.
2. Give a differential diagnosis for this condition.
3. How would you confirm your diagnosis?
4. What are the treatment options for this condition?

Answers

1 What is the most likely diagnosis in this case and why? Describe this condition and its aetiology.

The most likely diagnosis is polymyalgia rheumatica (PMR), as suggested by the neck, shoulder, and hip pain, with stiffness worst in the morning and improving during the day, accompanied by nonspecific systemic symptoms including feverishness, loss of appetite, tiredness, depression, and lethargy. The presence of anaemia, elevated inflammatory markers, unremarkable X-ray, and biochemistry results supported the diagnosis.

Onset of PMR is typically acute and patients usually experience marked stiffness in the mornings, lasting on average about one hour. Sometimes, the weakness is sufficiently severe as to make getting up or turning in bed difficult. The proximal muscles are usually affected symmetrically, but muscle atrophy is absent and weakness is attributable to pain. Other symptoms may include loss of weight, depression, and fever.

PMR only affects people aged over 55 years with the peak incidence occurring at age 75 years. Lifetime risk of PMR is 1.7% for men and 2.4% for women. The ageing of the neurohumoral regulatory systems, the tissues, and the immune system (immunosenescence—see case 17) are implicated in the onset of the disease, as is dysfunction of the hypothalamic-pituitary-adrenal axis. Although the cause of PMR is unknown, it has been suggested that infection may play a role (e.g. mycoplasma pneumonia, parvovirus B19, chlamydia pneumonia, parainfluenza virus type 1). Altered cellular immunity (reduced level of circulating CD8+T cells, elevated circulating immunoblasts, proliferative response of peripheral blood leucocytes against arterial and muscle antigens) has prompted speculation that the potential antigen driving the autoimmune reactions may be intimal elastin (often damaged with ageing). There are also changes in humoral immunity, elevated circulating immune complexes and cytokines, including IL-6, IL-2, IL-10 and TNF-α. The presence of HLA-DRB1*04 and *01 is associated with more severe forms of PMR, more relapses, and increased risk of giant cell arteritis (see case 39).

Patients with PMR have low-grade axial synovitis and magnetic resonance imaging studies have also shown extra-capsular inflammation (e.g. subdeltoid, subacromial bursitis).

2 Give a differential diagnosis for this condition.

The differential diagnosis includes:

- Infections (e.g. osteomyelitis, bacterial endocarditis—see case 10).
- Malignancy, paraneoplastic syndromes (e.g. metastatic disease, myeloma, other bone lesions—see case 24).

- Spondyloarthropathies—pain usually improves with rest.
- Crystal arthropathies—pain is usually severe, constant and sharp, with acute swellings, and redness of the affected joints, affecting sleep, and mobility.
- Connective tissue diseases (e.g. rheumathoid arthritis).
- Fibromyalgia syndrome—fatigue, generalized muscle aching, stiffness and tenderness, most commonly affecting neck, shoulders, thighs, and lower back, but with normal blood test results (uncommon in older people).
- Metabolic abnormalities (e.g. hypothyroidism).
- Myopathies (drug induced, e.g. by cholesterol lowering drugs, idiopathic), creatine kinase would usually be raised.

3 How would you confirm your diagnosis?

The diagnosis of PMR is a clinical one based on a typical presentation of the disease and the exclusion of other disorders. It is based on a 'stepped approach'. After examination, ESR, C-reactive protein, full blood count, urea and electrolytes, calcium, creatinine, thyroid function tests, creatine kinase, serum, and urine immunoglobulins should be performed. Depending on the differential diagnosis, further tests may be necessary, including electromyography, muscle biopsy, echocardiogram, joint fluid aspiration, and rheumatoid factor. Elevated C-reactive protein is characteristic as is an elevated ESR (>100mm/h) although ESR may occasionally be normal. There may be co-existent giant cell arteritis (see case 39).

4 What are the treatment options for this condition?

Oral steroids (e.g. prednisolone of 15mg per day) should be given after which there is a dramatic improvement in symptoms within a few days or even a few hours, although the response is not conclusive for a diagnosis of PMR since many conditions may improve with such treatment. In cases of partial improvement, further investigation for co-morbidities such as osteoarthritis is necessary. If there is a lack of response, an alternative diagnosis should be considered. All patients should be alert to the symptoms and signs of giant cell arteritis (scalp tenderness, chewing causing jaw claudication, headache and visual disturbances), and of the need to alert their physician urgently if such symptoms occur.

Patients should be monitored through clinical symptoms and inflammatory marker level (ESR and C-reactive protein—some authors consider the latter more helpful). Steroid doses are gradually reduced after symptoms subside. The length of treatment in most patients is around two years, although a minority requires small doses of steroids for many years. Steroid-sparing drugs have not been found beneficial, nor have anti-TNF drugs (e.g. rituximab).

Patients should be monitored for complications from corticosteroid use (e.g. diabetes, peripheral oedema, vascular disease), and bone protection medication (to prevent osteoporosis) should be considered.

Further reading

Alvarez-Rodriguez L, Lopez-Hoyos M, Mata C, *et al.* (2010). Circulating cytokines in active polymyalgia rheumatica. *Ann Rheum Dis*; **69**(1): 263–269.

Bird HA, Leef BF, Montecucco CM, *et al.* (2005). A comparison of the sensitivity of diagnostic criteria for polymyalgia rheumatica. *Ann Rheum Dis*; **64**: 626–629.

Leeb BF, Bird HA, Nesher G, *et al.* (2003). EULAR response criteria for polymyalgia rheumatica: results of an initiative of the European Collaborating Polymyalgia Group. *Ann Rheum Dis*; **62**: 1189–1194.

Mackie SL (2013). Polymyalgia rheumatica: pathogenesis and management. *Clin Med*; **13**(4): 398–400.

Salvarani C, Cantini F, Hunder GG (2008). Polymyalgia rheumatica and giant-cell arteritis. *Lancet*; **372**: 234–245.

Siebert S, Lawson TM, Wheeler MH, Martin JC, Williams BD (2001). Polymyalgia rheumatica pitfalls in diagnosis. *J R Soc Med*; **94**: 242–244.

Case 29

A 79-year-old man who had recently moved back to the UK from abroad was referred to the rapid access geratology clinic by his GP because of abnormal blood results. He had had type 2 diabetes diagnosed in middle age and managed his own insulin injections. Other past medical history included hypertension and a myocardial infarction 10 years previously. He was still driving and lived independently with his wife in a three-bedroom house and enjoyed gardening. Medications were aspirin 75mg od, simvastatin 40mg on, amlodipine 10mg od, ramipril 2.5mg od, bisoprolol 10mg od, furosemide 80mg od, insulin glargine 18 units at night, six units novorapid at breakfast, four units at lunch, and eight units with evening meal.

On examination, he looked well with a heart rate of 82bpm, blood pressure of 150/80mmHg, respiratory rate of 18 breaths per minute, and oxygen saturation 96% on air. On auscultation, the heart sounds were normal, and there were reduced breath sounds at the bases. Abdomen was soft and non-tender, bowel sounds were normal, and there were no palpable masses. There was some slight ankle swelling. Weight was 80 kg and BMI was 28 kg/m².

Blood test results revealed the following:

- Hb: 8.9g/dL
- MCV: 79fL
- WCC: 8.3×10^9/L
- Neut: 4.2×10^9/L
- HCt: 0.37L/L
- Na: 134mmol/L
- K: 6.2mmol/L
- Urea: 31mmol/L (25mmol/L, six months earlier, taken abroad)
- Creat: 300µmol/L (310µmol/L, six months earlier, taken abroad)
- Albumin: 29g/L
- CRP: 12mg/L

- CXR: small pleural effusions bilaterally
- Urine dip: – trace blood, + + protein
- ECG: sinus; narrow QRS with occasional ventricular ectopics; no changes of hyperkalaemia.

Questions

- How does normal ageing affect the kidneys and what are the implications for medical care?
- What is the estimated GFR in this patient?
- What stage chronic kidney disease (CKD) does this man have? What other test is required to further classify his renal disease stage?
- What is the most likely cause of his renal failure?
- Would you make any changes to his medications? What other blood tests should be requested?
- Would renal replacement therapy be appropriate for this older patient?
- What is the role for renal transplantation in older patients?

Answers

1 How does normal ageing affect the kidneys and what are the implications for medical care?

There is a gradual reduction in the estimated glomerular filtration rate (eGFR) from the fourth decade onwards. Renal blood flow decreases by about 10% per decade and by the age of 80 years, blood flow has fallen from 600ml/min to 300ml/min. There is also loss of renal mass, mostly from the cortex, with a reduction in number and size of nephrons, partly resulting from glomerulosclerosis. The declining number of nephrons and reduced blood flow cause a reduction in glomerular filtration rate. There is thickening of the basement membrane and renal arterial resistance increases. In patients with diabetes or systemic hypertension, these normal ageing changes can be accelerated and more prominent. Age-related changes in renal function may impact little on a day-to-day basis, but lead to a lack of renal reserve. In addition, the ageing kidney is less able to concentrate urine and to respond to hormones such as vasopressin. The questions of whether renal ageing is a physiological or pathological process, and whether CKD in older people is the same or different from CKD in younger individuals remains unclear (as it does for age-related cognitive decline).

The implications of renal ageing for medical care include:

- Decreased drug excretion and greater likelihood of drug toxicity (see cases 4 and 36)
- Increased likelihood of adverse drug effects, e.g. drowsiness/confusion from opiates
- Susceptibility to dehydration and hyponatraemia
- Covert renal impairment made critical by infection, medication, or dehydration
- Difficulties in managing co-morbid conditions, such as heart failure, or diabetes.

2 What is the estimated GFR?

Formal measurement of glomerular filtration requires the measurement of clearance of an exogenous marker, which is not practicable routinely. Surrogate techniques are thus used to give an eGFR derived from plasma creatinine, age, gender, and ethnicity, using the following equations:

a. Cockcroft and Gault equation

$$\text{CrCl (mL/min)} = \frac{Y \times [140 - \text{age (years)}] \times \text{weight}^* \text{(kg)}}{\text{Serum creatinine (micromol/L)}}$$

Where Y = 1.23 males, 1.04 females. *Ideal body weight should be used if actual weight is greater than 120% ideal body weight.

This gives a measure of clearance of 18.5mL/min in this patient.

b. Modified diet in renal disease study equation

This is more accurate, but is not easy to use in practice, unless with an automatic online calculator or similar:

$$\text{GFR} \left(\text{mL}/\text{min}/1.73\,\text{m}^2 \right) = 175 \times (\text{Cr})^{-1.154} \times (\text{Age})^{-0.203} \\ \times (0.742 \text{ if female}) \times (1.212 \text{ if black})$$

This gives an estimated GFR of 16mL/min/1.73 m².

c. CKD-Epi

This equation has been derived more recently and is now the recommended method for use by reference laboratories, which should report eGFR along with the serum creatinine:

$$\text{GFR} = 141 \times \min(\text{Scr}/\kappa, 1)^\alpha \times \max(\text{Scr}/\kappa, 1)^{-1.209} \\ \times 0.993^{\text{Age}} \times 1.018\, [\text{if female}] \times 1.159\, [\text{if black}]$$

Where Scr is serum creatinine (mg/dL), κ is 0.7 for females and 0.9 for males, α is −0.329 for females and −0.411 for males, min indicates the minimum of Scr/κ or 1, and max indicates the maximum of Scr/κ or 1.

This patient's eGFR was 18mL/min/1.73 m² derived by this method. eGFR calculated using cystatin C is recommended where more accurate risk stratification is required particularly for individuals at lower risk, according to eGFR estimated using the serum creatinine.

3 What stage chronic kidney disease (CKD) does this man have? What other test is required to further classify his renal disease stage?

This man has chronic kidney disease (CKD) stage G4 using just the eGFR. The urinary albumin:creatinine ratio is required to fully classify his renal disease stage, which is CKD G4 A3 (see Table 29.1).

The renal disease is chronic as shown by the previously elevated Cr and urea, anaemia, and the fact that he is clinically well, i.e. there is no overt precipitant of acute renal failure.

CKD describes abnormal kidney function (reduced GFR) and/or structure (albuminuria (albumin:creatinine ratio (ACR) more than 3mg/mmol), urine sediment abnormalities, electrolyte and other abnormalities due to tubular disorders, abnormalities detected by histology, structural abnormalities detected by imaging, or history of kidney transplantation) of greater than three months' duration. It is common, frequently unrecognized, and often exists together with other conditions, such as cardiovascular disease and diabetes, as seen in the current case. Moderate to severe CKD is associated with an increased risk of adverse outcomes including acute kidney injury, falls, frailty and mortality, and is an independent risk factor for cardiovascular disease. The risk of CKD increases with age, exceeding 20% in individuals older than 60 years and >35% in those older than 70 years in developed countries, although estimates are conflicting owing to variability of measurement methods. As kidney dysfunction progresses, some coexisting conditions become more common and increase in severity.

Table 29.1 shows the stages of CKD as defined by the Kidney Disease: Improving Global Outcomes (KDIGO) and UK NICE guidelines. In 2013, three ACR categories (ACR under 3mg/mmol, 3–30 mg/mmol, and over 30mg/mmol) were added for each GFR category in the updated classification in recognition of the additional importance of proteinuria.

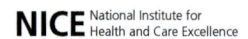

NICE National Institute for Health and Care Excellence

Table 29.1 Classification of chronic kidney disease using GFR and ACR categories

GFR and ACR categories and risk of adverse outcomes			ACR categories (mg/mmol), description and range		
			<3 Normal to mildly increased	3–30 Moderately increased	>30 Severely increased
			A1	A2	A3
GFR categories (ml/min/1.73 m^2), description and range	≥90 Normal and high	G1	No CKD in the absence of markers of kidney damage		
	60–89 Mild reduction related to normal range for a young adult	G2			
	45–59 Mild–moderate reduction	G3a[1]			
	30–44 Moderate–severe reduction	G3b			
	15–29 Severe reduction	G4			
	<15 Kidney failure	G5			

Increasing risk →

[1] Consider using eGFRcystatinC for people with CKD G3aA1 (see recommendations 1.1.14 and 1.1.15)

Abbreviations: ACR, albumin:creatinine ratio; CKD, chronic kidney disease; GFR, glomerular filtration rate

Adapted with permission from Kidney Disease: Improving Global Outcomes (KDIGO) CKD Work Group (2013) KDIGO 2012 clinical practice guideline for the evaluation and management of chronic kidney disease. Kidney International (Suppl. 3): 1–150

Both increased ACR and decreased GFR are associated with increased risk of adverse outcomes, but increased ACR and decreased GFR in combination multiply the risk (see Table 29.1).

Ageing and vascular disease are associated with low GFR and high albuminuria, and the possibility of over-diagnosis of CKD in older people using current definitions has been raised. However, both low eGFR and high albuminuria are independently associated with mortality and end stage renal disease regardless of age, and mortality shows a lower relative risk, but higher absolute risk differences at older age.

Despite higher risks for mortality and end stage renal disease in diabetes overall, the relative risks of these outcomes by eGFR and ACR are much the same irrespective of the presence or absence of diabetes, emphasizing the importance of kidney disease as a predictor of clinical outcomes. It should be noted that CKD predisposes to acute kidney injury and vice versa, as is seen in acute and chronic cognitive failure (delirium and dementia—see cases 1 and 46).

Acute kidney failure is also a predictor of poor outcome in systemic illness, as is seen for delirium.

Testing for CKD using eGFR creatinine and ACR should be offered to those with the following risk factors:

- diabetes
- hypertension
- acute kidney injury (monitor for at least two to three years, even if serum creatinine has returned to baseline)
- cardiovascular disease (ischaemic heart disease, chronic heart failure, peripheral vascular disease, or cerebral vascular disease)
- structural renal tract disease, recurrent renal calculi, or prostatic hypertrophy
- multisystem diseases with potential kidney involvement—for example, systemic lupus erythematosus
- family history of end stage kidney disease
- opportunistic detection of haematuria.

4 What is the most likely cause of his renal failure?

The most likely cause of the renal failure is diabetes. Diabetes causes around a quarter of end stage renal disease in the UK.

Membraneous nephropathy should be considered in view of the high level of proteinuria and low albumin. However, there is minimal ankle oedema so he is not nephrotic. A renal biopsy would confirm or refute this diagnosis.

5 Would you make any changes to his medications? What other blood tests should be requested?

The patient is taking aspirin 75mg od, simvastatin 40mg on, amlodipine 10mg od, ramipril 2.5mg od, bisoprolol 10mg od, furosemide 80mg od, insulin glargine 18 units at night, novorapid six units at breakfast, four units at lunch, and eight units with evening meal.

He is on appropriate secondary prevention for a patient with a past history of myocardial infarction (aspirin, simvastatin, beta-blocker, and angiotensin converting enzyme (ACE) inhibitor), but remains hypertensive.

In younger people with CKD and diabetes, or with an ACR of 70mg/mmol or more, the systolic blood pressure should be kept below 130mmHg (target range 120–129mmHg), and the diastolic blood pressure below 80mmHg, whereas less stringent targets of systolic pressure below 140mmHg (target range 120–139mmHg) and diastolic pressure below 90mmHg are recommended for non-diabetic patients. However, there is a lack of data to guide treatment of hypertension in older patients (especially those aged above 80 years). The UK NICE guidance gives no specific recommendations for the treatment of hypertension in this age group, irrespective of the presence of CKD. Available evidence suggests it may be prudent not to reduce the blood pressure much below 140/90mmHg since low blood pressure is associated with dizziness, orthostatic hypotension, falls, and fractures in this age group. Further, in those with CKD, the response to BP lowering drugs may be altered. As a general guide, BP should be lowered slowly and targets recommended for younger people should not be pursued aggressively in older patients with multiple co-morbidities.

Wu *et al.* performed a meta-analysis of randomized clinical trials of antihypertensive therapy involving ACE inhibitors, angiotensin receptor blockers (ARBs), alpha-blockers, beta-blockers, calcium channel blockers, diuretics, and their combinations) in patients with diabetes with a follow-up of at least 12 months, reporting all cause mortality, requirement for dialysis, or doubling of serum creatinine levels. Compared with placebo, only ACE inhibitors significantly reduced the doubling of serum creatinine levels (odds ratio 0.58) and only beta-blockers showed a significant difference in mortality (odds ratio 7.13). Although the beneficial effects of ACE inhibitors compared with ARBs did not reach statistical significance, ACE inhibitors consistently showed higher probabilities of being in the superior ranking positions among all three outcomes. Although the protective effect of an ACE inhibitor plus calcium channel blocker compared with placebo was not statistically significant, the treatment ranking identified this combination therapy to have the greatest probability (73.9%) for being the best treatment on reducing mortality, followed by ACE inhibitor plus diuretic (12.5%), ACE inhibitors (2.0%), calcium channel blockers (1.2%), and ARBs (0.4%). However, the bulk of trial data are from younger patients and the benefits of angiotensin antagonists are not as clear-cut in older patients, in whom the possibility of side effects is higher.

Therefore, in this patient with diabetes, one would usually try to maximize the dose of the ACE inhibitor, but the K is already at 6.2. Given the decrease in mortality with beta-blockers, there is an argument for continuing the bisoprolol. In general, renin-angiotensin system antagonists should not be stopped unless K levels rise above 6.0mmol/L and other K raising drugs have been stopped. Similarly, these drugs should not be discontinued unless the serum creatinine rises >30% or the eGFR to >25% above baseline levels. The patient should be informed of the increase in bleeding risk with antiplatelet agents in renal failure, but should remain on aspirin.

Haematinics, vitamin B_{12}, and folate should be measured to look for a contributing cause for the anaemia. The MCV is low, which would not be expected in anaemia associated with renal failure, suggesting iron deficiency. It is likely that an erythopoiesis stimulating agent will be required.

The calcium, phosphate, and parathyroid hormone concentrations should be measured, since the eGFR is less than 30ml/min/1.73 m² (GFR category G4 or G5). Vitamin D analogues, (1-alpha hydroxyl vitamin D or 1.25 OH vitamin D -calcitriol) should be given for vitamin D deficiency if present.

The serum bicarbonate should be measured and if less than 20mmol/L, oral supplementation should be considered. There is some evidence that sodium supplementation slows disease progression, but sodium overload may occur.

6 Would renal replacement therapy be appropriate for this older patient?

The patient should be referred to a renal specialist for further management, and discussion of the advantages and disadvantages of renal replacement therapy. The case history suggests that he has a good quality of life and remains active, but the renal disease is secondary to diabetes, and there is a history of ischaemic heart disease. US studies estimate a life expectancy of <2 years for patients with diabetes and end stage renal failure versus, 10.4 years for the person aged 75–79 years without these co-morbidities. In addition, this patient's diabetes and ischaemic heart disease puts him at higher than average risk of complications from dialysis. Besides medical factors, distance, and ease of travelling to a regional dialysis centre, the impact of the need for three to four times weekly day-long visits to the hospital, and availability and feasibility of home dialysis will impact on decisions regarding renal replacement therapy in older patients.

The overall impact of dialysis on quality of life may deter older patients from commencing therapy and careful consideration should be given to quality versus quantity of life in discussions with patients. Nevertheless, increasing numbers of older people are undergoing dialysis: in 2012, the median age of prevalent renal replacement therapy patients was 58 years, of haemodialysis patients was 66 years, and peritoneal dialysis was 63 years.

More recent data from 2012 (cohort of 2007), show that five-year survival of new renal replacement therapy patients aged >65 years was 32%, and for >75 years was 20%. There was no difference in survival between diabetics and non-diabetics in the 65 + age group.

7 What is the role for renal transplantation in older patients?

Traditionally, age has been thought of as a relative contraindication to renal transplantation. In 2012, the median age of transplant patients was 52 years, and only around 5% of patients aged over 65 years on renal replacement therapy go on to have a transplant. Common barriers to transplantation in older patients include the high prevalence of co-morbidities particularly vascular disease, which is associated with poorer graft survival and a shortage of transplantable kidneys, resulting in younger patients being prioritized. However, there are some data supporting the role of renal transplantation in carefully selected older patients. A study conducted by Otero-Ravina compared rates of graft survival for 137 patients over the age of 60 years with 484 patients under the age of 60 years. For those over 60 years, graft survival at 1 and 5 years was 73% and 56% respectively, compared with 82% and 70% for patients aged less than 60 years. However, when the results were adjusted to exclude patients who died from other causes (most commonly infections and cardiovascular disease) while the grafts were functioning, graft survival rates in the two groups were similar. The age of the donor also affected the survival of the graft; grafts from donors aged under 60 years survived better. Preliminary data from other studies demonstrate a survival benefit in older patients who undergo renal transplantation, compared with those who remain on dialysis.

Further reading

Eckardt KU, Coresh J, Devuyst O, *et al.* (2013). Evolving importance of kidney disease: from subspecialty to global health burden. Lancet; **382**(9887): 158–169.

Jassal S, Krahn M, Naglie G, *et al.* (2003). Kidney transplantation in the elderly: a decision analysis. *J Am Soc Nephrol*; **14**: 187–196.

Kidney Disease: Improving Global Outcomes (KDIGO) CKD Work Group (2013). KDIGO 2012 clinical practice guideline for the evaluation and management of chronic kidney disease. *Kidney Int*; (Suppl. 3): 1–150 (http:kdigo.org).

Lamping DL, Constantinovici N, Roderick P, *et al.* (2000). Clinical outcomes, quality of life, and costs in the North Thames Dialysis Study of elderly people on dialysis: a prospective cohort study. *Lancet*; 4; **356**(9241): 1543–1550.

Levey AS, Coresh J (2012). Chronic kidney disease. *Lancet*; 14; **379**(9811): 165–180.

Murtagh FE, Marsh JE, Donohoe P, Ekbal NJ, Sheerin NS, Harris FE (2007). Dialysis or not? A comparative survival study of patients over 75 years with chronic kidney disease stage 5. *Nephrol Dial Transplant*; **22**: 1955–1962.

Nitsch D, Grams M, Sang Y, *et al.* (2013). Associations of estimated glomerular filtration rate and albuminuria with mortality and renal failure by sex: a meta-analysis. *BMJ*; 29; 346: f324.

Otero-Ravina F, Rodriguez-Martinez M, Gude F, González-Juanatey J, Valdes F, Sánchez-Guisande D (2005). Renal transplantation in the elderly: does patient age determine the results? *Age Ageing*; **34**(6): 583–587.

Shlipak MG, Matsushita K, Ärnlöv J, *et al.* (2013). Cystatin C versus creatinine in determining risk based on kidney function. *N Engl J Med*; 5; **369**(10): 932–943.

Tangri N, Kitsios GD, Inker LA, *et al.* (2013). Risk prediction models for patients with chronic kidney disease: a systematic review. *Ann Intern Med*; 16; **158**(8): 596–603.

Treit K, Lam D, O'Hare AM (2013). Timing of dialysis initiation in the geriatric population: toward a patient-centered approach. *Semin Dial*; **26**(6): 682–689.

Rosenberg F, Isles C, Simpson K, Prescott G (2005). Renal replacement therapy in the over-80s. *Age Ageing*; **34**(2): 148–152.

Wu HY, Jenq-Wen Huang JW, Lin HJ (2013). Comparative effectiveness of renin-angiotensin system blockers and other antihypertensive drugs in patients with diabetes: systematic review and bayesian network meta-analysis. *BMJ*; 347: f6008.

Case 30

A 76-year-old man was referred by his GP with a one-month history of tiredness, day-time sleepiness, fever with temperatures up to 37.8°C, night sweats, and half a stone weight loss. In the previous two weeks, he had noted a widespread rash over his body, mostly on his trunk and hands. He denied any loss of appetite or pain. He had also had a sore throat for two weeks. There was a past history of seasonal asthma for many years and an inguinal hernia 20 years previously. He was not taking any medication except sildenafil (Viagra) occasionally. He was a non-smoker, and drank an occasional glass of wine. He lived alone, his wife having died of cancer 10 years earlier. In the past, he had travelled regularly to the Canary Islands, but denied travelling abroad in the last two years.

On examination, his throat was red and he had a non-itchy rash all over his body, including scalp, face, trunk, back, soles, and palms. The lesions were macular and nodular, and some were necrotic (Figs 30.1 and 30.2). Temperature was 36.8°C with a heart rate of 70bpm regular and a blood pressure of 130/70 mmHg. There was a high-stepping gait and bilateral weakness in ankle dorsiflexion, worse on the left, reduced joint position sensation in the toes, and reduced sensation to light touch, and pinprick below the knees. The rest of the examination was unremarkable.

Investigations showed the following:

- Hb 12.7g/dl; WCC 6.9 × 10^9/L (3.5 × 10^9/L neutrophils 2.07 × 10^9/L lymphocytes) platelets 307 × 10^9/L; APTT 40.9sec, PT 17.5sec
- CRP: 63mg/L
- Na 135mmol/L; K 4.8mmol/L; bilirubin 9μmol/L; ALP 350 IU/L; alb 34 G/L; adjusted calcium 2.38mmol/L
- Blood cultures and throat swabs: negative
- HBsAg—not detected; Hepatitis C antibody—not detected; Lyme disease (*Borrelia burgdorferi*) antibody negative; monospot test for infectious mononucleosis (Epstein–Barr virus)—negative
- Anti Nuc Abs—negative; serum electrophoresis—normal; urine electrophoresis—normal
- Tumour markers: normal
- CXR: normal.

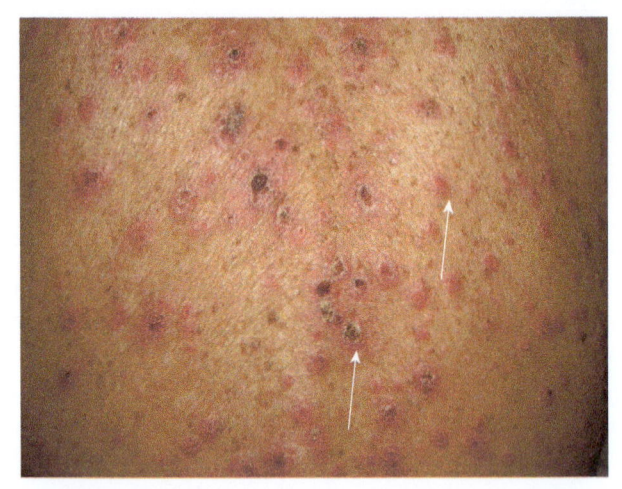

Fig. 30.1 Erythematous papular, nodular lesions, some with ulceration and crusting, arrows (patient's back).

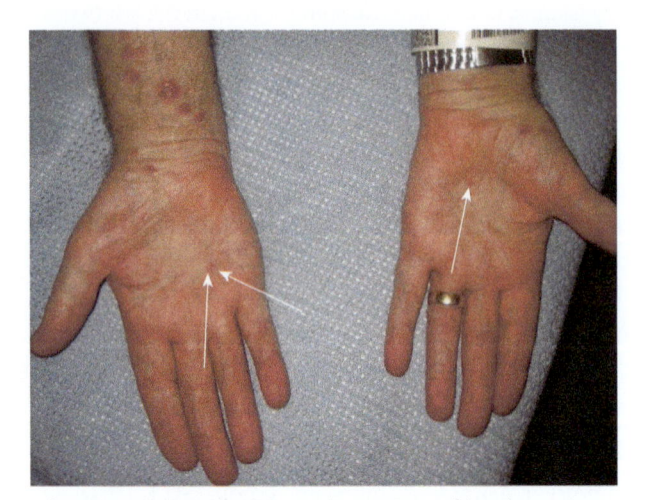

Fig. 30.2 Erythematous lesions involving palmar aspect of hands.

Questions

1. List the differential diagnosis you would consider.
2. What is the most likely diagnosis and how would you confirm it?

Answers

1 List the differential diagnosis you would consider.

The differential diagnosis in this case is wide and includes:

- *Hypersensitivity, inflammatory, and autoimmune disorders.* Drug eruption (unlikely since no new drugs were taken), erythema multiforme—usually a reaction to infection or to a drug, acute systemic lupus erythematosus.
- *Infection*—local or systemic, e.g. tuberculosis, tinea corporis, or other fungal infections, excoriated scabies, Lyme disease, AIDS—Acquired Immuno Deficiency Syndrome, syphilis, folliculitis, rickettsial infection.
- *Dermatitis* (e.g. contact, less likely atopic, or nummular).
- *Other primary skin disorders.* Lichen planus, psoriasis, parapsoriasis, pityriasis rosea, pityriasis lichenoides et varioliformis acuta (PLEVA)—a rare condition of unknown aetiology, which may present as acute papular lesions evolving into pseudo-vesicles with central necrosis, a chronic variant with scaling papules, or a severe ulcero-necrotic variant with fever.
- *Neoplasm or paraneoplastic skin disorder* (e.g. cutaneous lymphoma, paraneoplastic pemphigus).
- *Keratoses.*

2 What is the most likely diagnosis and how would you confirm it?

The history and clinical findings of a widespread maculopapular rash affecting trunk, limbs, face, scalp, but most characteristically palms and soles, with fever, redness of the pharynx, malaise and tiredness, are features of syphilis. This was the most likely diagnosis in this patient and was confirmed on skin biopsy, and serologic testing. Syphilis can mimic many conditions and should be considered in the differential diagnosis of skin eruptions (especially if affecting soles and palms), or lesions of the mucosal surfaces with lymphadenopathy. The patient's age should be disregarded.

The diagnosis of syphilis in older patients is difficult owing to its rarity, the wide variety of clinical presentations, and lack of awareness among clinicians. Syphilis has become again an important infection in Western Europe since the 1990s, its rising prevalence matching other acute sexually transmitted diseases in the older population.

Case development

The patient was told at the follow-up visit that he had syphilis.

Questions continued

3 Describe your further assessment and which other conditions might you expect to find in this patient?
4 How would you approach obtaining a sexual history from older people? Until what age are older people likely to be sexually active?
5 List the most common causes of sexual dysfunction in older people.
6 What contributes to the risk of sexually transmitted diseases in older people and why may diagnosis be difficult?
7 Does HIV infection differ in older versus younger patients?

Answers continued

3 Describe your further assessment and which other conditions might you expect to find in this patient?

A comprehensive sexual history should be taken although older patients are commonly reluctant to discuss their sexual life. A detailed travel history was sought and specific questions asked about unprotected sexual intercourse (without condom). He admitted that he took sildenafil (Viagra), but only for 'solitary use', and denied ever having had sexual contact other than with his wife. He also denied any other possible source of infection.

Unprotected intercourse is commoner among older adults, owing to:

- fear of poor sensation and impotence
- lack of fear of pregnancy
- lack of health education
- lack of experience with condoms
- religious beliefs.

Patients infected with syphilis must be tested for Human Immunodeficiency Virus (HIV) infection, as well as for other sexually transmitted diseases, since sexually transmitted diseases often co-exist and syphilis is an important facilitator of HIV transmission. There is a suggestion that syphilis follows an unusually aggressive course in patients who are also infected with HIV: the ulcers of primary syphilis are multiple, painful, and large, genital ulcers are more common in the secondary stage, and progression to tertiary syphilis and neurosyphilis is faster.

The true rates of sexually transmitted diseases in the elderly population are unknown, but the incidence of syphilis and HIV infection in the 'over 55' age group is increasing. HIV infection in later life is most commonly contracted through male to male sexual contact, but other common routes are heterosexual contact, and injecting illicit drugs as seen in younger age groups. The proportion of patients with an unidentified origin for their HIV infection appears higher at older than at younger ages. Suggested reasons include reluctance to admit to intravenous drug use, or sexual activities, as in the current case.

In the UK, around one third of all patients with HIV infection present late in the course of the disease. Late presentation is more common in older patients, in whom the diagnosis is more likely to be missed. There are reports of older patients experiencing an average delay of over three months after presenting with typical HIV related infection symptoms before referral for relevant testing. Older patients are less likely to be offered tests for sexually transmitted disease, but are more likely to accept them, if offered the opportunity.

This patient was indeed HIV positive with a CD4 count of 200 and a viral load of 101,614. because of his neurological findings, he was also tested for neurosyphilis, and his cerebro-spinal fluid serology was positive. New data suggest that widowerhood is associated with an increased risk of sexually transmitted diseases in older men. HIV testing should be considered in all patients, regardless of age, in whom HIV may be part of the differential diagnosis, e.g. diagnosis of any sexually transmitted infection, pyrexia of unknown origin (see case 16), weight loss of unknown cause, chronic diarrhoea, unexplained blood dyscrasia (e.g. thrombocytopenia, neutropenia), aseptic encephalitis/meningitis, and certain skin lesions, such as recurrent or multidermatomal herpes zoster.

Older patients with HIV or syphilis infection should be referred to a genito-urinary clinic or HIV specialist for further management. What constitutes best practice in looking after older patients with HIV or AIDS is unclear: geriatricians should probably be involved in most cases, together with genito-urinary medicine (GUM) specialists and infectious disease experts to help in the management of co-morbidities. This patient was counselled about the risks and methods of preventing transmission of his infections to others, and was referred to an infectious diseases specialist for further management.

4 How would you approach obtaining a sexual history from older people? Until what age are older people likely to be sexually active?

Taking a sexual history from older patients can be very difficult, owing to clinicians' lack of awareness of sexual activity in the elderly people, and both patients and clinicians may find the interview embarrassing. Older patients often dislike talking about problems related to sexuality and there is generally poor knowledge about reliability of sexual history in older patients. Clinicians should consider taking a sexual history from older patients presenting with a new rash and unexplained loss of weight. Older homosexual men and women, who grew up in societies where their sexual orientation was unacceptable, or even treated as a form of mental illness, may find it particularly difficult. There are only few published data on sexual function in older people who have moved out of their homes to live in residential care.

Despite research showing that interest in sex declines with age, data from the USA indicate that at the age of 55, men can expect another 15, and women 10, years of sexually active life. This period may become longer as drugs for erectile dysfunction come into greater use. The proportion of 70-year-olds participating in sexual intercourse and being satisfied with it appears to have increased from 1971 to 2000 to over 50% of those interviewed. Although sexual activity is more related to marital status, 31% of unmarried older men are sexually active.

5 List the most common causes of sexual dysfunction in older people.

The most common causes of sexual dysfunction in older people are:

- *Drugs*, e.g. benzodiazepines, beta-blockers, antiepileptics, anticholinergics, antidepressants, antipsychotics, digoxin, antiandrogens, oestrogens, antihypertensives, cancer chemotherapy.
- *Dyspareunia*—the most common sexual complaint of older female patients, often caused by low oestrogen levels causing urogenital atrophy, but also by local irritants, vaginitis, endometriosis, pelvic tumours, urinary tract infections, ovarian cysts, and postoperative adhesions.
- *Erectile dysfunction* may be multifactorial, reflecting vascular and neurological impairments, drugs, diabetes mellitus, and psychological factors.

6 What contributes to the risk of sexually transmitted diseases in older people and why may diagnosis be difficult?

The increased risk of sexually transmitted diseases and diagnostic difficulty may be caused by:

- Unsafe sexual practices ('safe sex fatigue').
- Older people not considering themselves to be at risk—or not caring.
- Lack of knowledge of risk factors for sexually transmitted diseases.
- Increase in foreign travel.
- Increase in internet use.
- Rising divorce rates.
- Increasing numbers of sexual partners.
- Effective treatment for impotence in old age ('Viagra restored sexual life').
- Not seeking medical attention at all, or only with significant delay.
- Sexually transmitted diseases symptoms (e.g. dysuria) being misinterpreted as due to urinary tract infection or age-associated conditions.
- Clinicians' lack of awareness.
- Clinicians' failure to elicit history of exposure to sexually transmitted diseases or risk factors.
- Clinicians' reluctance to test for sexually transmitted diseases.

7 Does HIV infection differ in older versus younger patients?

HIV diagnosis is more likely to be delayed in older patients for the reasons discussed earlier. Data suggest that the time to development of AIDS following HIV infection is shorter in older people because of ageing related reduction in CD4 T-cell counts. Following the introduction of Highly Active Antiretroviral Therapy (HAART) treatment (from which older people benefit at least as much as younger patients) and better treatment of opportunistic infections and malignancies, life expectancy among older HIV infected patients has increased. Reported increases in certain morbidities in older patients with HIV may be secondary to associated risk factors rather than the HIV itself. The US Senate Special Committee on Aging predicts that by 2015, 50% of patients infected with HIV/AIDS will be older than 50 years and that HIV/AIDS has therefore become a chronic disease.

Compared to younger people, HIV infection in older patients, is associated with:

- A wider differential diagnosis.
- Greater likelihood of opportunistic infections for a given CD4 count.
- Increased risk of death, e.g. from complications due to opportunistic infections.
- Cognitive impairment. This is more common in older people and thus older people with HIV or AIDS may be more susceptible than younger patients to HIV-associated causes of cognitive decline, including AIDS-associated dementia (incidence has reduced since the introduction of effective treatment for AIDS) and HIV-associated mild cognitive disorder, although reported higher prevalence may in part be caused by poorly matched controls.
- Higher cancer rates and increases in serious cardiovascular events. This may be related in part to routine health checks and thus earlier diagnoses of cancer of anus and lung, and Hodgkin's lymphoma. Screening for cardiovascular risk factors should be considered since protease inhibitors (HAART) increase total cholesterol, triglycerides, LDL cholesterol, and insulin resistance.
- Low bone mineral density and osteoporosis, which may also be related to smoking, alcohol, low BMI, low socioeconomic status, or some medications.

Further reading

Bhaskaran K, Hamouda O, Sannes M, *et al.* (2008). For the Concerted Action on Sero Conversion to AIDS and Death in Europe (CASCADE) Collaboration. Changes in the risk of death after HIV seroconversion compared with mortality in the general population. *JAMA*; **300**: 50–59.

Fisher M, Cooper V (2012). HIV and ageing: premature ageing or premature conclusions? *Curr Opin Infect Dis*; **25**: 1–3.

Goulet J, Fultz S, Rimlands D, *et al.* (2007). Aging and infectious diseases: do patterns of comorbidity vary by HIV status, age and HIV severity? *Clin Infect Dis*; **45**: 1593–1601.

Kearney F, Moore AR, Donegan CF, Lambert J (2010). The ageing of HIV: implications for geriatric medicine, *Age Ageing*; **39**: 536–541.

Kleinplatz PJ (2008). Sexuality and older people. *BMJ*; **337**: a239.

Lindau ST, Gavrilova N (2010). Sex, health, and years of sexually active life gained due to good health: evidence from two US population based cross sectional surveys of ageing. *BMJ*; **320**: c810.

May M, Gompels M, Delpech V, *et al.* (2011). Impact of late diagnosis and treatment on life expectancy in people with HIV-1: UK collaborative HIV cohort (UK CHIC) study. *BMJ*; **343**: d6016.

May M, Gompels M, Delpech V, *et al.* (2012). Life expectancy of HIV-1-positive individuals approaches normal, conditional on response to antiretroviral therapy: UK collaborative HIV cohort study. Eleventh International Congress on Drug Therapy in HIV Infection, Glasgow, abstract O133.

Sabin C (2012). Review of life expectancy in people with HIV in settings with optimal ART access: what we know and what we don't. Eleventh International Congress on Drug Therapy in HIV Infection, Glasgow, abstract O131.

Taylor A, Gosney MA (2011). Sexuality in older age: essential considerations for healthcare professionals. *Age Ageing*; **40**: 538–543.

Wöhrl S, Geusau A (2007). Clinical update: syphilis in adults. *Lancet*; **369**(9577): 1912–1914.

Case 31

An 83-year-old woman was admitted after a collapse in a supermarket witnessed by her son. He reported that she had suddenly fallen to the floor with her left arm shaking, and had been incontinent of urine. The episode lasted several minutes and she had gradually come round, but had been confused and disorientated afterwards.

Over the previous six weeks, she had complained of headaches and had begun taking regular paracetamol. The onset of double vision had prompted an optician's appointment, which was awaited, and over the previous two weeks she had had several episodes of urinary incontinence. She lived alone in a bungalow and did not go outside unaccompanied as she was frightened of falling, but she was otherwise independent. Her son lived nearby and took her shopping once a week. Past medical history included osteoporosis, diverticulitis, left breast mastectomy for breast carcinoma with spread to regional nodes three years previously, and hypothyroidism. Medications were Adcal D3, alendronate, levothyroxine, and paracetamol.

On examination, she was slightly drowsy and disorientated with AMTS of 6. Observations were otherwise unremarkable except for oxygen saturations of 94% on air. Blood pressure was 136/88mmHg. General systems were normal. Neurological examination revealed nuchal rigidity, with diplopia on looking to the left, unilateral hearing loss, and mild dysarthria. Limb tone was normal with power 5/5 in the upper limbs and 4/5 in the lower limbs. Reflexes were absent throughout with upgoing plantar responses.

Investigations revealed the following:

- CXR: unremarkable
- ECG: sinus rhythm 88bpm, no overt abnormality
- Hb: 10.2g/dL
- WCC: 7.3×10^9/L
- Neut: 3.7×10^9/L
- HCt: 0.42L/L
- Na: 142mmol/L

- K: 3.5mmol/L
- Urea: 9mmol/L
- Creat: 112μmol/L
- Calcium: 2.5mmol/L
- ALT: 38IU/L
- Bili: 25μmol/L
- Alp: 476U/L
- TSH: 2.2
- CRP: 10mg/L
- CT brain scan: periventricular changes in keeping with small vessel disease. No acute haemorrhage, mass, or space-occupying lesion. No signs of raised intracranial pressure.

Questions

1. What are the most common causes of new-onset seizures in older people? What are the common differential diagnoses in this age group? What are the essentials of management?
2. What is the most likely underlying cause of seizures in this patient given the clinical history and CT brain findings?
3. What is the pathophysiology of this condition and the clinical features?
4. What further investigations would you perform?
5. What is the most appropriate treatment and what is the prognosis?

Answers

1 What are the most common causes of new-onset seizures in older people? What are the common differential diagnoses in this age group? What are the essentials of management?

The most common causes of new-onset epilepsy in older people are shown in Table 31.1 (epilepsy is the term given when there are two or more seizures).

Table 31.1 Causes of seizures and epilepsy in older adults

	Relative proportion (%)
Acute seizures	
Acute stroke	50
Metabolic encephalopathy	6–30
Drugs	10
Others (trauma, infection)	5–20
Epilepsy	
Cerebrovascular disease	30–50
Dementia	9–17
Others (tumour, trauma)	5–15
Unknown	30–50

Primary epilepsy most commonly presents around puberty and very rarely presents *de novo* in older people. The onset of new seizure is highest in the older adult population (>70 years) owing to the higher prevalence of structural brain pathology. Most seizures in elderly patients are focal in onset, with or without evolution to a bilateral convulsive seizure.

Cerebrovascular disease is the most common known cause of epilepsy in older people, causing one-third to one-half of cases. Risk factors for post-stroke epilepsy (haemorrhage, cortical involvement, large size) are similar to those for acute symptomatic seizures. The risk of unprovoked seizures is highest in the first year after a stroke, but remains substantially elevated for at least seven years. Dementia is also a common cause of epilepsy in older populations: between 9 to 16% of patients with AD will develop seizures, a rate up to 10 times that of the age-matched population. Younger age at onset and more severe dementia have been identified as independent risk factors for incidental epilepsy. Conversely, epilepsy is associated with earlier onset of cognitive decline in patients with amnestic mild cognitive impairment and AD.

Metabolic or biochemical disturbances, including hyponatraemia hypocalcaemia, hypoglycaemia uraemic and hepatic encephalopathy, intercurrent illness, drugs (e.g. ciprofloxacin, cholinesterase inhibitors, antidepressants), alcohol withdrawal, thiamine deficiency (Wernicke's encephalopathy in alcoholic or malnourished patients), are also commonly associated with seizures in older people.

A witness account is the key to diagnosis, as was provided in the current case by the son and should be obtained if at all possible. Post-event confusion and drowsiness are highly suggestive of seizure, but incontinence and shaking are much less specific, and may occur in cerebral hypoperfusion associated with syncope (see case 11).

The diagnosis of seizure may be particularly difficult in older people because of the likelihood of co-morbid pathology and lack of a clear history, particularly in patients with dementia. Patients with seizure may be misdiagnosed as 'confusion', 'funny turns', blackouts, memory disturbance, syncope, dizziness, dementia, transient ischaemic attack (TIA), depression, or psychiatric disorder. Distinguishing brain ischaemia, which produces reduced neural activity and 'negative' symptoms, e.g. hemiparesis or hemisensory loss from seizures causing neural overactivity, and 'positive' symptoms, e.g. tingling or shaking, should not usually be a problem. However 'limb-shaking' TIAs occurring in the setting of high-grade carotid stenosis (see TIA and stroke *Oxford Case Histories*) may cause diagnostic difficulty. An interictal EEG has limited utility, with low sensitivity and specificity for the diagnosis of epilepsy.

The cause of the seizure must be determined and any reversible causes treated. Owing to the high prevalence of side effects and drug interactions, antiepileptic medications are often not prescribed until after a second seizure has occurred. Treatment should start at low doses and titrate up slowly with target therapeutic doses and drug levels lower than in younger populations. Antiepileptic drugs polypharmacy should be avoided. Lamotrigine and levatericetam are common first line choices in older people. Carbamezepine often causes drowsiness. The presence of gross brain structural abnormality or a wish to return to driving may favour early treatment. If the patient is a driver, they must be told to stop driving and to inform the DVLA.

2 What is the most likely underlying cause of seizures in this patient, given the clinical history and CT brain findings?

The most likely diagnosis is leptomeningeal carcinomatosis, secondary to breast carcinoma as suggested by the history of relatively recent breast cancer with positive lymph nodes, recent onset of headaches without overt CT brain scan abnormality, nuchal rigidity, diplopia, unilateral deafness, incontinence, upgoing plantars, and the absence of evidence for an alternative cause of seizure.

The differential diagnosis includes that for seizures in general in older people, as cited in answer 1. Cerebral metastasis was not supported by the CT brain scan findings, although occasionally brain deposits may be missed on plain CT being visible only after administration of contrast. Blood tests did not suggest any metabolic or infective cause and there was no obvious history suggestive of dementia, although this would need to be assessed further if appropriate. The low AMTS is likely to be caused by the postictal state, but would need to be rechecked. The brain scan showed evidence of small vessel disease as is commonly the case in older people, but there was no previous history of TIA or stroke that would raise the risk of cerebrovascular disease-associated seizure. The history of headache raises the possibility of temporal arteritis (see case 39) that may occasionally cause seizure, usually in the context of stroke, but there were no other features to suggest this diagnosis.

3 What is the pathophysiology of this condition and the clinical features?

Leptomeningeal carcinomatosis occurs in approximately 5% of advanced cancers, particularly adenocarcinomas of the breast, lung, and gastrointestinal tract, and also lymphoma, leukaemia, and melanoma. The incidence is increasing as neuroimaging techniques advance diagnosis and newer cancer therapies extend patient life expectancy.

Cancers arising from outside the central nervous system can metastasize to any intracranial structure. Metastatic seeding to the leptomeninges can occur via haematogenous spread of malignant cells through the choroid plexus or the arachnoid vessels, or via direct invasion from existing central nervous system tumours. Direct tumour invasion can give rise to specific cranial nerve and spinal root lesions. Systemic malignancies can also spread via the peripheral nerves or seed to the subarachnoid space during surgical resection of intraparenchymal tumours. *De novo* tumours can also arise in the leptomeningies in lymphoma, sarcomas, and melanomas.

Symptoms and signs in leptomeningeal carcinomatosis are usually consistent with multiple areas of nervous system involvement. The diagnosis should always be considered in patients with a history of cancer presenting with isolated cranial nerve lesions, cerebral, and/or spinal cord symptoms. In a series of 150 patients with solid tumour leptomeningeal carcinomatosis, the most common presenting signs and symptoms were:

- headache (39%)
- nausea and vomiting (25%)
- leg weakness (21%)
- cerebellar dysfunction (17%)
- altered mental status (16%)
- diplopia (14%)
- facial weakness (13%).

Overall prevalence of clinical signs and symptoms in leptomeningeal carcinomatosis are as follows:

- cranial nerve palsy (75%)
- cerebral signs (66%)
- headache (66%)
- spinal nerve deficits (60%)
- altered mental status (45%)
- limb weakness (44%)
- gait disturbances (33%)
- meningism (21%)
- sensory abnormalities (21%)
- nausea and vomiting (20%)
- cerebellar signs (16%)
- seizures (12%)
- dizziness (9%)
- autonomic dysfunction (1%).

Partial seizures with or without secondary generalization can be caused by cortical irritation from adjacent leptomeningeal deposits, invasion of brain parenchyma, or local oedema. Headache can be caused by increased intracranial pressure or meningeal irritation, which is suggested by neck pain or stiffness exacerbated by head movements. Nuchal rigidity may be present, with or without headache. Pain with straight leg raising suggests spinal meningeal irritation. In radiculopathy, the roots of the cauda equina supplying the lower extremities, bowels, and bladder are most often affected. Cauda equina involvement can be manifested as leg pain, leg weakness or numbness, urinary incontinence or retention (see case 7), and/or an asymmetry of deep tendon reflexes.

4 What further investigations would you perform?

The following further investigations should be performed:

- lumbar puncture and cerebrospinal fluid (CSF) examination
- brain MRI with gadolinium.

Gadolinium-enhanced MRI of the brain and spine usually provides evidence of disease. Although MRI is probably more sensitive (70–85%) than a single CSF specimen for cytology, it is less specific because false positive cytologies are rare.

Characteristic CSF findings are raised opening pressure, and elevated cell count (lymphocytic pleocytosis) and protein, with low glucose. Normal CSF examination is extremely rare although not all parameters are always abnormal. Cytology is positive in 50% of cases on first CSF sampling, rising to 85% on repeat. Unsurprisingly, extensive meningeal involvement is more likely to be associated with positive CSF cytology.

Typical brain MRI changes include thin, diffuse leptomeningeal contrast enhancement following the contours of the gyri and sulci, or multiple nodular deposits in the subarachnoid space. Common sites of abnormal leptomeningeal enhancement include the cerebellar folia, the cortical surface (Fig. 31.1), and the basal cisterns, particularly along the ventral surface of the brainstem. Enhancement of the cranial nerves may occur (Fig. 31.2) as well as secondary hydrocephalus (Fig. 31.3). In addition, the cisternal segments of the cranial nerves may be abnormally thickened and enhancing. High-resolution contrast-enhanced skull base MRI can sometimes show cranial nerve abnormalities that are not seen on routine MRI. Fluid-attenuated inversion recovery images may show hyperintensity within the subarachnoid space, indicative of high protein content.

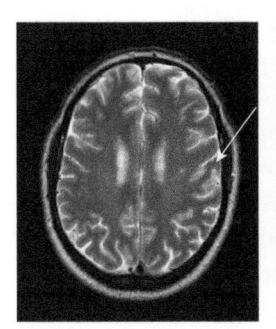

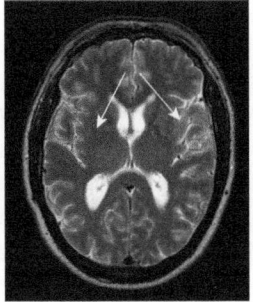

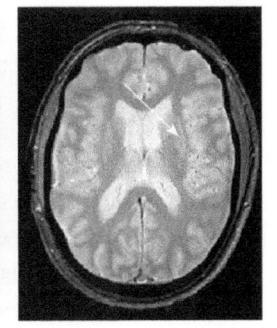

Fig. 31.1 Axial MRI brain slices with gadolinium showing right cortical and left temporal meningeal enhancement (arrows).

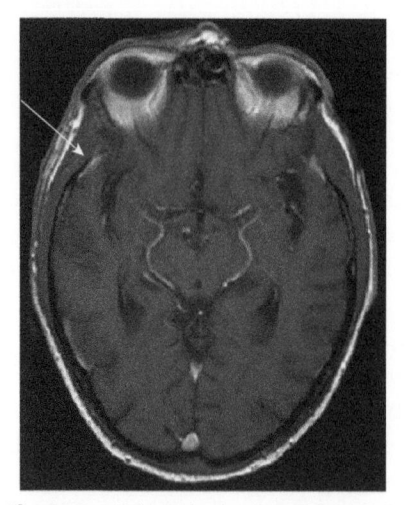

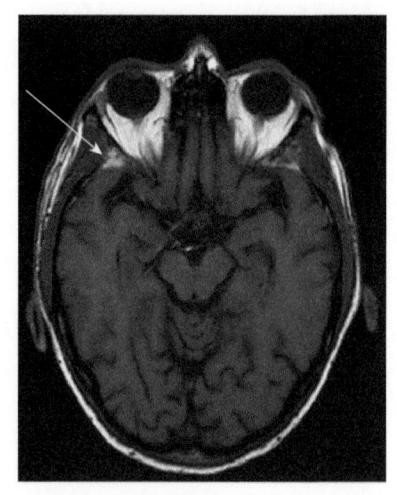

Fig. 31.2 Axial MRI brain slice with gadolinium showing thickening and enhancement of the oculomotor nerve (arrows).

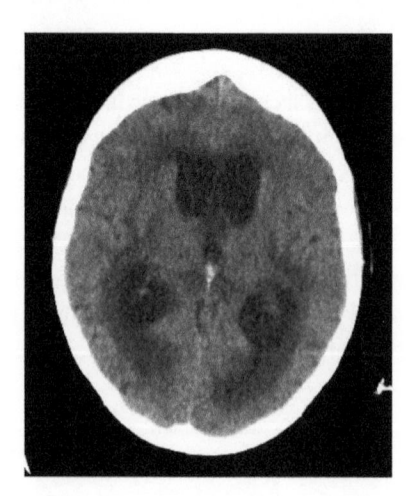

Fig. 31.3 Axial CT brain slices showing secondary hydrocephalus associated with meningeal carcinomatosis.

Any or all of these findings may be accompanied by ventriculomegaly in the absence of, or out of proportion to the degree of sulcal enlargement (i.e. hydrocephalus). In older patients, it may be difficult to distinguish hydrocephalus from *ex vacuo* enlargement of the ventricles. Imaging findings that suggest true hydrocephalus include abnormal periventricular T2 hyperintensity (suggesting transependymal CSF absorption) and sulcal effacement (see case 6). CT with contrast may be considered if MRI is contraindicated, but sensitivity is considerably lower.

5 What is the most appropriate treatment and what is the prognosis?

The primary tumour will need to be identified in those cases where it is not already known.

In general, treatment is aimed at increasing life expectancy, stabilizing neurological status, and reducing neurological disability, although the prognosis is poor with life expectancy around two to four months on average. In exceptional cases where the primary tumour is a responsive adenocarcinoma or haematological malignancy with minimal neurological deficit and good performance status, survival with treatment can be six to eight months, and a few patients have a good long-term response. The appropriate therapeutic approach for an individual patient is dependent upon the risk categories shown in Table 31.2.

Table 31.2 Risk categories in patients with leptomeningeal metastases

Poor risk	Good risk
Poor performance status	Good performance status
Multiple, fixed neurological deficits	Minimal or no fixed neurological deficits
Extensive systemic cancer without good treatment options	Effective systemic treatment of cancer possible
Encephalopathy or bulky CNS disease	

In the current case, the patient should be considered for treatment aimed at the underlying primary tumour. High dose radiotherapy, intrathecal, and systemic chemotherapy are possible therapeutic options, although should not be undertaken lightly. Careful assessment of the cancer burden, patient's performance status, and degree of frailty is needed before discussions with the patient regarding the risks and benefits of any therapy.

Further reading

Cavanna L, Rocchi A, Gorgni S, et al. (2011). Cerebrospinal fluid cytology diagnosis of HER2-positive leptomeningeal carcinomatosis from HER2-positive metastatic gastric cancer: case report. *J Clin Oncol*; **29**(13): e367–e368.

Fisher S, et al. (2014). Neuroborreliosis mimicking leptomeningeal carcinomatosis in a patient with breast cancer. A case report. *Journal of Investigative Medicine*; **2**: DOI 10.117712324709614529417.

Grossman S, Krabak M (1999). Leptomenigeal carcinomatosis. *Cancer Treat Rev*; **25**: 103–119.

Pentheroudakis G, Pavlidis N (2005). Management of leptomeningeal malignancy. *Expert Opin Pharmacother*; **6**(7): 1115–1125.

Case 32

A 74-year-old woman was seen in the rapid access out-patient clinic with new onset diarrhoea and faecal incontinence. The GP referral letter stated that she 'has frequent passage of small amounts of soft faeces and is not coping at home'. She had been admitted with a stroke four months earlier, with weakness in her right arm and leg, but had recovered well and returned home. Past medical history included depression, hypertension, myocardial infarction, and surgery for haemorrhoids three years previously. Medications were aspirin, citalopram, ramipril, amlodipine, furosemide, isosorbide mononitrate, and simvastatin. The GP had started oxybutynin in the last six weeks for long-standing increased urinary frequency, urgency and occasional incontinence, associated with difficulty in reaching the toilet in time. She was a non-smoker who did not drink alcohol, and lived in a ground floor flat with her husband. A carer came each morning to assist with washing and dressing.

On examination, she appeared well, and was able to mobilize slowly but independently with a tripod stick. The temperature was 36.5°C, pulse was 72bpm regular, and blood pressure was 120/70mmHg. General systems examination was unremarkable but during the examination, she became incontinent of soft watery stool of which she was not aware. On neurological examination, power was 3/5 in the right arm and 4/5 in the right leg with brisk reflexes and right-sided extensor plantar, unchanged since discharge following the stroke.

Investigations showed the following:

- FBC, ESR, U&E, TFT, LFT, calcium, B_{12}, glucose, cholesterol, folate: normal
- CXR: slightly enlarged heart
- ECG: sinus rhythm; heart rate 72bpm; left bundle branch block; long-standing
- Urine dipstick: negative for blood; nitrates; leucocytes.

Questions

1 What further details should be established from the history to further evaluate this patient's faecal incontinence?
2 List further examinations that are necessary in this case and explain why these are important.
3 Discuss the relevance of a history of stroke to faecal incontinence.
4 Describe the risk factors for faecal incontinence in this case and list other common risk factors.

Answers

1 What further details should be established from the history to further evaluate this patient's faecal incontinence?

A comprehensive history should be taken from the patient and, if she agrees, from husband and carer to establish details about past and present patterns of defaecation: the duration; frequency; stool type; the use of underwear or incontinence pads; the awareness of need to open the bowels; the duration of symptoms; precipitating events; diet and fluid intake; toilet access; history of anorectal surgery; obstetric history (including the number of vaginal deliveries, the deliveries of high-birth-weight babies, obstetric forceps—in this patient not relevant as she did not have children); history of other neurological disease; diabetes mellitus; and all medications. The impact of the incontinence on the patient's (and husband's) lifestyle should be documented.

It is also important to establish whether there is functional or true incontinence, i.e. the presence of frequency and urgency without the loss of bowel contents. The history should guide further examination.

A history of frequent passage of small quantities of soft faeces suggests faecal impaction and overflow, especially in a patient with physical impairment, as in the current case.

2 List further examinations that are necessary in this case and explain why these are important.

Further examination should include:

- The inspection of underwear for faecal staining, inspection of perineal and anal area for skin tags, scars, haemorrhoids, and rectal prolapse, to exclude leakage from perianal fistulas, abscesses, and fissures as causes of 'pseudo-incontinence'. The presence of dermatitis suggests chronic incontinence.
- Digital anorectal examination, assessment of anal tone, and perianal sensation.
- Abdominal examination
- MoCA or similar cognitive test (in this case—22/30)
- Bimanual digital examination of rectum and vagina should be considered.

A history of frequent passage of small quantities of soft faeces suggests faecal impaction and overflow, especially in a patient with physical impairment. Abdominal examination may reveal colonic faecal loading and faecal impaction can usually be confirmed on rectal examination. If the rectum is empty, high impaction can be confirmed with a plain abdominal X-ray (Fig. 32.1).

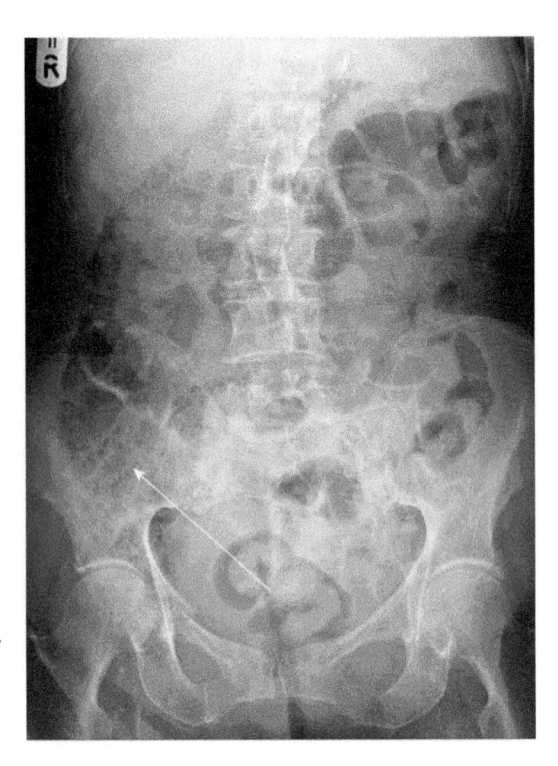

Fig. 32.1 Plain abdominal X-ray showing faecal loading of the whole colon particularly on the right side (white arrow), consistent with severe constipation (image from a different patient).

Digital anorectal examination is also important to exclude masses and to assess anal tone: lack of or reduced resistance to the examining finger is indicative of a dysfunctional anal sphincter.

Bimanual digital examination with one digit in the vagina and another in the rectum may be considered to determine perineal body thickness and characteristics of the anal sphincters. The external anal sphincter is a moderately firm 2cm thick mass within the perineal body. If during the examination, the anal sphincter is not palpable or the examiner's fingers are not separated by significant tissue, it is likely that the sphincter is damaged. This can be further evaluated by asking the patient to tighten the sphincter around the examining finger.

Perianal sensation and pudendal motor function can be tested by evoking the anocutaneous reflex ('anal wink sign') by gently stroking the skin surrounding the anus and observing a reflex contraction of the external anal sphincter. The anal wink sign should be elicited bilaterally; absence suggests nerve damage and interruption of the spinal arc.

A brief cognitive screen should be performed as part of any comprehensive geriatric assessment. Significant cognitive impairment may be associated with urinary and faecal incontinence owing to loss of central control of continence function and/or lack of understanding of the need to find a toilet or in locating one.

3 Discuss the relevance of a history of stroke to faecal incontinence.

Faecal incontinence in patients who have suffered a stroke is associated with:

- Advanced age (ageing is associated with lower anal sphincter pressures)
- Greater severity of stroke and resulting impairment of higher cortical centres
- Presence of diabetes mellitus (associated with abnormal anal sphincter function)
- Presence of other disabling diseases
- Prescription of anticholinergic drugs
- Impaired vision
- Impaired affect (anxiety or depression)
- Impaired cognition
- Impaired communication
- Presence of dehydration or inadequate food intake
- Impaired dexterity and mobility
- The need for assistance in using the toilet is the strongest risk factor for post-stroke faecal incontinence, increasing the risk more than three-fold.

Faecal incontinence in stroke patients is associated with increased use of district nurse services, institutionalization, and death. Post-stroke faecal incontinence may be transient with high rates of up to 40% on admission, falling to around 20% at the time of discharge and less than 10% at six-month follow-up. The vast majority (at least 80%) of post-stroke patients with faecal incontinence also have urinary incontinence.

Recent data suggest that a significant number of patients with faecal incontinence three years post-stroke, were continent one year post-stroke, indicating the need for vigilance in detecting delayed faecal incontinence in post-stroke patients.

4 Describe the risk factors for faecal incontinence in this case and list other common risk factors.

The risk factors for faecal incontinence in this patient are:

- Age older than 70 years. Decrease in anal resting pressure and anal squeeze pressure after the menopause suggests a possible role for oestrogen in faecal incontinence. Slower pudendal nerve conduction, perineal descent at rest, and decreased anorectal sensory function are also frequently found in old age.

- Urinary incontinence
- Neurological disease (stroke)
- Poor mobility
- Surgery for haemorrhoids
- Medications altering anal sphincter tone—nitrates, calcium channel antagonists, as well as SSRI (citalopram), and anticholinergic drugs (oxybutynin).

Other risk factors for faecal incontinence include:

- Poor general health
- Obstetric trauma
- High parity
- Diabetes mellitus
- Severe cognitive impairment or learning difficulties
- Drugs: broad spectrum antibiotics (penicillins, cephalosporins, macrolides); sedating agents including antipsychotics, benzodiazepines, tricyclic antidepressants; and agents altering bowel habit including metformin, laxatives, iron, digoxin, antacids containing magnesium, loperamide, opioids, and anticholinergic drugs (e.g. antiemetics).
- Medical conditions causing diarrhoea, e.g. inflammatory bowel disease, irritable bowel syndrome, intestinal cancer.
- Obesity
- Mass effect (e.g. carcinoma of the rectum, foreign body)
- Pelvic radiotherapy; radiation proctitis
- Rectal prolapse; cauda equina syndrome; acute disc prolapse.

Case progression

Anorectal examination of this patient revealed a rectum full of hard, dry stool causing faecal impaction consistent with the history of frequent passage of small quantities of soft faeces. The faecal impaction was likely to have been exacerbated by the prescription of anticholinergic medication (oxybutynin).

Questions continued

5 Discuss the management strategies for this patient.
6 Discuss management of faecal incontinence in general and list criteria for referrals to a specialist incontinence service.
7 What is the prevalence of faecal incontinence among older people?

Answers continued

5 Discuss management strategies for this patient.

Faecal impaction promotes mucus production and fluid accumulation, with distension of the anal sphincters causing loss of tone and control. Constant inhibition of the internal anal sphincter, permitting leakage of liquid stool around the impaction results in 'spurious diarrhoea', of which patients usually have no awareness. Faecal impaction is associated with older age, neurological disorders, immobility, rectal hyposensitivity, cognitive impairment, and inadequate intake of dietary fibre and fluids. Common symptoms include abdominal pain, nausea, vomiting, delirium (see case 1), and general clinical deterioration. Possible complications include bleeding and intestinal wall perforation.

This patient's treatment consisted of removal of faecal material by enemas and the administration of oral polyethylene glycol solutions to clear stool from the proximal colon. She tolerated this treatment well and the bowel was cleared without need for further intervention.

Maintenance therapy included avoiding constipating drugs and dehydration, regular use of fibre supplements and laxatives, and weekly enemas as required. She was given dietary advice and her medications were reviewed: amlodipine and isosorbide mononitrate were stopped, as the blood pressure was consistently low with significant symptomatic postural hypotension. Glyceryl trinitrate (GTN) tablets were prescribed on demand basis for chest pain. She was not felt to be depressed and so the citalopram, which she had been taking for almost two years, was stopped. Oxybutynin was continued as it improved her urinary frequency.

6 Discuss management of faecal incontinence in general and list criteria for referrals to the specialist incontinence service.

The cause of any underlying diarrhoea should be established and treated. Older patients presenting with faecal incontinence and loss of weight, new onset constipation, anaemia, or positive faecal occult blood tests should have further investigations for cancer, or other bowel pathology.

In the absence of any treatable cause, the following should be offered:

- advice on dietary modification, fluid intake, and bowel habit
- availability of continence products
- where to get counselling if needed.

Practical issues may include:

- disposable pads
- skin care

- disposable gloves
- odour control
- improved toilet access
- review of medication.

Prescription of anti-diarrhoeal drugs that slow motility of the gut (e.g. loperamide hydrochloride) is appropriate in certain cases of non-infectious diarrhoea. In patients intolerant of loperamide, codeine phosphate should be used. No other medications have been shown to be of benefit.

Specialist incontinence management should be offered to patients who fail to improve after initial input, but will usually be ineffective in those with severe cognitive impairment in whom behavioural factors, such as inability to remember the location of a toilet should be considered.

Specialist assessment may include endoanal ultrasound, anorectal physiology studies, and proctography. Patients may be considered for:

- Biofeedback regimen of anal sphincter strength training and rectal co-ordination. (However, a systematic review found no therapeutic benefits from the few available randomized controlled trials).
- Rectal irrigation. In constipation and faecal incontinence, a study of 348 patients showed success in just under half of patients at 21 months, as an empty rectum meant no incontinence.
- Bowel retraining through a management programme focused on regular defaecation.
- Pelvic floor muscle training
- Specialist dietary assessment and management.

Invasive treatment may be considered for some, but is not an option for many older patients in whom surgery is high risk and evidence for superiority of surgical versus conservative therapy is lacking, but some data are emerging on injecting local bulking agents. Surgical outcomes of sphincter repairs have been shown to be poorer in older female patients.

7 What is the prevalence of faecal incontinence among older people?

The true prevalence of faecal incontinence among community-dwelling people older people is uncertain. It has been estimated that around two-thirds of all patients avoid discussing it with their medical practitioners and available data vary in the definitions and methods of ascertainment. It is thought that between 3% and 7% of people aged over 65 in the community suffer occasional or frequent episodes of faecal incontinence, compared with around 62% of older people in nursing homes. There are no clear data to suggest that the frequency of faecal incontinence differs between the sexes although women might be expected to be at higher risk owing to the association with childbirth-associated injury.

Further reading

Ahmad M, McCallum IJD, Mercer-Jones M (2010). Management of faecal incontinence in adults. *BMJ*; **340**: 1350–1355.

Brown SR, Nelson RL (2007). Surgery for faecal incontinence in adults. *Cochrane Database Syst Rev*; **2**: CD001757.

Christensen P, Krogh K, Buntzen S, Payandeh F, Lauberg S (2009). Long-term outcome and safety of transanal irrigation for constipation and faecal incontinence. *Dis Colon Rectum*; **52**: 286–292.

Cheetham MJ, Brazzelli M, Norton CC, Glazener CMA (2003). Drug treatment for faecal incontinence in adults. *Cochrane Database Syst Rev*; **3**: CD002116.

Edwards NI, Jones D (2001). The prevalence of faecal incontinence in older people living at home. *Age Ageing*; **30**: 503–507.

Harari D, Coshall C, Rudd AG, Wolfe CDA (2003). New-onset fecal incontinence after stroke: prevalence, natural history, risk factors, and impact. *Stroke*; **34**: 144–150.

Macmillan AK, Merrie AE, Marshall RJ, Parry BR (2004). The prevalence of faecal incontinence in community-dwelling adults: a systematic review of the literature. *Dis Colon Rectum*; **47**: 1341–1349.

Maeda Y, Lauberg S, Norton C (2010). Perianal injectable bulking agents as treatment for faecal incontinence in adults. *Cochrane Database Syst Rev*; **5**: CD007959.

Case 33

Case 33.A

A 74-year-old retired teacher was admitted after a fall that occurred because of weakness in the left leg. He had sustained a fracture of the right femur and went on to have right hemiarthroplasty. He was subsequently transferred from the surgical ward to the rehabilitation ward. His recovery was slow, and he had difficulty in mobilizing; two weeks post surgery, he was only able to stand with the use of a walking frame and the help of two people.

Previous medical history was unremarkable other than falls over the past year, in which he had 'tripped in the street'. He often felt tired and had found fast walking and climbing stairs more difficult over recent months. There was no family history of note.

On examination on the rehabilitation ward, he was thin with poor muscle bulk. The wound on the right hip was well healed. The muscles of the right hand were wasted. Tone was normal in all limbs, but there was hyper-reflexia in the legs and upgoing plantars. The rest of the examination was unremarkable.

Case 33.B

A 72-year-old retired nurse was referred by her GP to the TIA clinic with a six-week history of left-sided weakness, difficulty in swallowing, and tiredness. She had noted that in recent months she had difficulty opening bottles, writing, and was increasingly clumsy, often dropping objects. There was some weight loss, but otherwise she felt well. There was a history of hypertension.

A general system examination was normal. There was wasting in the small intrinsic muscles in her hands. Tone was normal, but fasciculations were noted over the arms and thighs. The power in the left leg was reduced to 4/5. There was hyper-reflexia in the left arm and both legs, with upgoing left plantar.

Case 33.C

An 82-year-old retired woman was referred by the GP to the day hospital with a history of falls and right leg weakness. Over the preceding two years, she had shown a tendency to stumble, which she attributed to her right foot 'not clearing the floor' and gradually worsening right leg weakness. She denied blackouts, pain, or sensory symptoms, but had lost weight despite a good appetite. The GP had organized an MRI of the lumbar spine, which revealed osteoporotic wedge fracture of L2 with minor disc degeneration (Fig. 33.1), and a CT brain scan, which showed no major abnormality (Fig. 33.2). Physiotherapy had not proved beneficial and the patient had been given a right lower leg splint. She had previously been very active and had looked after her disabled husband for many years.

There was a past medical history of kidney stones, hypertension, hypercholesterolaemia, and diabetes mellitus.

Fig. 33.1 The T1 weighted sagittal MRI images of the lumbar and sacral spine from patient in case C revealed osteoporotic wedge fracture of L2, with minor disc degeneration.

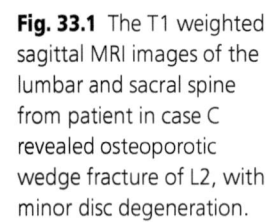

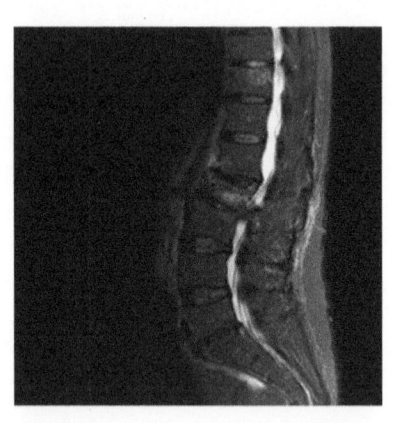

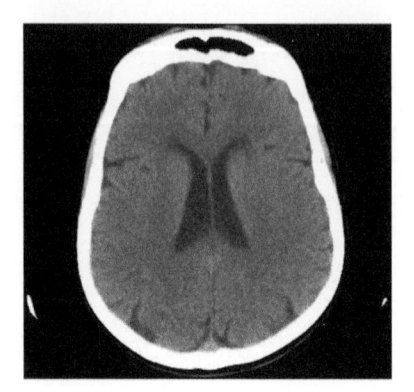

Fig. 33.2 Plain CT brain scan, axial slice from patient in case C.

Questions

1. In case C, are the MRI findings relevant to the clinical presentation?
2. What is the most likely underlying diagnosis in all three cases?
3. What specific clinical features should be looked for on examination?
4. What investigations would you consider?
5. What specific management issues might arise?
6. Describe the role of rehabilitation in this condition and the characteristics of rehabilitation in older versus younger patients.

Answers

1 In case C, are the MRI findings relevant to clinical presentation?

In case C, the patient's symptoms were gradual in onset and principally affected the right lower limb, which could not be explained by the MRI abnormalities. The falls may have contributed to the osteoporotic wedge fracture.

In spinal stenosis or disc herniation with compression of the lumbosacral nerve roots, patients usually complain of lower back pain. Pain frequently extends to the thigh and to below the knee in around a half of patients. Patients have difficulties with walking, and depending on the affected root will have abnormal knee or ankle jerks, and altered sensation in the calf or foot.

Cervical spine disease (e.g. from degenerative cervical spine disease or tumour) with myelopathy and radiculopathy may result in upper motor neuron signs in the lower limbs. There may be co-existent lower motor neuron signs in the upper limbs and presentation may include vague numbness or tingling in affected limbs, weakness, poor balance, gait disturbance, clumsy hands, or falls.

2 What is the most likely underlying diagnosis in all three cases?

The most likely diagnosis is motor neurone disease (MND). All three patients presented with progressive neurological weakness, and upper and lower motor neuron signs in the different regions. The three cases illustrate that MND may present atypically in older people including with:

- falls as seen in the above cases
- stroke-like symptoms, e.g. dysarthria, leg weakness, as seen in case B
- respiratory failure
- swallowing difficulties
- dementia
- weight loss
- functional decline
- aspiration and chest infection.

MND is a neurodegenerative disease, which usually affects older adults, with over 20% of patients first diagnosed at age >70 years and the incidence is 2/100,000. Risk factors include male gender, age, athleticism, and family history. MND is a progressive and fatal disorder of unknown cause with clinical evidence of denervation (muscle weakness, wasting, and fasciculation), and upper motor neuron dysfunction (brisk reflexes, extensor plantar response, spasticity). Patients may present with a mixture of lower and upper neuron features, or pure lower or pure upper motor neuron signs, or bulbar features, or isolated respiratory failure. Around 15% have frontotemporal dementia, but around half have evidence of executive dysfunction on testing. The average time from onset of first symptoms to diagnosis is one year and weakness in one limb is the most common presentation.

Clinically, there are four main subgroups of MND:

- *Amyotrophic lateral sclerosis* is associated with progressive weakness with lower and upper motor neurone signs, muscle wasting, fasciculations, and brisk reflexes (brisk jaw jerk, jaw clonus, and extensor plantar reflexes). Emotional lability is often present.
- *Progressive bulbar palsy* is associated with early onset of speech and swallowing problems, with a poor prognosis.
- *Progressive muscular atrophy* usually starts in one leg with asymmetrical weakness and wasting.
- *Primary lateral sclerosis* is very rare, and slowly progressive, with late speech problems, and early onset of ascending tetraparesis.

Median survival in patients with MND varies with approximate linear progression of the disease: 50% of patients die within 30 months of the first symptoms, around 20% survive for five years after the first symptoms, and only a small number survive beyond 10 years. Poor prognostic factors include old age, and bulbar and respiratory failure at disease onset, and dementia. A minority of all patients die suddenly and most commonly during sleep, possibly from pulmonary embolism, or cardiorespiratory arrest.

Besides stroke, multiple sclerosis and spinal disease, other conditions that may mimic MND or cause diagnostic difficulty include:

- Myopathies, which may cause weakness, fever, malaise, recurrent falls, dysphagia, and aspiration. Causes include drug and toxin induced (e.g. statins, steroids, choloroquine, colchicine, alcohol, cocaine) inclusion body myositis (an inflammatory muscle disorder causing symmetrical or asymmetrical weakness, or atrophy of forearms, long finger flexors, quadriceps, and neck flexion weakness as well as dysphagia), endocrine disorders, polymyositis/dermatomyositis, and, rarely, mild forms of myotonic dystrophy.
- Myasthenia gravis typically causes limb(s), diplopia, ptosis and bulbar weakness, and respiratory crisis may occur.
- Benign cramp fasciculation syndrome, in which there is cramp or fasciculations in large muscles (e.g. calves), but no weakness or wasting.
- Dual pathologies, e.g. peripheral neuropathy and cervical myelopathy.
- Radiation-induced lumbar radiculopathy, Infections (HIV), corticobasal degeneration.

3 What specific clinical features should be looked for on examination?

If MND is suspected; a thorough examination to look for the following should be performed:

- Impairment of sensation, MND does not affect the sensory system
- Lower motor neuron signs:
  - weakness
  - hypotonia
  - hyporeflexia
  - areflexia
  - fasciculations including of tongue
  - wasting, atrophy including of tongue
- Upper motor neuron signs:
  - hyper-reflexia
  - clonus
  - spasticity
  - extensor plantar motor response
  - jaw jerk
- Dysphagia, dysarthria, sialorrhoea, pseudobulbar affect, tongue atrophy.
- Preservation of extraocular movements.
- Frontal lobe dysfunction (e.g. using the MoCA or ACE III).

4 What investigations would you consider?

There is no diagnostic test for MND, so the diagnosis is clinical and requires a history of progression of symptoms with upper motor neuron (UMN) and lower motor neuron (LMN) signs present in bulbar territories and/or in the limbs.

The following investigations may be useful, mainly to exclude other causes, some of which are treatable:

- Full blood count; erythrocyte sedimentation rate; full biochemical profile; creatine kinase; serum/urine electrophoresis.
- Electromyography may be useful to detect presence of sub-clinical LMN dysfunction in the presence of UMNs in the same territory.
- Nerve conduction studies are not diagnostic, but may show evidence of disorders of neuromuscular transmission (or demyelination, which is not consistent with MND).

- MRI brain/spine to exclude other conditions, e.g. multiple sclerosis, stroke, tumours, and degenerative spinal disease.
- Depending on the clinical features: B_{12}, Serum Venereal Disease Research Laboratories test; Lyme and HIV serology; AChR antibodies; anti-GM1 antibodies; antineuronal antibodies for paraneoplastic syndrome; muscle biopsy; lumbar puncture.
- CSF is normal in MND so abnormalities suggest an alternative diagnosis.

5 What specific management issues might arise?

The management of patients with chronic, long-term, progressive conditions requires a multidisciplinary team, which might include a clinician, physiotherapist, nurse, occupational therapist, psychologist, speech and language therapist, dietitian, pharmacist, and in some cases orthotist/prosthetist. Specialist neurologist input was sought in all the mentioned cases. The drug Riluzole is licensed for the treatment of MND and prolongs life expectancy on average for around three to four months, but requires specialist guidance.

Specific symptomatic treatment may be required for:

- hypersalivation: hyoscine patch
- spasticity: botulinum toxin
- fasciculation and cramps: exercise, physiotherapy
- increased emotionality: drugs, e.g. SSRIs
- neck weakness and head drop may need specialist collars
- breathlessness when lying flat, morning nausea and headache, day-time fatigue, and tiredness should all prompt assessment for non-invasive ventilation.

Nutritional support (see case 5) is needed in around 70% of patients and enteral feeding may be necessary. End-of-life issues should be discussed at an appropriate stage.

6 Describe the role of rehabilitation in this condition and characteristics of rehabilitation in older versus younger patients.

The World Health Organization defines rehabilitation as 'a process aimed at enabling people to reach and maintain their optimal physical, sensory, intellectual, psychological, and social functional levels, as well as providing the tools they need to attain independence and self-determination'.

Although MND is a progressive, irreversible condition, rehabilitation has an important role in maintaining the patient's independence and wellbeing for as long as possible. Complete restoration of physical capacity is not possible, but mental and social function can be optimized. In the mentioned cases, the multidisciplinary team assessed all three patients, including for assistive devices (e.g. walking stick, wheelchair), and for the presence of depression, the need for carers/spouses support, and the adaptation of the home environment.

Rehabilitation in older versus younger patients:

- Is required more commonly when compared to the younger population (many conditions requiring rehabilitation are more common in the elderly, e.g. cerebrovascular disease).
- Is required more commonly following acute admission to hospital. Acute hospitalization may cause decline in the function of older patients, from baseline with reductions in the functional capacity of both cardiovascular and musculoskeletal system, and deconditioning as early as day two of admission. Rehabilitation should therefore be part of the acute care of older patients from the start of acute illness.
- The home environment may need altering (e.g. stair rails, commodes) in particular if rehabilitation is to take place in the home, which has been shown to be as effective as hospital rehabilitation, e.g. after stroke.
- The time in rehabilitation may be extended, since recovery from an illness may take longer in older patients.
- May commonly be complicated by dementia or delirium. Rehabilitation is made difficult by delirium, but may aid recovery of cognition.
- Evidence suggests that long-term care residents are less likely to regain previous level of function.
- Prevention of complications (e.g. pressure ulcers, contractures) is more often needed.
- Co-morbidities are more common, e.g. poor vision, difficulties in hearing, receptive dysphasia, and a need for the optimization of nutrition, hydration.
- More likely to have medically complex needs.
- More likely to require carer's support, e.g. advanced planning for respite care.
- More often need active measures to prevent de-conditioning after successful rehabilitation, e.g. because of overly helpful carers.

Further reading

Crocker T, Young J, Forster A, Brown L, Ozer S, Greenwood DC (2013). The effect of physical rehabilitation on activities of daily living in older residents of long-term care facilities: systematic review with meta-analysis. *Age Ageing*; **42**(6): 682–688.

Cameron ID, Kurrie SE (2002). Rehabilitation and older people. *Med J Austr*; **177**: 387–391.

Deutch A, Granger CV, Heinemann AW, *et al.* (2006). Poststroke rehabilitation: outcomes and reimbursement of inpatient rehabilitation facilities and subacute rehabilitation programs. *Stroke*; **37**(6): 1477–1482.

Brooks BR. El Escorial World Federation of Neurology criteria for the diagnosis of amyotrophic lateral sclerosis (1994). *J Neurol Sci*; **124**(Suppl): 96–107.

Halar EM, Bell KR (1998). Immobility, physiological functional changes and effects of inactivity on body functions. In: DeLisa JA, Gans BM (eds). Rehabilitation Medicine Principles and Practice, 3rd edition. Philadelphia, USA: Lippincott-Raven: 1015–1034.

Newrick PG, Langton-Hewer R (1984). Motor neurone disease: can we do better? A study of 42 patients. *Br Med J (Clin Res Ed)*; **289**(6444): 539–542.

Meyer FA, von Känel R, Saner H, Schmidt JP, Stauber S (2015). Positive affect moderates the effect of negative affect on cardiovascular disease-related hospitalizations and all-cause mortality after cardiac rehabilitation. *Eur J Prev Cardiol*; **22**:1247–53.

Poynter L, Kwan J, Sayer AA, Vassalo M (2008). Do cognitively impaired patients benefit from rehabilitation? *Rev Clin Gerontol*; **18**; 53–64.

Talbot K (2009). Motor neuron disease: the bare essentials. *Pract Neurol*; **9**: 303–309.

Case 34

An 86-year-old woman was seen in the out-patient clinic with a history of poor appetite and poor sleep. She had been discharged from hospital six weeks earlier following a six-month long hospital admission for myocardial infarction, worsening heart failure, urinary tract infection, and two episodes of chest infection, during which she had been delirious on several occasions. Prior to that admission, she had lived alone in an old house without heating and her only relative, a niece, lived abroad. She had been receiving four visits a day from carers who helped with almost all daily activities. Owing to further physical and cognitive decline during her hospital stay, she was discharged to a nursing home for which her niece provided financial support.

She had a past history of hypertension, TIA, and a stroke two years previously, which had left her with slight left hand and leg weakness, and she had subsequently been diagnosed with vascular dementia. She was able to mobilize with a frame for a few steps only. Her medications included paracetamol, aspirin, clopidogrel, atenolol, ramipril, simvastatin, omeprazole, furosemide, and spironolactone.

On examination, the chest was clear, and the abdomen was soft with no tenderness or palpable masses. There was bilateral soft tissue oedema of her feet. During the examination, frequent scratching was observed, and she complained of itching. The care home staff member who accompanied her to hospital reported that she frequently awoke during the night complaining of itch.

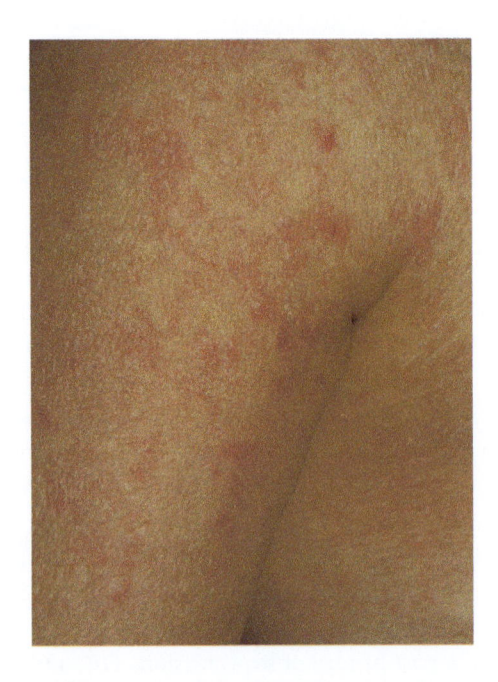

Fig. 34.1 Photograph of patient's upper arm and back.

Questions

1 Describe skin changes seen in Figure 34.1 and list the differential diagnosis for pruritus in older people.
2 How would you further investigate this patient?

Answers

1 Describe skin changes seen in Figure 34.1 and list the differential diagnosis for pruritus in older people.

Figure 34.1 shows asteatotic eczema, dry skin, scaly erythema, and excoriations. This patient suffers from generalized pruritus (itching), which is a common symptom in older patients. Older people are more prone to dry (itchy) skin owing to physiological changes in the structure of the skin with ageing (e.g. reduced secretion from sebaceous glands, changes in epidermis cells structure) causing reduced moisture retention. Also, older people are more likely to have co-morbidities associated with itch. The prevalence of pruritus rises with age, from ~10% at 16–30 years old to over 20% at ages 61–70 years, with some epidemiological data showing a prevalence of over 40% in the older population. Mechanisms of pruritus include:

- neuropathic, from nervous system pathology such as multiple sclerosis
- dermatological (e.g. dry skin)
- psychogenic (e.g. depression)
- systemic (e.g. chronic renal failure, anaemia).

The differential diagnosis for pruritus in older people includes:

- *A primary skin disorder,* such as dry skin xerosis, an abnormal dryness of the skin and asteatosis, characterized by a deficiency of sebaceous gland secretion, is the most common cause of pruritus in old age. Other common primary skin disorders include seborrhoeic dermatitis, contact dermatitis, psoriasis, and lichen planus. Bullous pemphigoid presents most commonly in older patients. Itchy 'urticated' skin may present before the blisters. Diagnosis is by skin biopsy and blood test for auto antigens. Treatment involves immunosupression. Aquagenic pruritus is a condition of unknown pathogenesis affecting older people following contact with water, however it is unlikely in the current case since it does not produce a rash.
- *Infection.* Scabies is easily missed and should always be considered in older people with generalized pruritus. In this case, the patient had moved to a nursing home and it seems that the itch had started subsequently. In view of her memory impairment, a careful history should be taken from her carers, to establish whether others in the nursing home or visitors were affected, and whether the itch was worse at night (common in scabies). Skin lesions in scabies (see Fig. 34.2) are characterized by linear excoriations and papules, often subtle, and burrows are best seen in the

web spaces of hands and feet, in intertriginous areas in the neck, axillae, genitals, around the nipples, or on the wrist flexor areas. In some cases, eczematization or secondary infection can hide burrows or papules. Other common infections include dermatophytosis (usually in the inguinal folds and upper thighs), pediculosis corporis, and folliculitis. In older patients with relevant risk factors and generalized pruritus, HIV-associated scabies should be considered (see case 30).

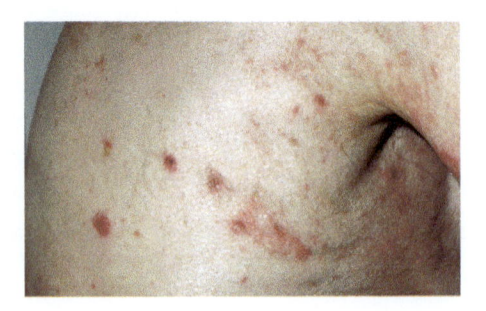

Fig. 34.2 Dry, itchy skin in an older patient with scabies.

- *Renal disease*: the uraemic pruritus of chronic renal failure (Fig. 34.3) is common among dialysis patients (see case 29). It is usually most prominent on the back, or around arterio-venous fistula sites, is worse at night-time, and sometimes during the dialysis procedure. Renal transplantion cures the itch.

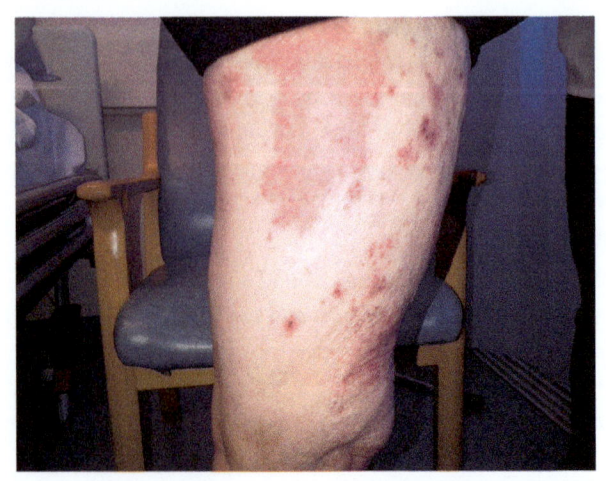

Fig. 34.3 Skin in an 84-year-old patient with chronic renal failure and long-standing pruritus, causing excoriations and eczematous changes.

- *Mixed causes, including drugs*: one recent study found that one in eight patients with drug reactions have pruritus without skin lesions. Recently started new drugs should be particularly scrutinized including statins (which also cause skin dryness), ACE inhibitors, opiates, barbiturates, plasma volume expanders, penicillins, and antidepressants.
- *Endocrine disease* (e.g. diabetes mellitus, hypothyroidism, hyperthyroidism).
- *Haematological diseases* (e.g. iron deficiency).
- *Liver and biliary diseases* (so-called cholestatic pruritus). This is usually generalized, but may involve sites otherwise uncommonly affected by pruritus, e.g. palms and soles.
- *Malignancies*—pruritus may precede the presentation of various neoplasms, sometimes by several years. It is less common with solid tumours, the most common associated malignancies are haematological, e.g. Hodgkin and non-Hodgkin lymphoma, leukaemias, multiple myeloma, and polycythaemia vera (PV). In PV, patients may have warm water-induced itch appearing within minutes after taking a bath. Patients with malignancy may also present with eruptive seborrhoeic keratosis, malignant acanthosis nigricans, or erythroderma. Pruritus is less common with solid tumours and may occur in brain tumours.
- *Neurological conditions* (neuropathic pruritus for which diagnostic clues may be the presence of burning sensations, pain, or sensory loss): cerebrovascular accidents; Creutzfeldt–Jakob disease; postherpetic neuralgia (around 60% of patients have pruritus at the site of herpes zoster); brachioradial pruritus; notalgia paraesthetica.
- *Connective tissue diseases* (e.g. dermatomyositis, systemic sclerosis, and systemic lupus erythematosus).
- *Burns, scars*.
- *Psychogenic* (e.g. in patients with depression, anxiety, delusional parasitosis). The diagnostic clue can be that pruritus in these conditions rarely disturbs patients' sleep. Such patients often complain of anogenital pruritus and candidosis should be considered in such cases.

The cause may not always be found despite extensive investigations. Age-related changes to skin affecting nerve fibres have not been well researched, but the loss of input from pain fibres may have a significant role in the pathogenesis of pruritus in later life.

2 How would you further investigate this patient?

A comprehensive history should be taken including from the carers in the present case, detailing the length of symptoms (pruritus is classed as chronic if lasting more than six weeks), generalized or localized nature, presence of nocturnal symptoms, and whether there are identifiable causal factors in drug or travel history, or contacts. Allergies should be considered and urticaria may be easily missed since the wheals are transient, lasting less than 24 hours. Constitutional symptoms including chills, fatigue, tiredness, weight loss, fever and night sweats, or history of psychiatric condition should be elicited.

The examination includes general systems, as well as the skin in which changes may be primary or secondary (excoriations). In some cases, the examination of the skin for dermographism may be useful, and a skin biopsy may need to be considered.

Investigations for generalized pruritus include:

- Full blood count, erythrocyte sedimentation rate
- Liver function tests, renal function tests, thyroid function tests, iron studies, serum and urine electrophoresis, blood glucose (in some cases PSA, plasma viscosity)
- Chest X-ray if indicated
- Urine examination, stool examination (depending on history—for ova and parasites, or occult blood)
- Hepatitis B and C serologies (in some cases HIV serology, autoimmune screen).

Further investigations may include endoscopy, CT, or MRI scans if underlying malignancy is considered.

Case development

It was established that no new drugs had been started at the time of onset of the pruritus.

Investigations showed the following:

- Hb 13.2g/dL; WCC 4.2 × 10^9/L Neut 2.4 × 10^9/L; HCt 0.55L/L
- Na 136mmol/L; K 3.6mmol/L; urea 6mmol/L; creat 120μmol/L; ALT 35IU/L; bili 6μmol/L; alp 250U/L; albumin 40g/L; iron 12mmol/l; ferritin 30glc 6mmol/L; CRP <6mg/L
- Urine dipstick: negative
- Stool: negative for ova, parasites, and cysts
- Urine and blood cultures: negative
- CXR: enlarged heart
- ECG: 55bpm, AF, LVH.

Questions continued

3 What is the most likely cause of her pruritus?
4 Describe how you would manage this patient and the general principles of managing older patients with pruritus.

Answers continued

3 What is the most likely cause of her pruritus?

The most likely cause of this patient's pruritus with associated poor sleep pattern, poor appetite, and normal investigations is xerosis (dry skin) with fine scaling, and epidermal cracking. The patient's symptoms became much more prominent after admission to the care home, probably because of the low humidity from the home's central heating (older people are less able to cope with rapid changes of environment from a warm home to very cold outdoors in winter months).

The patient had dry and scaly skin, most prominent on the extensor aspects of the arms, dorsum of hands, and on the shins, and did not have any typical signs of scabies. Xerosis is a common cause of pruritus in older patients and typically gets worse during the winter months. It is often seen after admission to hospital because of enthusiastic washing. It may develop into asteatotic eczema, which is characterized by dryness as well as inflammation.

4 Describe how you would manage this patient and the general principles of managing older patients with pruritus.

The main aim of treatment is to correct skin dryness and she and her carers were advised to use aqueous cream instead of soap or gel for washing. The cream (any type of moisturizing cream may be used) should be applied to the skin before contact with water. A generous amount of moisturizing cream with menthol was applied to the skin with excellent results.

Data on the efficacy of pruritus treatments are scarce. Treatment involves identifying the cause and applying aetiological therapy (if possible). General measures include trimming nails to prevent scratching, the use of cotton clothing and the avoidance of alcohol, spices, and some drugs (e.g. allopurinol) which might intensify the sensation.

In asteatotic eczema/xerosis, the skin dryness and irritation should be minimized by the use of soap substitutes since the sebaceous glands of older people are less active and the resulting asteatosis is made worse by soaps and over-frequent washing. Emollients (moisturizing lotions and creams, e.g. cetraben, aqueous cream with 1% menthol) and bath oil should be sufficient to settle irritation in most patients. Further measures may include covering skin with a paste bandage or Zipsoc stocking, which sooths and protects skin from finger nails—thus reducing the itch/scratch cycle.

Depending on the cause of pruritus, the following may be appropriate:

- Avoiding contact allergen (patch testing may be indicated)
- Discontinuing culprit medications

- Pursuing anti-microbial or antifungal therapy
- Treating any underlying condition (depression, tumour, renal failure)
- Drugs including:
  - topical corticosteroids (usually for localized pruritus)
  - topical capsaicin—despite poor evidence of efficacy, it is often used in cases with neuropathic pruritus
  - topical antihistamines—only some available evidence for topical doxepin in atopic dermatitis
  - oral antihistamines—despite poor evidence these are often used for generalized pruritus. They may be useful for patients with poor sleep, but may cause confusion and falls
  - μ-opioid receptor antagonists (e.g. naltrexone) for cholestatic pruritus
  - antidepressants—SSRIs; tricyclic antidepressants; there is some evidence that mirtazapine may have H1 antihistaminic and serotonergic effects, and might be effective in pruritus associated with uraemia, atopic dermatitis, neurotic excoriations, and some malignancies
  - anticonvulsants—some evidence (e.g. gabapentin, pregabalin)
  - immunosuppressants for atopic dermatitis
  - phototherapy—may be useful for the older patients taking multiple medications
  - systemic steroids in cases of intractable pruritus.

Further reading

Fett N, Haynes K, Propert KJ, Margolis DJ (2014). Five-year malignancy incidence in patients with chronic pruritus: a population-based cohort study aimed at limiting unnecessary screening practices. *J Am Acad Dermatol*; **70**: 651–658.

Ikoma A, Steinhoff M, Ständer S, Yosipovitch G, Schmelz M (2006). The neurobiology of itch. *Nat Rev Neurosci*; **7**: 535–547.

Raksha MP, Marfatia YS (2008). Clinical study of cutaneous drug eruptions in 200 patients. *Indian J Dermatol Venereol Leprol*; **74**: 80.

Ständer S, Schäfer I, Phan NQ, *et al.* (2010). Prevalence of chronic pruritus in Germany—results of a cross-sectional study in a sample working population of 11,730. *Dermatology*; **221**: 229–235.

Ständer S, Weisshaar E, Mettang T, *et al.* (2007). Clinical classification of itch: a position paper of the International Forum for the Study of Itch. *Acta Derm Venereol*; **87**: 291–294.

Case 35

A 78-year-old retired banker was reviewed by the GP for breathlessness, which had gradually worsened over the past four years. He now found himself breathless on minimal exertion around his flat, which he shared with his wife. He had a maximum exercise tolerance of 40 yards on the flat.

He had had many falls over the previous few months, with a frequency of around one every fortnight occurring when rising from a chair or manoeuvring backwards with his Zimmer frame. He had not had any loss of consciousness but had been admitted to hospital briefly following the most recent fall, as he was unable to get up unaided.

He had been started on galantamine six months previously for presumed Alzheimer's dementia but his wife had not noticed any significant improvement in his short-term memory. He slept a lot in the day, and was reluctant to go outside the house.

Other medical history included type 2 diabetes, postural hypotension, gout, renal impairment, previous left total hip and knee replacement, thrombocytopenia, and depression.

Medications were aspirin 75mg od; simvastatin 20mg od; furosemide 80mg; metformin 500mg td; tamsulosin MR 400mcg od; citalopram 20mg od; ferrous gluconate 600mg od; allopurinol 300mg bd od; loperamide 2mg bd; omeprazole 20mg od and galantamine.

He was a lifelong non-smoker and drank minimal alcohol. He had had around 20kg of unintentional weight loss over the previous two years. He mobilized with a Zimmer frame indoors and a four-wheeled walker outside.

On examination, heart rate was 68bpm, and pulse was slow rising in character. His blood pressure was 148/88 with no significant postural drop. His JVP was not raised and there was no pedal or sacral oedema. There was an ejection systolic murmur with radiation to the carotids and the second heart sound was very soft. Abdomen was soft and non-tender with no palpable masses. There was some wasting of the quadriceps muscles and postural sway on standing. Grip strength was decreased. MMSE was 22/30 and MoCA was 18/30.

Questions

1 What is the cause of his breathlessness and what further investigations would you perform?
2 Discuss the prognosis and management options for this patient.

Answers

1 What is the cause of his breathlessness and what further investigations would you perform?

This patient's breathlessness is caused by severe aortic stenosis (AS), as evidenced by the systolic murmur radiating to the carotids, slow rising pulse, and quiet second heart sound.

AS affects 2–7% of patients over 65 years in Europe and North America, and 10% of patients over 80 years. The most common cause in older people is calcification of the aortic valve. AS may also be caused by rheumatic valve disease or a congenital bicuspid valve, commonly seen in men in their sixth decade. AS is progressive and as the valve tightens, the blood flow from the left ventricle is restricted. This causes a rise in left ventricular pressure, leading to an increase in cardiac workload, and subsequent left ventricular hypertrophy.

The classic triad of symptoms seen in patients with AS are: angina due to concomitant coronary artery disease, dyspnoea and dizziness, or syncope. These symptoms are all related to exertion. The normal response to exercise is to increase cardiac output, however, severe aortic stenosis prevents this response. Blood pressure then falls, coronary ischaemia and cardiac arrhythmias develop, causing angina, dyspnoea, and syncope. In the initial stages, patients are often asymptomatic, and it may take up to 10 years before patients develop symptoms.

Patients with AS are at risk of collapse and sudden death due to ventricular tachycardia, although this is rare in truly asymptomatic patients (<1%). However, the risk increases as symptoms develop.

The investigation of choice is an echocardiogram to visualize an often thickened, calcified, and immobile valve. It also provides information regarding left ventricular function and size and can be used to screen for other valve disease or additional aortic pathology. It can provide prognostic information and allows estimation of the valve gradient if left ventricular function is reasonable. Valve gradients ≥50mmHg and valve areas of ≤0.5cm^2 indicate severe stenosis. Cardiac catheterization is rarely done as a first line investigation but is useful for further management as of the patient, as it can provide additional information such as left ventricular function and presence of coronary artery disease.

CXR and ECG are useful to assess evidence of left ventricular failure, hypertrophy, and conduction abnormalities.

2 Discuss the prognosis and management options for this patient.

Once symptoms develop in aortic stenosis, prognosis is poor with survival of only two to three years if left untreated. Asymptomatic patients should be re-assessed regularly so that progression of AS may be managed promptly. Medical management does not alter prognosis of the disease but is aimed at relieving symptoms. It is also important to treat atherosclerotic risk factors, so while statins have not been shown to be useful in halting the progression of AS, they should be used in combination with ACE inhibitors, diuretics, and digoxin to address vascular risk factors if required. Antihypertensive medications should be titrated with care to avoid hypotension.

It is difficult to predict the rate of progression of AS in individual patients, however, studies have indicated that the valve area decreases on average at a rate of 0.1–0.3cm^2 per year and the gradient across the valve can increase by 10–15mmHg per year. Rate of progression is increased in older patients with chronic renal impairment and coronary artery disease.

Definitive management for AS is open heart surgery to replace the diseased aortic valve. However, this is a substantial procedure and is not without significant risk of morbidity and mortality, and will involve a significant period of postoperative recovery. In patients <70 years, operative mortality is 1–3%. This rises to 4–8% in selected older patients. Risk factors for increased perioperative mortality include older age, increased number of co-morbidities especially coronary heart disease, pulmonary hypertension, emergency procedure, female sex, evidence of left ventricular dysfunction, and previous cardiac surgery. Successful valve replacement leads to improved symptoms and quality of life, and long-term survival may be close to age-matched controls. Despite this, older patients tend to be under-referred for consideration of surgery.

In the current patient, aortic valve replacement carries a high perioperative risk. The patient has multiple co-morbidities and has a frailty syndrome.

The term *frailty* is difficult to define, but is closely related to the ageing process where multiple body systems lose their inbuilt reserves. Often frail patients have multiple co-morbidities and a relatively minor insult can lead to major change in their functional ability and care needs. The Fried clinical phenotype of frailty scores patients for five different characteristics:

- unintentional weight loss
- fatigue or exhaustion
- low energy expenditure
- reduced gait speed
- reduced muscle strength.

Patients scoring 0/5 are termed robust, 1–2/5 pre frail and 3–5/5 frail. However, patients with MMSE of <18 were excluded in the original classification study, so the relationship between this model of frailty and cognition is uncertain. However, patients who have underlying physical frailty tend to have lower cognitive reserves, and are more susceptible to delirium and dementia.

This patient would score at least 3 if using the Fried criteria and his history of Alzheimer's disease, depression, and polypharmacy (currently taking 10 medications) make him susceptible to delirium during the perioperative period (see case 1). He also has poor mobility with a number of recent falls. This together with his decreased muscle strength and probable sarcopenia (see case 5) would make rehabilitation lengthy and challenging. His diabetes and thrombocytopenia also increase the risk of conventional surgery. Figure 35.1 shows the decision-making flow chart for the treatment of severe AS.

In the current patient, a transcatheter aortic valve implantation (TAVI) procedure would be more suitable. A TAVI is usually carried out under a general anaesthetic or a local anaesthetic with sedation. The aortic valve is accessed transluminally, often via the subclavian, or femoral artery. The aortic valve ring is then dilated with a balloon catheter and the new prosthetic valve is positioned over the existing aortic valve. Recovery and length of stay post procedure is substantially reduced in patients undergoing TAVI, compared to those who have surgical aortic valve replacement.

The 30-day mortality rate is between 5–15% and complications include stroke (1–5%); need for permanent pacemaker (PPM-7% in patients with a balloon expanded system and 40% with a self-expanding system); and vascular complications (20%). Paravalvular regurgitation is common, although it is often mild, rarely of clinical significance, and does not affect long-term survival. 1–2% of patients undergoing a TAVI require emergency heart surgery due to life-threatening complications during the procedure. At one year, survival is around 60–80%, despite these patients frequently being frail with multiple co-morbidities. Most patients report a substantial improvement in symptoms following the procedure, although the long-term durability of the procedure is still being assessed. Preliminary three to five-year follow-up data are promising.

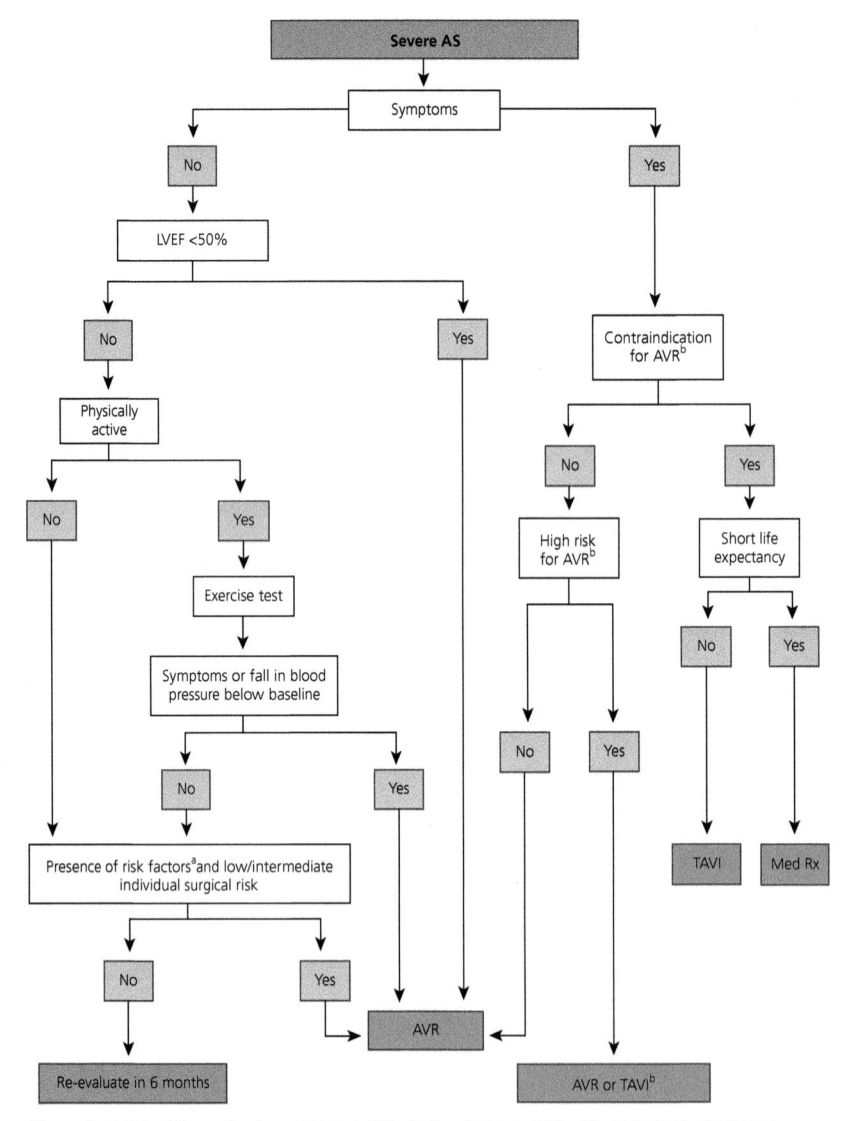

AS = aortic stenosis; AVR = aortic valve replacement; BSA = body surface area; LVEF = left ventricular ejection fraction; Med Rx = medical therapy; TAVI = transcatheter aortic valve implantation.

[a]Surgery should be considered (IIaC) if one of the following is present: peak velocity >5.5 m/s; severe valve calcification + peak velocity progression ≥0.3 m/s/year: Surgery may be considered (IIbC) if one of the following is present: markedly elevated natriuretic peptide levels; mean gradient increase with exercise >20 mmHg: excessive LV hypertrophy.

[b]the decision should be made by the 'heart team' according to individual clinical characteristics and anatomy..

Fig. 35.1 Flow chart for the management of severe aortic stenosis.

(Vahanian, Alec *et al.*, Guidelines on the management of valvular heart disease (version 2012). *European Heart Journal* (2012), 33:19: p2451–2496. With permission of Oxford University Press (UK) © European Society of Cardiology, http://www.escardio.org/guidelines.)

Further reading

Guidelines on the management of valvular heart disease (version 2012). The Joint Task Force on the Management of Valvular Heart Disease of the European Society of Cardiology (ESC) and the European Association for Cardio-Thoracic Surgery (EACTS).

NICE guidance: Transcatheter aortic valve implantation for aortic stenosis (March 2012). NICE interventional procedure guidance [IPG421].

British Geriatrics Society (2015). Fit For Frailty Guidance.

Case 36

A 74-year-old man was brought to the emergency department by his wife and son, who were worried about his odd behaviour. He had been well until two days before when he had become confused and disorientated. There was a past history of left total knee replacement, osteoarthritis of the right knee, and a stroke two years earlier, from which he had recovered physically, but had required treatment for depression. He did not smoke, was teetotal, and was usually independent and self-caring, working twice a week in a local charity shop. Medications were aspirin, amlodipine, paracetamol, sertraline, and tramadol. Trazodone had recently been prescribed by his GP for difficulty sleeping.

On examination, he was shivering and restless with rambling speech, and pyrexia of 38.5°C. Pulse was 110bpm regular, blood pressure was 190/90mmHg, respiratory rate was 22 per minute, and oxygen saturations on room air were 98%. General systems were unremarkable. There was tremor in the right hand and arm, increased rigidity and brisk reflexes in all limbs, and occasional myoclonus. His AMTS was 0/10 and CAM was positive at 4/4.

Initial investigations showed the following:

- Blood tests, including full blood count, electrolytes, liver and renal function tests, TFTs, coagulation studies, glucose and creatine kinase: all normal
- Urine myoglobin, urine dipstick: normal
- Blood and urine cultures: results awaited
- Acetaminophen, ethanol, and salicylate: not detected
- ECG: sinus rhythm, heart rate 110bpm, regular
- CXR: normal
- CT brain scan: no abnormalities seen
- EEG: non-specific changes, no evidence of seizure activity
- Lumbar puncture: normal.

The admitting doctor prescribed erythromycin for a presumed chest infection, but overnight he deteriorated further, and by morning he was hallucinating and sweating excessively. The muscular rigidity was worse, temperature was over 41°C, and blood pressure was 210/100mmHg.

Subsequently, blood and urine cultures were reported as negative.

Questions

1 What is the most likely diagnosis in this patient and why may older patients be particularly at risk of developing this syndrome?
2 Which alternative diagnoses would you have considered?
3 Why did the patient develop this syndrome?
4 Describe common features of this syndrome and the markers of severity.
5 How would you make the diagnosis?
6 How would you treat this patient?

Answers

1 What is the most likely diagnosis in this patient and why may older patients particularly be at risk of developing this condition?

The most likely diagnosis is serotonin syndrome, a hyperserotonergic state in which there is hyperstimulation of 5-HT1A and 5-HT2 receptors in the brain stem and spinal cord. This is not an idiosyncratic reaction, but is a result of serotonin toxicity caused by drugs that increase serotonin production or its release, inhibit serotonin reuptake and metabolism, or increase postsynaptic receptor sensitivity.

The incidence of serotonin syndrome is increasing (although it remains under-diagnosed) owing to increased availability and use of serotonergic drugs (most frequently selective serotonin reuptake inhibitors), and the ageing population. Older patients are more often on multiple drugs that may include other serotoninergic medications.

Serotonin syndrome usually starts within the first 24 hours (usually within six to eight hours) of:

- initiating a serotonergic drug.
- increasing the dose of serotonergic drug(s).
- combining two or more serotonergic drugs, including lithium.
- combining serotonergic drugs with others that affect their metabolism. For example, selective serotonin reuptake inhibitors with drugs that inhibit the cytochrome P450 2D6 and/or 3A4 isoenzymes, or with monoamine oxidase inhibitors, which inhibit the breakdown of serotonin.
- overdose of a serotonergic agent. Serotonin syndrome occurs in around 15% of cases of selective serotonin reuptake inhibitors overdose, and in the case of venlafaxine (serotonin-norepinephrine reuptake inhibitor), the rate is around twice as high.

2 Which alternative diagnoses would you have considered?

The alternative diagnoses to consider include:

- *Delirium secondary to underlying infection*, intracerebral pathology (see cases 1 and 31) alcohol or drug withdrawal, but investigations were normal.
- *Neuroleptic malignant syndrome* can cause a similar clinical picture and is particularly difficult to differentiate from serotonin syndrome if dopamine antagonists and serotonergic drugs are being used in combination. In neuroleptic malignant syndrome, creatine phosphokinase is usually elevated, leucocytosis is common, and there may be a history of abrupt

withdrawal of a dopamine agonist. Level of consciousness is usually reduced and patients are akinetic with prominent rigidity and bradyreflexia, and myoclonus is not seen. Neuroleptic malignant syndrome usually develops and recovers more slowly than serotonin syndrome, over days or weeks.

- *Lethal (malignant) catatonia*—(see case 26, *Case Histories in Acute Neurology and the Neurology of General Medicine*). Patients with catatonia usually have pre-existing psychosis and symptoms including extreme negativism, mutism, immobility, echolalia or echopraxia, excessive motor activity, and peculiar involuntary movements may occur.
- *Anticholinergic toxicity*—agents that block central and peripheral muscarinic cholinergic receptors may cause red skin colour changes, dry mouth, urinary retention, hyperthermia, agitation, altered mental status, mydriasis, and dry mucous membranes. However, muscular tone and reflexes are normal.
- *Overdose* with sympathomimetic drugs.
- *Migraine coma*—(see case 34, *Case Histories in Acute Neurology and the Neurology of General Medicine*), but this is unlikely in a patient with no history of migraine.
- *Non-convulsive status epilepticus*—(see case 31, *Case Histories in Acute Neurology and the Neurology of General Medicine*) may cause reduced consciousness, motor activity and stupor, but is unlikely in the absence of a history of epilepsy. The diagnosis can be excluded with EEG.

Other conditions which may produce a similar clinical picture, but which could not have been the cause in this case, include:

- *Malignant hyperthermia*. This may be accompanied by elevated creatine phosphokinase, potassium, and magnesium, disseminated intravascular coagulation, acidosis, and rhabdomyolysis. However, there was no recent exposure to anaesthetic agents in this case.
- *Thyrotoxic storm*—(see case 20, *Case Histories in Acute Neurology and the Neurology of General Medicine*).
- *Amphetamine overdose*.
- *Alcohol or drug withdrawal (see case 27)*. This typically causes agitation, confusion, and restlessness, but the increased tone would not be expected.
- *Heat stroke*—(see case 48).
- *CNS infection*.
- *Tetanus*.

3 Why did the patient develop this syndrome?

This patient had been taking two serotonergic drugs: sertraline (a selective serotonin reuptake inhibitor) and the analgesic, tramadol. The latter has opioid agonist and serotonin reuptake inhibitor characteristics, and is metabolized by the cytochrome P (CYP)-450 iso-enzyme 2D6 and CYP3A4. The combination of tramadol and selective serotonin reuptake inhibitors has been reported to cause serotonin syndrome. The patient was then given trazodone, which further inhibited serotonin reuptake. After admission to hospital, the patient's clinical condition deteriorated, as all medications were continued and erythromycin was prescribed, which would have further inhibited cytochrome P450.

Drugs that can cause serotonin syndrome include:

- *Monoamine oxidase inhibitors (MOIs)*, e.g. tranylcypromine, phenelzine, moclobemide, particularly dangerous in combination with selective serotonin reuptake inhibitors, and may cause fatalities. When switching from a selective serotonin reuptake inhibitor to a monoamine oxidase inhibitor, a washout period of at least five times the half-life of the selective serotonin reuptake inhibitor is recommended. In the majority of cases with severe serotonin syndrome, MOIs were involved.
- *Selective serotonin reuptake inhibitors*, e.g. citalopram, fluoxetine, fluvoxamine, paroxetine, sertraline.
- *Serotonin and norepinephrine reuptake inhibitors*, e.g. venlafaxine, duloxetine.
- *Tricyclic antidepressants*, e.g. clomipramine, imipramine.
- *Bupropion*—has a weak selective serotonin reuptake inhibitor activity.
- *Lithium*.
- *Over-the-counter drugs, herbs, and weight-loss medications*, e.g. nutmeg, Panax ginseng, or St. John's Wort (Hypericum perforatum), which contains hypericin and hyperforin that inhibit the synaptic uptake of monoamines, nefazodone, fenfluramine.
- *Analgesics*, e.g. dextromethorphan, tramadol, fentanyl, pethidine, oxycodone, buprenorphine, methadone, dextropropoxyphene, pentazocine.
- *Atypical antipsychotics*. Serotonin syndrome has been reported in combinations of risperidone with paroxetine; olanzapine with mirtazapine and tramadol; olanzapine with lithium and citalopram.
- *Antibiotics* that significantly inhibit cytochrome P450 enzymes that metabolize serotonergic agents, e.g. clarithromycin and ketoconazole.

Linezolid causes monoamine oxidase inhibition and cases of serotonin syndrome have been reported when linezolid was taken with paroxetine, sertraline, and some over-the-counter drugs.

- *Miscellaneous drugs.* Manufacturers may place warnings based on theoretical concerns, e.g. sumatriptan and ondansetron are serotonergic agents, but they work through distinct 5-HT receptor systems probably unrelated to serotonin syndrome. Other drugs that have been implicated include: antihistamines; psychedelic drugs (LSD, MDA, MDMA 'ecstasy'); CNS stimulants and serotonin releasers (amphetamine, cocaine, methamphetamine); anticonvulsants such as carbamazepine, valproate, antiretroviral drugs (in combination with fluoxetine).

4 Describe common features of this syndrome and the markers of severity.

The following symptoms and signs characterize serotonin syndrome, but not all are necessarily present simultaneously:

- *Mental status changes.* Restlessness, disorientation, hypervigilance, anxiety, confusion, agitation, delirium, hallucinations, lethargy, drowsiness, and coma.
- *Autonomic instability.* Hyperthermia (in severe cases the temperature may be over 41°C), tachycardia, hypertension, hypotension, tachypnoea, dilated pupils, excessive lacrimation, flushing, excessive sweating, shivering, diarrhoea, abdominal cramps, and vomiting.
- *Neurological/neuromuscular abnormalities.* Tremor, rigidity (can be more prominent in lower than in upper limbs), hyper-reflexia, akathisia, motor restlessness, myoclonus, spontaneous or inducible clonus (usually easily induced by ankle dorsiflexion), ocular myoclonus (rapid contractions of the eye muscles, 'ping-pong gaze' or oscillations of gaze in all directions), nystagmus, ataxia/incoordination, and bilateral upgoing plantars.

Serotonin syndrome varies widely in severity, but may be life-threatening, and a case-fatality of over 10% has been reported.

Indicators of severity include:

- increasing tone and progressive rigidity, particularly truncal rigidity
- high-grade fever (> 38.5°C)—usually rapid rising
- compromised respiratory function with rising pCO_2.

Potentially lethal complications of serotonin syndrome include:

- rhabdomyolysis
- adult respiratory distress syndrome

- hypotension
- ventricular tachycardia
- metabolic acidosis
- renal failure
- disseminated intravascular coagulopathy
- seizures
- coma.

5 How would you make the diagnosis?

The diagnosis of serotonin syndrome requires recognition of the clinical syndrome and exclusion of alternative diagnoses. The Hunter Toxicity Criteria Decision Rules (high specificity and sensitivity for the diagnosis) present the best available diagnostic criteria for serotonin syndrome and include the following:

- The use of serotonergic agents (including amphetamine and its derivatives) or certain dietary supplements within the past five weeks. Fluoxetine and paroxetine have half-lives of up to five weeks and are potent inhibitors of CYP2D6, as well as being substrates, and can thus prolong the half-lives of many other drugs for weeks after being stopped.
- The presence of one of the following:
  - tremor and hyper-reflexia
  - hypertonia and body temperature >38.5°C
  - spontaneous clonus, or inducible clonus and agitation, or diaphoresis.

6 How would you treat this patient?

Once the diagnosis of serotonin syndrome was made, all serotonergic drugs were stopped immediately. The patient was given oxygen, intravenous fluids, intravenous nitroprusside for blood pressure control and active external cooling was applied with ice, fans, and a cooling blanket. He recovered well over the next 24 hours.

Treatment of serotonin syndrome is based on anecdotal reports, as no prospective studies evaluating pharmacological treatments exist. Treatment generally includes:

- Stopping all serotonergic drugs.
- Supportive care—oxygen, cardiac monitoring, intravenous fluids.
- Intravenous chlorpromazine for severe toxicity (serotonin antagonist—most commonly used for severe toxicity).

- Control of specific features: hypertension and tachycardia are treated with short-acting agents; hyperthermia with external cooling measures (e.g. ice, as antipyretic agents are ineffective). Benzodiazepines are given for treatment of rigidity, seizures, and agitation. For patients with severe manifestations cyproheptadine (5-HT2 antagonist) could be considered, despite lack of evidence for its efficacy.
- In cases where there is severe rigidity and hyperpyrexia, ventilating the patient with neuromuscular blockade can achieve rapid resolution of hyperpyrexia suggesting that at least some of the elevated temperature may be driven by peripheral muscle rigidity.
- After recovery the risks and benefits of reintroducing serotonergic agent(s) should be carefully assessed.

Further reading

Ables AZ, Nagubilli R (2010). Prevention, recognition, and management of serotonin syndrome. *Am Fam Physician*; **81**(9): 1139–1142.

Bleakley S. Review of choice and use of antidepressants (2009). *Progress in Neurology and Psychiatry*; **13**(1): 14–20.

Boyer EW, Shannon M (2005). The serotonin syndrome. *N Engl J Med*; **352**: 1112–1120.

Buckley NA, Dawson AH, Isbister GK (2014). Serotonin syndrome; *BMJ*; **348**: g1626.

Dunkley EJ, Isbister GK, Sibbritt D, Dawson AH, Whyte IM (2003). The Hunter Serotonin Toxicity Criteria: simple and accurate diagnostic decision rules for serotonin toxicity. *QJM*: **96**: 635–642.

Gillman PK (2006). A review of serotonin toxicity data: implications for the mechanisms of antidepressant drug action. *Biol Psychiatry*; **59**: 1046–1051.

Case 37

Case 37.A

A GP referred a 74-year-old woman to the rapid access clinic with decreased mobility, tiredness, and long-standing severe left knee pain that became worse at night. She was persistently sleepy during the day and awake all night, and had sustained two falls over recent months. She was usually independent in all daily activities and lived with her partner in a ground floor flat. There was a history of osteoarthritis of the knees, a right total knee replacement, and she was awaiting left knee replacement. There was no history of anxiety or depression. She drank an occasional glass of sherry, and medication was paracetamol and ibuprofen. On examination, she was apyrexial, pulse was 80bpm, and blood pressure was 120/65mmHg without postural drop. The rest of the examination was normal.

Investigations showed the following:

- FBC, U&Es, LFTs, TFTs, CRP, urine dipstick: normal
- Ferritin 35µg/L; folate 8µg/L; vitamin B_{12} 880ng/L
- ECG; sinus rhythm; heart rate 72bpm regular
- CXR: normal.

Case 37.B

A 76-year-old man was referred by his GP to the geratology out-patient clinic with a history of tiredness, loss of energy, poor appetite, and poor sleep. He reported frequently waking up his partner by getting up owing to painful sensations in his legs in the evenings, relieved by movement. Past medical history included myocardial infarction four years earlier, and hypercholesterolaemia. He was taking paracetamol, aspirin, simvastatin, lisinopril, and bisoprolol. The examination was unremarkable.

Investigations showed the following:

- FBC, U&Es, LFTs, TFTs, CRP, urine dipstick: normal
- Ferritin 30µg/L; folate 7µg/L; vitamin B_{12} 680ng/L
- ECG-HR 55/min regular; Q wave in I, II, and aVF leads
- CXR: normal.

Case 37.C

A 68-year-old man was referred to the out-patient clinic with poor concentration and a need for frequent rests during the day with poor, unrestorative sleep. Past medical history included hypertension and diabetes mellitus, and his GP had recently diagnosed depression. His wife had stopped sleeping in the same room with him several years previously on account of his loud snoring. Medications were metformin, gliclazide, ramipril, bendroflumethiazide, amlodipine, and aspirin. The examination was unremarkable except for obesity (BMI was 33).

Investigations were all normal except for HBA1C of 10% and random glucose of 14mmol/L.

Questions

1 What is the group of disorders exemplified by these cases?
2 What is the most likely underlying diagnosis in each case?
3 List at least two other examples of these disorders.
4 How would you investigate patients presenting with these conditions?
5 How would you manage these patients?

Answers

1 What is the group of disorders exemplified by these cases?

All these patients have a sleep disorder. Sleep disorders are often under-diagnosed and are only rarely spontaneously reported by older patients, despite being common. The prevalence of sleep disorders increases with age and more often affects women. The condition is more common among residents of long-term care facilities than in the general older population owing to exposure to night-time noise, higher prevalence of physical and mental conditions (e.g. dementia), incontinence, lack of exposure to daylight, and reduced exercise. Sleep disorders are also more likely to affect people exposed to acute or chronic stress, with anxiety-prone personality, or who have a personal or family history of insomnia.

The impact of physiological brain ageing on sleep is not well understood, nor are the effects of sleep on memory in older people. It is known that in older individuals, reduction in pineal gland production of melatonin and in the number of neurons in the supra-chiasmatic nucleus of the hypothalamus probably contributes to reduced sleep efficiency, shorter sleeping time, early morning waking, night-time wakefulness, longer sleep latency, and more day-time napping.

Sleep disorders are associated with:

- poor health
- poor quality of life
- increased day-time sleepiness
- increased accidents and falls
- increased functional impairment
- increased healthcare costs
- increased rate of institutionalization
- increased mortality
- difficulties with concentration and memory
- depression, anxiety, dementia, Parkinson's disease, heart failure
- poor balance
- risk of delirium in hospitalized patients
- three to five-fold increased overall risk of hypertension
- in some cases (e.g. obstructive sleep apnoea) with an increased risk of stroke.

2 What is the most likely underlying diagnosis in each case?

In case A, the diagnosis is insomnia associated with poor control of knee pain.

Insomnia is the most common sleep disorder in older people (around 6–10% of all sleep disorders) and is defined as impaired day-time function in patients complaining of poor quality sleep, difficulties in initiating and maintaining sleep or early waking, despite having good circumstances for sleep. Insomnia often presents as a symptom of other sleeping disorders. Insomnia may be acute (<1 month), sub-chronic (1–3 months), or chronic (>3 months). Insomnia may occur spontaneously, for example owing to inadequate sleep hygiene, or in relation to co-existing disorders—medical (e.g. back pain), or psychiatric (e.g. depression). It has been estimated that around 50% of people >60 years old experience insomnia and associations have been reported with increased risk of cognitive decline, mood disorder, and depression.

In case B, the diagnosis is restless legs syndrome, a subcategory of sleep-related movement disorder.

Restless legs syndrome is found in around 10% of older people (>70 years). There may be a family history of restless leg syndrome and it is more common in patients with peripheral neuropathy, end-stage renal failure, and iron deficiency. Patients have the urge to move their legs, which relieves the unpleasant, sometimes painful, leg sensations. Commonly these symptoms occur prior to or at onset of sleep, causing difficulty with falling asleep or waking during the night on account of leg discomfort. A recent study assessed possible mechanisms underlying this condition and apart from dopaminergic dysfunction identified involvement of the glutamatergic system.

In case C, the diagnosis is most probably obstructive sleep apnoea (OSA), a subcategory of sleep-related breathing disorder.

Sleep apnoea may be:

- obstructive (caused by increased airways resistance during inspiration, caused by pharyngeal collapse)
- central (loss of ventilatory drive caused by primary neurological disease, drugs, high altitude).

OSA is characterized by snoring and episodic obstruction to airflow for 10 seconds or more during sleep (apnoea). Patients may awake gasping, but in the majority of cases, snoring is the main symptom. The prevalence of sleep apnoea increases with age and obesity. There is some evidence that patients with Alzheimer's and vascular dementia have higher incidence of snoring and obstructive sleep apnoea.

3 List at least two other examples of these disorders.

The most common other sleep disorders are:

- *Drug related*, caused by withdrawal of some drugs, e.g. opioids, alcohol, antidepressants (some SSRIs, TCA) or intake of other including alcohol, steroids, thyroid hormone preparations, and some antidepressants.
- *Circadian rhythm sleep disorder*, caused by mismatch between the person's sleep-wake cycle and the environment, e.g. early morning awakening and difficulty staying up until bedtime (commoner in older patients).
- *Periodic limb movement disorder* in which the legs kick or jerk, with rhythmic, repetitive, stereotyped movements during sleep over 20 to 40 seconds, waking the patient, and causing day-time sleepiness.
- Rapid-eye-movement (REM) sleep behaviour disorder (RBD). There may be a family history and/or history of self-injury during sleep or injury to a bed partner during REM sleep, which may be associated with violent behaviour and vivid dreams. Movements range from simple jerks to running, swearing, punching, kicking, and usually occur towards the end of the night. The prevalence of this sleep disorder rises with age and is more common in men than in women. It is present in up to 50% of patients with Parkinson's disease, around 70% of patients with Lewy body dementia (see case 25) and more than 90% of patients with multiple system atrophy (see case 40), and may antedate these conditions by several years. One small study has shown that over 80% of patients with idiopathic RBD developed a synucleinopathy during median follow-up of six years. REM sleep disorder may also be associated with some drugs including selective serotonine uptake inhibitors, anticholinergics, monoamine oxidase inhibitors, and tricyclic antidepressants.

There are more than 70 other sleeping disorders, according to the *International Classification of Sleep Disorders (ICSD-2)*, 2nd edition.

4 How would you investigate patients presenting with these conditions?

A comprehensive history should be obtained, including a daily sleep diary with particular reference to the following:

- A thorough history of sleep patterns and day-time functioning including day-time naps, recent stressors such as retirement, sleep history (e.g. sleep pattern at night, the number of awakenings) and information from a bedroom partner (snoring, limb movements, interrupted breathing, shortness of breath, confusion on wakening, sleepwalking).

- History of medical symptoms (e.g. headaches, pain at night, orthopnoea, gastroesophageal reflux, nocturia) and of psychiatric conditions (e.g. dementia, depression, panic attacks). Patients may need formal assessment for cognitive impairment or depression.
- Identification of drugs (newly started or recently stopped) that may contribute to sleep disorders: decongestants; diuretics; antihypertensives (e.g. calcium channel blockers, beta-blockers); xanthines-theophylline; analgesics; anti-Parkinsonian drugs; over-the-counter and herbal medications.
- Alcohol, caffeine and nicotine intake, and food eaten towards bedtime.
- Laboratory tests: glucose; haemoglobin A1C (HBA1C); iron studies; renal function in cases of suspected restless legs syndrome or periodic leg movement disorder; and thyroid function tests (e.g. hypothyroidism predisposes to obstructive sleep apnoea).
- Polysomnography is indicated in cases of suspected sleep-related movement disorders or sleep-related breathing disorders, in potentially self-injurious behaviour during sleep and in patients resistant to sleep interventions. A snoring history may also warrant ear, nose, and throat specialist examination to look for nasal pathology or excessive oropharyngeal tissue.

Patients A and B did not need further investigation since the diagnoses could be made with confidence from the clinical history. Patient C had height, weight, and neck circumference measured, and was referred for polysomnography.

5 How would you manage these patients?

All patients should have underlying conditions treated. For case A, better pain control was the priority. For case B with restless legs syndrome, dopaminergic agents (e.g. dopamine agonists, levodopa) were recommended. Treatment of iron deficiency, where present, may also help. For case C, treatment with nocturnal continuous positive airway pressure (CPAP) was initiated with good effect. Mandibular devices may be considered in cases of intolerance to CPAP (e.g. where there is claustrophobia from tight fitting masks). A possible novel treatment involves electrical stimulation of the hypoglossal nerve by a pacemaker that is synchronized with chest inspiration, causing the tongue to be pulled forwards, and this may prove helpful in patients for whom present devices are ineffective or not tolerated.

In general, treatment should be initiated if a sleep disorder causes impairment of quality of life and functioning. General measures include:

   i. A trial of improved sleep hygiene and elimination of day-time naps. Sleep hygiene calls for a routine of preparation for bed and a comfortable night-time environment in terms of temperature, quietness, and darkness. Daily exercise and, where appropriate, weight loss should be encouraged together with reduction or elimination of alcohol, caffeine, and nicotine before bedtime.

ii. Cognitive behavioural therapy delivered individually or in small groups may be considered for primary or co-morbid persistent insomnia in older patients. A recent meta-analysis indicates that cognitive behavioural therapy and drug treatment produce similar improvement during the treatment period, but cognitive behavioural therapy confers longer-term benefit.

iii. Drugs: there is a lack of evidence for hypnotic drugs in older people and current recommendations emphasize starting at low dose with frequent regular review and short-term use. The most commonly used drugs are benzodiazepines, non-benzodiazepine benzodiazepine receptor agonists ('Z-drugs' zopiclone, zolpidem, zaleplon) and other hypnotics. In some cases sedating antidepressants are used as are sedating antihistamines (e.g. diphenhydramine).

The dose and the choice of drugs prescribed for older people will depend on:

- age (lower dose for older patients)
- co-morbidities (e.g. renal, hepatic, or pulmonary disease)
- response to previous treatment
- the nature of sleep disorder symptoms.

Hypnotic agents may be effective in secondary insomnia, caused by pain for example, and if given with selective serotonin reuptake inhibitor in insomnia related to depression and anxiety. All hypnotics increase the risk of falls in older people and those with very short half-lives (zaleplon and zolpidem) may not maintain sleep through the night. Systematic reviews for adverse events show these to be less common and less severe with Z-drugs than with long acting benzodiazepines. Long-term hypnotic treatment should be avoided, on account of tolerance, and the risk of dependence. The effect from sedative drugs in older patients is more likely to be more harmful than beneficial in the longer term. Melatonin agonists have reportedly shown modest benefit in delayed sleep phase syndrome with fewer serious side effects compared to hypnotics, but data are few. Herbal preparations have not been shown to improve quantitative measures of sleep in meta-analyses. Currently, there is no evidence for effective therapy in dementia-related sleep disorders.

Further reading

Allen RP, Barker PB, Horská A, Earley CJ (2013). Thalamic glutamate/glutamine in restless legs syndrome: increased and related to disturbed sleep. *Neurology*; **80**(22): 2028–2034.

Ancoli-Israel S, Ayalon L (2009). Diagnosis and treatment of sleep disorders in older adults. *Focus*; **7**: 98–105.

Arnuff I (2015). Sleep: what the day owes the night. *Lancet Neurol*; **14**(1): 19–20.

Chung F, Subramanyam R, Liao P, Sasaki E, Shapiro C, Sun Y (2012). High STOP-Bang score indicates a high probability of obstructive sleep apnoea. *Br J Anaesth*; **108**: 768–775.

Cricco M, Simonsick EM, Foley DJ (2001). The impact of insomnia on cognitive functioning in older adults. *J Am Geriatr Soc*; **49**(9): 1185–1189.

Iranzo A, Tolosa E, Gelpi E, et al. (2013). Neurodegenerative disease status and postmortem pathology in idiopathic rapid-eye-movement sleep behaviour disorder: an observational cohort study. *Lancet Neurol*; **12**(5): 443–453.

Morin CM, Benca R (2012). Chronic insomnia. *Lancet*; **379**: 1129–1141.

Morin CM, LeBlanc M, Daley M, Gregoire JP, Merette C (2006). Epidemiology of insomnia: prevalence, self-help treatments, consultations, and determinants of help-seeking behaviors. *Sleep Med*; **7**(2): 123–130.

Redline S, Yenokyan G, Gottlieb DJ, et al. (2010). Obstructive sleep apnea-hypopnea and incident stroke: the sleep heart health study. *Am J Respir Crit Care Med*; **182**: 269–277.

Riemann D, Perlis ML (2009). The treatments of chronic insomnia: A review of benzodiazepine receptor agonists and psychological and behavioral therapies. *Sleep Med Rev*; **13**: 205–214.

Santamaria J, Iranzo A (2014). Sleep disorders matter in neurology. *Lancet Neurol*; **13**(1): 18–20.

Strollo PJ Jr, Soose RJ, Maurer JT, et al. (2014). Upper-airway stimulation for obstructive sleep apnea. *N Engl J Med*; **370**: 139–149.

Roepke SK, Ancoli-Israel S (2010). Sleep disorders in the elderly. *Indian J Med Res*; **131**: 302–310.

Unruh ML, Redline S, An MW, et al. (2008). Subjective and objective sleep quality and aging in the sleep heart health study. *J Am Geriatr Soc*; **56**: 1218–1227.

West S, Prudon B (2013). Sleep medicine—prevalent and relevant. *Clin Med*; **13**(5): 492–494.

Yaggi HK, Concato J, Kernan WN, Lichtman JH, Brass LM, Mohsenin V (2005). Obstructive sleep apnea as a risk factor for stroke and death. *N Engl J Med*; **353**: 2034–2041.

Case 38

A 67-year-old retired cleaner was admitted with increasing lethargy, abdominal fullness, and a painful right leg ulcer. The ulcer had not improved despite eight weeks' regular treatment and dressing by the district nurse. Past medical history included a myocardial infarction five years previously, and a right total knee replacement 18 months before.

On examination, she was pale. Heart rate was regular at 88bpm, respiratory rate 18 breaths per minute, oxygen saturation 97% on air, and temperature 36.2°C. Cardiovascular and respiratory examination was unremarkable. Abdominal examination revealed an enlarged spleen. The ulcer on the right leg was deep with a well-defined bluish edge, and was approximately 6cm in length with some surrounding erythema (Figs 38.1 and 38.2).

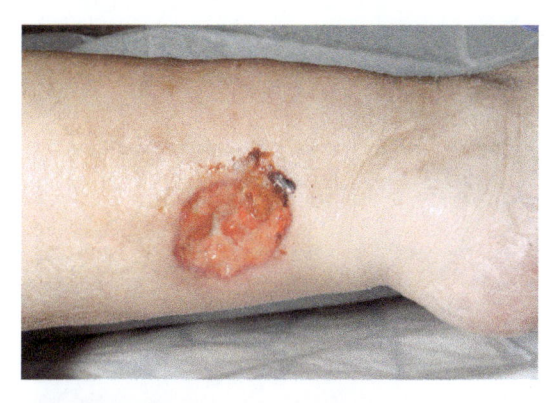

Fig. 38.1 Ulcer on the right lower leg.

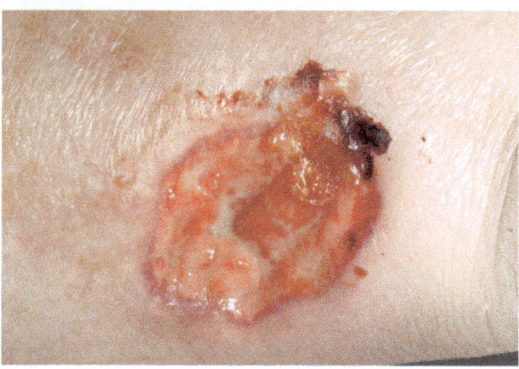

Fig. 38.2 A close-up of the ulcer shown in Fig. 38.1.

Investigations showed the following:

- Hb 8.2g/dL; WCC 14×10^9/L; neutrophils 8.0×10^9/L; lymphocytes 2.27×10^9/L; platelets 136×10^9/L
- U&E and LFT normal
- CRP: 27mg/L
- CXR: normal
- Abdominal ultrasound showed massive splenomegaly, as well as an enlarged liver (Fig. 38.3).

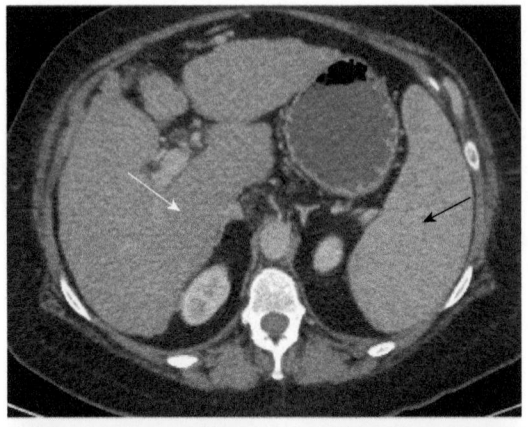

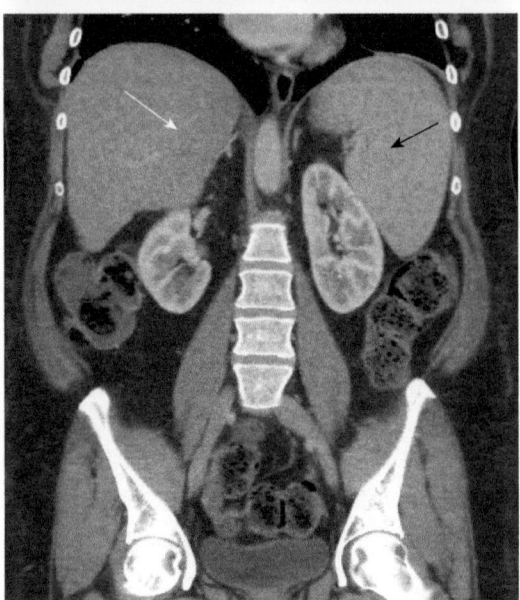

Fig. 38.3 Axial and coronal reconstruction of a portal phase contrast enhanced CT scan showing irregular liver (white arrow) with enlarged spleen (black arrow).

Questions

1 What are the possible causes of leg ulcers?
2 What is the most likely cause for the leg ulcer in this case and what is the underlying diagnosis? Which other conditions are associated with this type of leg ulcer?
3 How would you manage this type of leg ulcer?

Answers
1 What are the possible causes of leg ulcers?
Leg ulcers may be caused by a wide variety of pathologies including:
- Infection
  - bacterial, e.g. streptococcal, syphilitic (see case 30)
  - viral, e.g. herpes viruses
  - parasitic, e.g. amoebae
  - mycobacterial
- Malignancy
  - squamous cell carcinoma
  - basal cell carcinoma
  - cutaneous lymphoma
  - Kaposi's sarcoma
  - melanoma
- Vascular disease
  - arterial
  - venous
- Vasculitis
  - antiphospholipid syndrome
  - Behçet's disease
  - rheumatoid arthritis
  - systemic lupus erythematosus
  - Wegener's granulomatosis
- Blood diseases
  - sickle cell anaemia
  - polycythaemia, thrombocythaemia
- Neuropathic
  - diabetes
  - leprosy
  - alcohol
  - trauma
- Pressure (see case 14)
- Pyoderma gangrenosum
- Necrobiosis lipoidica.

2 What is the most likely cause for the leg ulcer in this case and what is the underlying diagnosis? Which other conditions are associated with this type of leg ulcer?

In older patients, the most common causes of ulcers are vascular and pressure-related.

The most likely cause of this patient's leg ulcer is pyoderma gangrenosum (PG) associated with underlying myelofibrosis. PG was first described in 1930. It is an uncommon cause of leg ulcers, but is important to recognize, as it is associated with an underlying systemic condition in around 50% of cases. The exact pathophysiology of the condition remains poorly understood, but it is thought that alterations in neutrophil chemotaxis within the immune system play a key role. The lesion starts as a small papule in the dermis, which goes on to break down and necrose the epidermis, eventually forming a well-defined painful ulcer with a violet or blue border. There are four types of PG:

- *classic ulcerative*, most commonly occurring on the legs
- *bullous*, usually occurring on the upper limbs and face often in association with haematological malignancies
- *pustular* is found on the trunk and extensor surfaces of the limbs almost exclusively in patients with concomitant inflammatory bowel disease
- *vegetative*, less aggressive than the other sub-types, is usually found as a single lesion in healthy patients. Vegetative PG normally responds better to local treatment than the other sub-types.

Histopathological findings in PG are nonspecific, but demonstrate neutrophil infiltration, epidermal necrosis, and haemorrhage. Although not diagnostic, skin biopsy is important to exclude other causes of slow-healing or chronic ulceration.

As stated earlier, approximately half all PG cases are associated with an underlying systemic condition. Commonly these include:

- Inflammatory bowel disease
  - ulcerative colitis
  - Crohn's disease
- Arthritic disease
  - seropositive rheumatoid arthritis
  - spondyloarthropathy
  - psoriatic arthritis
  - osteoarthritis

- Haematological disease
  - myeloid leukaemias
  - myelofibrosis
  - monoclonal gammopathy of unknown significance (often raised IgA)
- Immunological disease
  - Sjögrens syndrome
  - systemic lupus erythematosus.

The level of activity of underlying bowel or rheumatologic disease does not correspond to the severity and activity seen in the PG.

3 How would you manage this type of leg ulcer?

Once PG has been identified, investigations should be performed to look for an underlying systemic condition, and may include:

- FBC, U&E, LFT
- Inflammatory markers
- Protein electrophoresis
- ANA/ANCA and antiphospholipid screen
- Swab and culture
- Bone marrow biopsy
- Gastrointestinal imaging
- Skin biopsy (Fig. 38.4)
- Any underlying systemic condition should be treated.

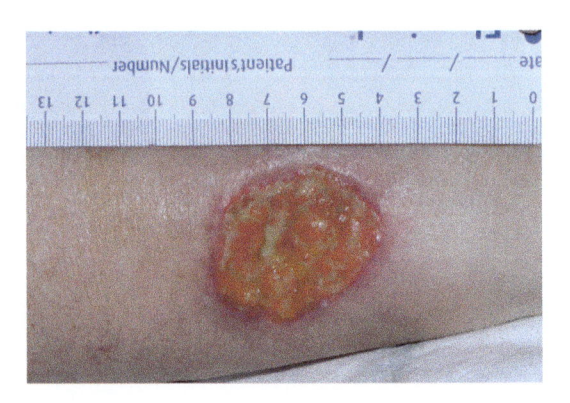

Fig. 38.4 Preparation for skin biopsy.

Specific PG therapy involves immunosuppressive agents. Topical treatments include corticosteroid creams and local injections of triamcinolone around the edge of the ulcer. There is some evidence to suggest benefit with topical tacrolimus, but this may cause immunosuppression even within a couple of weeks.

If topical measures are ineffective, then systemic treatment with oral corticosteroids such as prednisolone may be necessary. There is emerging evidence for the use of intravenous methylprednisolone once daily over a period of three to five days, and some trials have shown benefit of minocycline in addition to oral prednisolone. Ciclosporin may be considered in resistant cases. Most patients show a good response within three weeks of starting ciclosporin, but should be closely monitored for adverse effects. Recent randomized control trials have shown an improvement in PG with the use of the TNF-α blocker infliximab.

Further reading

Brooklyn TN, Dunnill MG, Shetty A, *et al.* (2006). Infliximab for the treatment of pyoderma gangrenosum: a randomised, double blind, placebo controlled trial. *Gut*; **55**(4): 505–509.

Callen JP (1998). Pyoderma gangrenosum. *Lancet*; **351**(9102): 581–585.

Chow RK, Ho VC (1996). Treatment of pyoderma gangrenosum. *J Am Acad Dermatol*; **34**(6): 1047–1060.

Kaur MR, Lewis HM (2005). Severe recalcitrant pyoderma gangrenosum treated with infliximab. *Br J Dermatol*; **153**(3): 689–691.

Case 39

A 74-year-old woman was seen in the out-patient clinic with a recent history of general deterioration, anaemia, poor appetite, tiredness, and fever. Colonoscopy and gastroscopy requested by the GP to investigate anaemia had found no abnormality. The past medical history included hypertension and decreased mobility caused by multiple fractures and a head injury sustained in a road traffic accident (RTA) a decade earlier. However, she was able to mobilize with a stick and lived independently with her husband. Medications were paracetamol, amlodipine, furosemide, and omeprazole prescribed in the last few weeks. She smoked five cigarettes per day, having recently cut down from 20, but took no alcohol.

On examination, she was pale, temperature was 37.5°C, with a respiratory rate of 16 breaths per minute, heart rate was 65bpm and regular, oxygen saturation was 98% on room air, and blood pressure was 130/70mmHg. Examination was otherwise unremarkable, except for longstanding scars on the legs and head, and reduced movement in the right leg from the previous RTA injuries.

Investigations showed the following:

- Hb 9.2g/dL; plts 550 × 10^9/L; MCV 90fL
- C-reactive protein (CRP) 44mg/L; erythrocyte sedimentation rate (ESR) 80mm/hour
- Biochemistry results, vitamin B_{12}, folate and iron studies: all normal, except albumin 33g/L
- Serum electrophoresis: polyclonal hyper-gamma-globulinaemia
- Urine electrophoresis: traces of protein; no Bence Jones protein detected
- Urine dipstick: negative
- Urine and blood cultures: negative
- CXR: enlarged heart
- ECG: 65bpm, sinus rhythm
- Echocardiogram, except for aortic sclerosis: results unremarkable
- Abdominal ultrasound: unremarkable.

Questions

1 What is the most likely cause of her symptoms?
2 How would you proceed in further assessment and confirm the diagnosis?
3 Which complications are associated with this condition?
4 How would you manage this patient? Which investigations are useful in this condition?

Answers

1 What is the most likely cause of her symptoms?

The history, examination, blood tests (elevated CRP, ESR, thrombocytosis, normocytic normochromic anaemia, moderately decreased serum albumin) and normal results of other investigations, suggest giant cell arteritis (GCA), also called temporal or cranial arteritis. The clinical features of GCA are variable and symptoms may be transient, or non-specific. The onset is usually gradual, but may occasionally be sudden. The differential diagnosis may include infection (e.g. infective endocarditis, see case 10), malignancy, and connective tissue/rheumatological disorders (see case 17). The risk factors for GCA are older age and female sex (two to four times more common than in males), smoking, and a lower number of pregnancies compared with controls.

GCA should be considered in patients aged 50 years or older, presenting with headache, or unexplained constitutional symptoms including fever, anaemia, visual disturbances, fatigue, depression, loss of weight, or any symptom of polymyalgia rheumatica (PMR—case 28). More rare clinical manifestations include:

- Tongue and throat pain, tongue infarction
- Pleural and/or pericardial effusions
- Aortic dissection or aneurysm, myocardial infarction, stroke
- Intestinal infarction
- Tumour-like masses in breasts, ovaries, and uterus
- The syndrome of inappropriate antidiuretic hormone secretion
- Peripheral neuropathy, mononeuritis multiplex
- Affective or psychotic symptoms
- Memory impairment
- Visual hallucinations
- Raynaud's phenomenon
- Sensorineural hearing loss
- Scalp necrosis.

GCA is a chronic granulomatous systemic inflammatory vasculitis of large and medium vessels usually affecting older Caucasians, being less common in Asians and African Americans. The incidence is 44.7 per 100,000 per year for >90 years, with the highest incidence in Scandinavia and among Americans of Scandinavian origin. The aetiology is not known, but may involve age-related changes of the immune system (see case 17) and blood vessels, the presence of HLA-DR4 or certain polymorphisms (ICAM-1), atheromatous disease, and previous infection with parvovirus B19, parainfluenza type 1, chlamydia pneumonia, and mycoplasma pneumoniae. Heavy smoking has been found to increase the risk of GCA in older women, but not men. Histological findings include necrotizing arteritis involving T-lymphocytes, macrophages, multinucleated giant cells, plasma cells, neutrophils, and eosinophils, in a granulomatous process. Thrombosis may develop at sites of active inflammation. GCA may affect almost any artery, and may rarely also involve veins, and can be classified into:

- Cranial artery GCA, the most common form; median age of onset is 72 years.
- Large-vessel GCA; patients usually present with arm 'claudication', without headache. The median age of onset is 66 years and temporal biopsy is less likely to be positive.

The diagnostic criteria for GCA from the American College of Rheumatology have a sensitivity and specificity of at least 90%, and require three or more of the following:

- Age at onset >50 years
- New onset of localized headache
- Tenderness or decreased pulse of the temporal artery
- ESR greater than 50mm/h by the Westergren method
- Temporal artery biopsy revealing vasculitis.

2 How would you proceed in further assessment and confirm the diagnosis?

This patient should have further history taken and be further examined. She should be asked about the presence of:

- Fever (present in up to 50% of cases). This is usually low grade, but rarely may be up to 39°C, making misdiagnoses of infection more likely.
- Headache (presence, character, location, progression).
- Visual disturbances (e.g. amaurosis fugax, diplopia, partial or complete vision loss—unilateral or bilateral).
- Eye, face, throat, or tongue pain (e.g. jaw 'claudication'—pain while eating). This should always be asked for directly as patients rarely volunteer this information.
- Arm claudication.

- Cough (usually non-productive), present in around 10% of patients with GCA, thought to be caused by vasculitis affecting the cough receptors.
- Shoulder, neck, upper arm, torso, and hip girdle stiffness and aching, suggestive of co-existent PMR. Around 15-20% of patients with PMR have GCA on temporal artery biopsy while symptoms of PMR are present in 40-60% of patients with GCA.
- Sore throat, hoarse voice.
- Visual hallucinations.

Further examination should include:

- Careful examination of temporal arteries, looking for the absence of pulses, presence of pain on palpation, increased thickness, and nodularity.
- Auscultation for bruits over the axillary fossa, carotid arteries, supraclavicular, or brachial areas indicating vasculitis.
- Examination for ocular muscle paresis.
- Examination of the fundi for optic disc oedema, indicating involvement of the optic nerve.
- Blood pressure measurement in both arms. A systolic blood pressure difference of more than 10 or 15mmHg may indicate vasculitis causing stenosis.
- Peripheral arterial pulses (looking for the absence of carotid, brachial, radial, femoral, and pedal pulses).
- Examination of the tongue for ulcers and of the scalp for necrosis.
- Examination for the distal extremities for swelling and synovitis, especially in the wrists and knees.

On more detailed questioning, this patient admitted having new pain in the right side of her jaw on eating, which was gradually getting worse. On examination, there was increased thickness of the right temporal artery. A temporal artery biopsy was requested for definitive diagnosis.

3 Which complications are associated with this condition?

Complications may develop at any stage of the disease and include:

- Unilateral or bilateral irreversible loss of vision (owing to involvement of the ophthalmic artery and anterior ischaemic optic neuropathy is the most common cause of vision loss) and is the most feared complication of GCA. Older age, optic disc swelling, and elevated CRP level are risk factors for progressive visual loss, despite appropriate therapy.

- Aneurysm formation (e.g. new murmur of aortic regurgitation in cases of an ascending aortic aneurysm causing secondary dilatation of the aortic valve—more common than descending aortic aneurysm).
- Aortitis.
- Aortic dissection.
- Central nervous system involvement from vasculitis.
- Cranial ischaemic events including TIA, stroke (e.g. progressive brainstem and cerebellar neurologic deficits may reflect vertebral artery disease—see case 19).

Some authors suggest screening all patients with GCA with computed tomography (CT) in order to exclude asymptomatic aneurysms of the aorta or other vessels (Fig. 39.1). In a small number of patients with claudication or absent pulses, MR angiography, or CT angiography may be needed, and echocardiography may be useful in cases of suspected ascending aortic aneurysm.

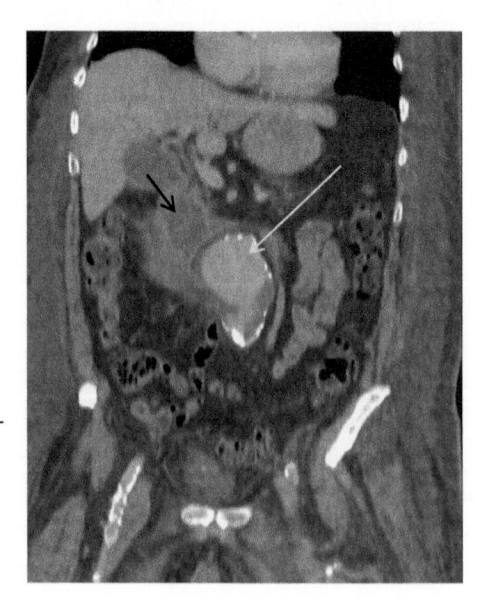

Fig. 39.1 A large aortic aneurysm (white arrow) with retroperitoneal haemorrhage and secondary infection (black arrow) from a different patient with GCA and aortic aneurysm.

4 How would you manage this patient? Which investigations are useful in this condition?

Treatment for GCA should start as soon as the condition is suspected owing to the risks of complications from untreated disease. Where clinical symptoms are consistent with GCA, elevated CRP has >95% sensitivity and ESR 75–85%, although ESR may rarely be normal. If both are elevated, the sensitivity for GCA is 99%. However, one large population-based GCA study has shown that thrombocytosis and elevated CRP levels together are a better predictor for the diagnosis than ESR. Also, a normal platelet count is more reliable than a normal ESR in ruling out GCA. Around 25–35% of GCA cases also have elevated aspartate aminotransferase and alkaline phosphatase at presentation.

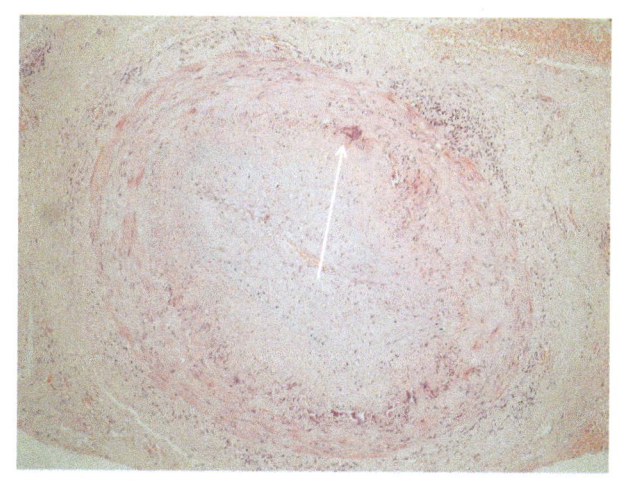

Fig. 39.2 Haematoxilin and Eosin staining of a medium-size artery with Giant Cell Arteritis. There are inflammatory cells on the edge of the tunica media. Arrow indicates a giant cell.

A temporal artery biopsy should be organized in the meantime, and this is the gold standard for diagnosis (Fig. 39.2). Temporal artery ultrasound may also be useful: one recent meta-analysis of ultrasound versus temporal artery biopsy found a sensitivity for ultrasound of ~70% and a specificity of ~80%. If a classic halo sign is seen around the artery on colour duplex ultrasonography, this has a specificity of 80–100% for the diagnosis and is comparable to magnetic resonance imaging. The role of positron emission tomography (PET) scanning with 18-fluorodeoxyglucose uptake requires further evaluation, but appears promising (see *Oxford Case Histories in Rheumatology*).

Temporal biopsy should preferably be performed in an expert centre where the diagnostic yield is higher. A biopsy will evidence the need for long-lasting steroid therapy, which may be associated with serious complications and thus should not be undertaken in the absence of diagnostic certainty. The choice of site to biopsy is straightforward in cases of painful or visibly changed temporal arteries, but may be problematic in the 40% of atypical cases in which the arteries appear normal. In such cases, it remains unclear whether unilateral or bilateral temporal artery biopsy should be undertaken, or whether in cases of negative unilateral biopsy, biopsy of the contralateral temporal artery should be performed.

One third of patients with biopsy-proven GCA have normal temporal arteries on clinical examination and biopsy may be negative, even in the presence of active disease (~10% cases) owing to:

- The presence of skip lesions, as the inflammation spares some arterial segments
- The sample taken is too small (usually <2cm)
- The clinically normal temporal artery is biopsied in error
- The GCA is confined to non-cranial vessels (e.g. axillary, subclavian arteries).

Typical changes of GCA will usually persist in the temporal arteries for up to two weeks after the start of glucocorticoid treatment. In biopsy negative cases where clinical suspicion is high, glucocorticoid treatment should continue. The most efficient starting dose of prednisolone is unknown and 20mg/day may be sufficient for some patients. However, concern regarding the potential consequences of under-treatment means that 40–60mg of prednisone for two to four weeks, with subsequent dosage being determined by level of response is the most usual therapy. Dramatic clinical improvement usually occurs within 24 to 48 hours, with ESR or CRP falling within a few days of therapy. Where response to glucocorticoid therapy is poor, the diagnosis of GCA should be re-visited. The clinical condition and inflammatory markers should be monitored regularly on follow-up with the steroid dosage adjusted accordingly.

Glucocorticoid dose should be reduced once good control of the disease is achieved with the awareness that over-rapid reduction may result in a relapse of the disease. Treatment usually lasts one to two years, but can be much longer and in a small number of patients, low dose prednisone may be required for many years to control symptoms. All patients with GCA should be advised to take aspirin unless there are contraindications in order to prevent platelet activation and to reduce thrombotic risks: studies have shown significant reduction in risk of visual loss and cerebral ischaemic events in patients with GCA on aspirin. Care must be taken regarding the risk of gastrointestinal bleeding on aspirin/steroid combinations however and ppi cover may be required.

Trials of steroid-sparing drugs in the treatment of GCA have shown conflicting results, but drugs such as cyclosporine and methotrexate may have a role in steroid-resistant cases.

Patients on long-term glucocorticoid treatment should take calcium supplements, vitamin D, and bisphosphonate to counteract osteoporosis. A very small number of cases with subclavian steal syndrome have been successfully treated with revascularization. All patients should be advised to seek urgent review should symptoms return.

Further reading

Ball EL, Walsh SR, Tang TY, Gohil R, Clarke JM (2010). Role of ultrasonography in the diagnosis of temporal arteritis. *Br J Surg*; **97**(12): 1765–1771.

Borchers AT, Gershwin ME (2012). Giant cell arteritis: a review of classification, pathophysiology, geoepidemiology and treatment. *Autoimmun Rev*; **11**(6–7): A544–A554.

Karassa FB, Matsagas MI, Schmidt WA, Ioannidis JPA (2005). Meta-analysis: test performance of ultrasonography for giant-cell arteritis. *Ann Intern Med*; **142**(5): 359–369.

Koenigkam-Santos M, Sharma P, Kalb B, *et al.* (2011). Magnetic resonance angiography in extracranial giant cell arteritis. *J Clin Rheumatol*; **17**(6): 306–310.

Pipitone N, Boiardi L, Bajocchi G, Salvarani C (2006). Long term outcomes of giant cell arteritis. *Clin Exp Rheumatol*; **246**(suppl 41): 565–570.

Salvarani C, Cantini F, Hunder GG (2008). Polymyalgia rheumatica and giant-cell arteritis. Lancet; **372**(9634): 234–245.

Tomasson G, Peloquin C, Mohammad A, *et al.* (2014). Risk for cardiovascular disease early and late after a diagnosis of giant-cell arteritis: a cohort study. *Ann Intern Med*; 21; **160**(2): 73–80.

Case 40

A 68-year-old retired English teacher was seen in the out-patient clinic with an eight-month history of progressive 'slowing-up', difficulty dressing, particularly with fastening buttons, and with cutting up meat during meals. His muscles were 'stiff', and he could not walk or turn quickly. He had an intermittent tremor affecting his arms, which became worse when holding objects, and his handwriting had deteriorated. There was occasional urinary incontinence. His wife reported that he had begun snoring and talking in his sleep, and that his voice had become quieter in recent months. He had longstanding constipation, but denied any other previous medical history. There was no family history of note. He had been taking privately obtained sildenafil for several years.

General system examination was unremarkable. He was alert, orientated, with slightly bent forward posture, and low volume voice. His face was expressionless and he was slow to start walking. Cranial nerves were normal. Gait was wide-based with small steps and absent arm swing, and he was unsteady when turning. There was bilateral cogwheel rigidity, which was slightly more pronounced in the right arm, and bradykinesia on finger and foot-tapping. Plantars were upgoing bilaterally.

MoCA score was 26/30 and GDS score was 4/15.

Investigations showed the following:

- FBC, ESR, urea, and electrolytes, TFTs, LFTs, glucose, cholesterol, calcium, CRP: normal
- B_{12}, folate: normal
- CXR: normal
- CT head: normal
- ECG: sinus rhythm, heart rate 72bpm
- Urine dipstick: negative for blood, nitrates, and leucocytes.

A diagnosis of idiopathic Parkinson's disease was made and he was started on levodopa/carbidopa 100/25mg three times per day, increased after an interval to 100/25mg four times per day. Although he and his wife felt there was some initial improvement, his mobility had deteriorated by the next follow-up visit six months later and he had had several falls, always falling backwards. On examination, gaze evoked nystagmus was noted, and he had resting tremor in his hands. There was increased rigidity in the left arm. Blood pressure was 140/70mmHg lying, falling to 100/55mmHg on standing, which was associated with feeling dizzy. Fludrocortisone was prescribed and he was provided with pressure stockings.

His levodopa/carbidopa was increased gradually to six tablets of 100/25mg per day, but his mobility did not improve.

Questions

1 What is the most likely diagnosis and why? Describe this condition.
2 List the diagnostic criteria for this condition and the poor prognostic factors.
3 List the differential diagnosis that you would have considered in this case.
4 How would you investigate this patient further?
5 How would you further manage this patient?

Answers

1 What is the most likely diagnosis and why? Describe this condition.

The most likely diagnosis is multiple system atrophy (MSA). This patient had early symptoms of erectile and bladder dysfunction, which is typical of MSA in which autonomic symptoms, including orthostatic hypotension and gastrointestinal symptoms often precede the onset of parkinsonism or ataxia, and are the presenting feature in 20–40% of cases. The MoCA score was 26/30 indicating no major cognitive impairment and the GDS was below the cut-off for depression.

MSA is a progressive neurodegenerative disease (akinetic-rigid syndrome), of unknown aetiology with a prevalence of around two to five per 100,000, and around 0.11 rate per 100,000/year for age-standardized incidence. The mean age of onset is 60 years. MSA is a sporadic disorder (with genetic factors conferring increased susceptibility) characterized by parkinsonian features, cerebellar ataxia, autonomic failure, urogenital dysfunction, and corticospinal disorders. Dementia was regarded as an exclusion criterion according to the consensus diagnostic criteria for MSA, although the recent prospective European MSA (EMSA) study showed that significant cognitive impairment may occur even early in the disease.

The clinical features of MSA were recently characterized in the prospective EMSA study, which examined over 400 patients with MSA in 19 different European study sites and found the following:

- Autonomic and urogenital dysfunction, e.g. urinary dysfunction (~80%), impotence, symptomatic orthostatic dysregulation (~75%), chronic constipation (~30%).
- Cerebellar dysfunction: gaze evoked nystagmus; gait ataxia; ataxia of limb movements; speech ataxia (67%).
- Pyramidal signs: hyper-reflexia (~40%); extensor plantars (~30%).
- Parkinsonism (~90%).
- Sleep disorder, particularly of rapid eye movement (REM) sleep (~70% see case 37).
- Restless legs syndrome (~30%) (see case 37).
- Depression and anxiety (in up to 50% see case 18).
- Pain, particularly 'coat hanger' aches in the shoulders and neck.
- Reduced genital sensitivity in around half of female patients compared to <5% with idiopathic Parkinson's disease.

α-Synuclein is the main component of the inclusion pathology in MSA as in dementia with Lewy bodies (see case 25), classifying these two disorders with Parkinson's disease as α-synucleinopathies. The hypothesis that REM sleep behaviour disorder presents a prodromal phase of the synucleinopathies has been supported by recent research findings.

MSA is sub-divided into MSA-P (parkinsonism predominant) and MSA-C (cerebellar predominant) although features of the disease may evolve with time such that early extrapyramidal signs may become dominated by cerebellar and autonomic features.

This patient was suffering from the MSA-P form of MSA as illustrated by bradykinesia, rigidity, hypokinetic speech, postural instability, and tremor. Data from the EMSA Study Group show that MSA-P is slightly more common (~58%) than MSA-C although in the Japanese population over 80% of patients have the cerebellar sub-type.

2 List the diagnostic criteria for this condition and the poor prognostic factors.

Diagnostic criteria from the second consensus statement on the diagnosis of MSA are as follows:

Definite MSA

Requires neuropathological samples showing synuclein–positive glial cytoplasmic inclusions with neurodegenerative changes in striatonigral, or olivopontocerebellar structures in association with striatonigral degeneration, or olivopontocerebellar ataxia.

Probable MSA

Autonomic failure (e.g. blood pressure falling within three minutes of standing by at least 30mmHg systolic or 15mmHg diastolic), urogenital dysfunction (e.g. involving urinary incontinence, urgency, erectile dysfunction in males) with either:

- poorly levodopa-responsive parkinsonism (bradykinesia with rigidity, tremor, or postural instability), or
- cerebellar dysfunction (e.g. gait ataxia with cerebellar dysarthria, limb ataxia, or cerebellar oculomotor dysfunction).

Possible MSA

Parkinsonism (bradykinesia with rigidity, tremor, or postural instability), or a cerebellar syndrome (gait ataxia with cerebellar dysarthria, limb ataxia, or cerebellar oculomotor dysfunction), and at least one feature suggesting autonomic dysfunction (urogenital dysfunction, significant orthostatic blood pressure drop, but not to the level required for the diagnosis of probable MSA), and at least one of the following:

- upgoing plantars with hyper-reflexia or stridor (possible MSA-P or MSA-C)
- rapidly progressive parkinsonism; poor response to levodopa; dysphagia within five years of motor onset; postural instability within three years; gait ataxia; hypometabolism in putamen; brainstem; or cerebellum on FDG-PET
- cerebellar oculomotor dysfunction; atrophy on MRI of middle cerebellar peduncle, pons, cerebellum, or putamen.

Inspiratory stridor, autonomic dysfunction, antecollis, or oculomotor abnormalities may occur before parkinsonism or ataxia.

Poor prognostic factors include:

- older age at the onset of the disease
- female sex
- frequent falling
- autonomic failure at the onset of disease
- short period before urinary catheter insertion
- early wheelchair dependence
- early speech disorder and dysphagia
- early onset of cognitive impairment.

3 List the differential diagnosis that you would have considered in this case.

The differential diagnosis includes:

- *Idiopathic Parkinson's disease.* This was the diagnosis made on the patient's first visit to the clinic. However, there were a number of features that appeared early in the course of the disease that would not be expected in the first stages of idiopathic Parkinson's disease: rapid progression; falls and voice change; new onset of snoring; impotence (hence sildefanil); urinary incontinence; marked postural hypotension; postural instability; early antecollis; the presence of cerebellar signs; upgoing plantars, and poor response of motor symptoms to levodopa treatment.
- *Progressive supranuclear palsy (PSP).* However, the typical features of PSP including slowing of vertical saccades, vertical supranuclear palsy, early

cognitive impairment, and personality change were not present in this patient. Figure 40.1 illustrates atrophy of the midbrain ('hummingbird sign') on MRI of a patient with PSP. This MRI finding appears relatively specific for PSP, but is not always present.

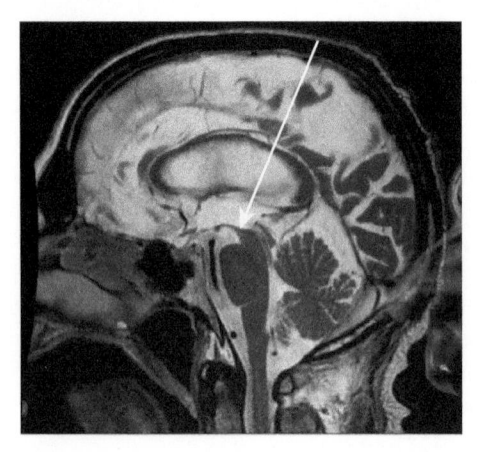

Fig. 40.1 MRI scan of the brain, T2-weighted sagittal midline section showing 'Hummingbird sign' (arrow), caused by prominent atrophy of the mesencephalon.

- *Creutzfeld–Jakob disease.* This may sometimes cause parkinsonism, but there was no cognitive disturbance, myoclonus, or sensory signs.
- *Vascular parkinsonism.* This is usually accompanied by vascular risk factors and/or history of symptomatic vascular disease, which were absent in this patient. Distinguishing between vascular parkinsonism and neurodegeneration may be difficult in older patients in whom vascular disease is present. Onset may be acute following basal ganglia stroke or insidious and associated with prominent diffuse subcortical white matter changes.
- *Corticobasal degeneration.* This is associated with higher cortical function abnormalities (apraxia, aphasia), frontal lobe neurological signs (e.g. pout/snout reflexes), asymmetric limb dystonia, myoclonus (stimulus sensitive), alien-limb syndrome, and sensory deficits.
- *Normal pressure hydrocephalus* (see case 6) was excluded by the CT scan findings.
- *Drugs* (e.g. neuroleptics, some calcium channel blockers—diltiazem, sodium valproate) and toxins may cause parkinsonism, but there was no relevant history in this case.
- *Space occupying lesion:* excluded by imaging.
- *Inherited disorders* (e.g. Huntington's disease, late onset spinocerebellar ataxia) may occasionally cause diagnostic difficulty, but in the current case there was no family history and no relevant clinical findings.

- *Dementia with Lewy bodies* (see case 25). Although this is associated with parkinsonism, it was unlikely in this case, given the absence of cognitive impairment or visual hallucinations.
- *Wilson's disease.* This should not be forgotten as a cause of movement disorders since it is treatable. Although it usually presents in children or young adults, cases have been reported in older people. However, it usually causes dysarthria and autonomic features would not be typical.

4 How would you investigate this patient further?

The diagnosis of MSA is a clinical one. Some specific features for and against the diagnosis are as follows:
- *Pros:* severe dysphonia; severe dysarthria; orofacial dystonia; inspiratory sighs; jerky; myoclonic postural or action tremor; antecollis; camptocormia (severe anterior flexion of the spine); Pisa syndrome (severe lateral flexion of the spine); new or increased snoring; pathological laughter or crying; contractures of hands or feet; cold hands and feet.
- *Cons:* dementia; hallucinations not induced by drugs; family history of ataxia or parkinsonism onset after age 75 years; white matter lesions that suggest multiple sclerosis; pill-rolling rest tremor; neuropathy.

Magnetic resonance imaging is not diagnostic, but may show atrophy of putaminal, pontine, and middle cerebellar peduncle in both MSA-P and MSA-C, particularly in advanced disease. The basal ganglia and brainstem may show posterior putaminal hypointensity, a hyperintense lateral putaminal rim or 'hot cross bun sign' (see Fig. 40.2).

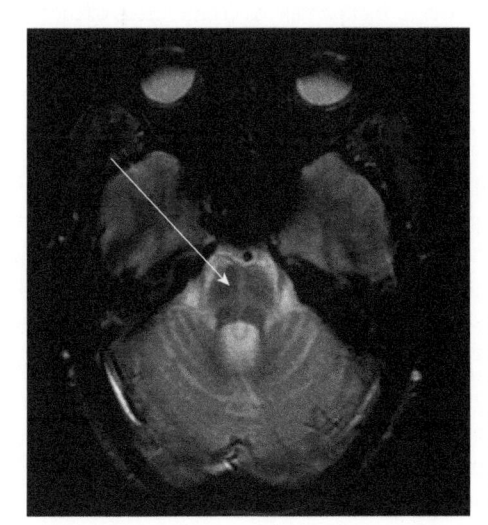

Fig. 40.2 MRI head T2-weighted axial image at the level of the brainstem/cerebellum showing the 'hot cross bun sign', i.e. cruciform hyperintensity in the pons (arrow).

Evidence of sleep disorder from formal sleep studies may be supportive of MSA diagnosis as these are included in the new consensus diagnostic criteria. Functional presynaptic and postsynaptic dopaminergic imaging using PET (fluorodeoxyglucose) and single-photon emission computed tomography (SPECT) show similar findings of decreased dopaminergic function in the striatal system in idiopathic Parkinson's disease, dementia with Lewy bodies and MSA, and are thus not diagnostic (see case 25 and Fig. 40.3).

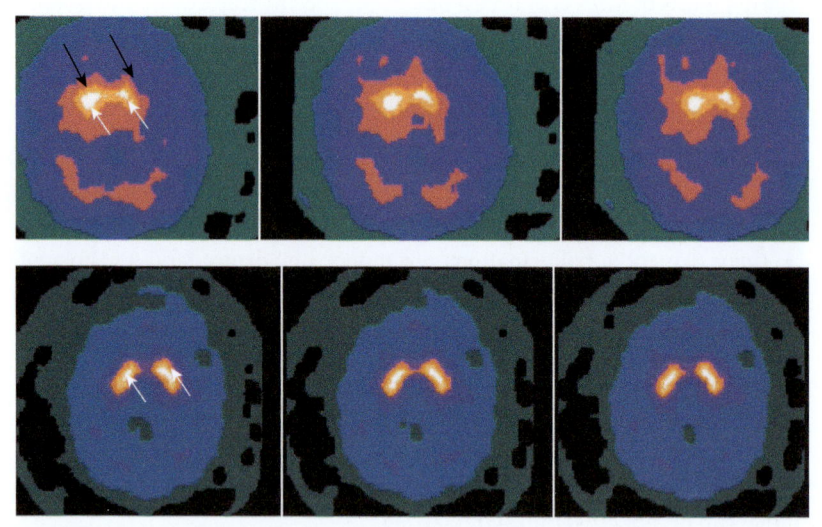

Fig. 40.3 Top images: PET DAT scan showing asymmetric loss of tracer uptake in both lentiform nuclei (white arrows) with further partial loss in both heads of caudate nuclei (black arrows) from this patient. Bottom images: normal scan with symmetric uptake within both heads of caudate and lentiform nuclei giving a normal 'comma' appearance.

Bladder function assessment in MSA often shows detrusor hyper-reflexia and abnormal urethral sphincter function and later, increased residual urine volume (see case 7). However, it is not pathognomic, and may be found in idiopathic Parkinson's disease. External urethral or anal sphincter denervation may be seen on electromyography in MSA early after disease onset, so these investigations may occasionally be helpful. Cardiovascular autonomic function tests, including cardiac response to deep breathing, Valsalva manoeuvre, tilt testing, and the axon reflex sweat test, do not appear to distinguish reliably between MSA and idiopathic Parkinson's disease.

5 How would you further manage this patient?

Treatment of MSA is supportive, but a trial of dopaminergic medication may be given for patients with parkinsonism despite the lack of any supportive randomized controlled trial data. Levodopa/carbidopa should be increased gradually from 25/100mg three times daily up to 800–1000mg/day, as tolerated with particular attention to postural symptoms. If levodopa/carbidopa has no effect, other dopaminergic drugs will usually also be ineffective. Levodopa/carbidopa can result in motor improvement in about 30% of patients, but only around 10% of these have a sustained response. Some patients do not respond to acute administration of levodopa or develop peak-dose related (craniocervical) dystonia without motor benefit, but deteriorate following withdrawal.

There is no effective treatment for ataxia. Patients may benefit from physical therapy (e.g. to prevent contractures), speech therapy, and occupational therapy (e.g. for appropriate equipment) input. Dysphagia may need dietitian input and ultimately, consideration of percutaneous endoscopic gastrostomy tube insertion. Discussion of power of attorney (see case 13) and advance directives should be considered, as for any degenerative neurological disorder. Palliative care management may be needed in end stage disease.

Management of autonomic dysfunction includes:

- Stopping or reducing antihypertensive drugs.
- Increased salt and water intake.
- Pressure stockings.
- Drugs for orthostatic hypotension (e.g. fludrocortisone, see case 11).
- An anticholinergic agent may be considered for urinary symptoms (e.g. solifenacin) or intranasal desmopressin for problematic nocturia.
- Treatment for constipation.

Dystonia may be treated with local botulinum injections. Loss of weight and dysphagia should be assessed with input from a speech and language therapist and a dietitian. In some patients, consideration of PEG insertion may be necessary.

Patients with MSA may also have postprandial hypotension (see case 11). Such patients should:

- avoid salt restriction
- avoid standing after meals
- be encouraged to walk between meals
- avoid large carbohydrate-rich meals.

The mean survival of patients with MSA is between six and nine years, and is therefore much shorter than survival with idiopathic Parkinson's disease, which is only around two years less than that of the general population if adequately treated. A significant number of patients with MSA die from infections related to lower urinary tract infections, and around 50% from bronchopneumonia. However, sudden death in patients with MSA may be prefaced by stridor. Patients with respiratory stridor should be assessed for continuous positive airway pressure and tracheostomy.

Further reading

Boesch SM, Wenning GK, Ransmayr G, Poewe W (2002). Dystonia in multiple system atrophy. *J Neurol Neurosurg Psychiatry*; **72**(3): 300–303.

Gilman S, Wenning GK, Low PA, *et al.* (2008). Second consensus statement on the diagnosis of multiple system atrophy. *Neurology*; **71**: 670–676.

Iranzo A, Tolosa E, Gelpi E, *et al.* (2013). Neurodegenerative disease status and post-mortem pathology in idiopathic rapid-eye-movement sleep behaviour disorder: an observational cohort study. *Lancet Neurol*; **12**: 443–453.

Jecmenica-Lukic M, Poewe W, Tolosa E, Wenning GK (2012). Premotor signs and symptoms of multiple system atrophy. *Lancet Neurol*; **11**: 361–368.

Riley DE, Chelimsky TC (2003). Autonomic nervous system testing may not distinguish multiple system atrophy from Parkinson's disease. *J Neurol Nerosurg Psychiatry*; **74**; 56–60.

Stefanova N, Bücke P, Duerr S, Wenning GK (2009). Multiple system atrophy: an update. *Lancet Neurol*; **12**(8): 1172–1178.

Watts L, Thompson S (2014). Atypical parkinsonian disorders. CME Journal Geriatric Medicine; **15**(1): 22–30.

Wenning GK, Colosimo C, Geser F, Poewe W (2004). Multiple system atrophy. *Lancet Neurol*; **3**: 93–103.

Winter Y, Bezdolnyy Y, Katunina E, *et al.* (2010). Incidence of Parkinson's disease and atypical parkinsonism: Russian population-based study. *Mov Disord*; **25**(3): 349–356.

Case 41

A 77-year-old man was admitted to the trauma ward after a fall at home in which he sustained a cervical spine fracture. He was subsequently transferred to the community hospital for palliative care input and discharge planning. He had a previous medical history of Alzheimer's dementia and benign prostate hypertrophy, and had a long-term urinary catheter. Three months earlier, he had been diagnosed with metastatic lung cancer involving the liver and thoracic spine. He was an ex-smoker and never drank alcohol. He had a live-in carer and a supportive son who informed the medical team that the patient had in the past expressed the wish to die at home. Medication included paracetamol, senna, donepezil, and morphine sulphate.

On examination, he was cachectic with poor muscle bulk. He called repeatedly for help and appeared distressed. Temperature was 36.5°C, pulse 72bpm regular, and blood pressure was 100/65mmHg. The rest of general systems examination was unremarkable, except for some suprapubic tenderness on palpation without urinary retention. Nervous system examination showed increased tone and reduced power of 1/5 in the right arm and both legs, and 3/5 in the left arm. Plantars were upgoing. AMTS was 5/10.

The discharge letter from the trauma ward stated that prior to transfer to the community hospital, the urinary catheter had to be reinserted four times in 48 hours as it had fallen out after each successful insertion.

The daughter, normally resident in the USA, arrived on the ward on the day of transfer to the community hospital, and asked the medical team for her father to be started on 'a pump' so that he could 'die quickly, in peace, without any further interventions'. However, the son was keen that his father should not be 'sedated too much' and wanted him to go home to die. They both wished to know for how long their father would survive.

Investigations showed the following:

- FBC, U&Es, Ca, PO_4: normal; CRP 18g/L; alkaline phosphatase 675 IU/L and albumin 33mg/L
- Urine dipstick: positive for leucocytes and erythrocytes
- Urine and blood culture: no growth

- ECG: sinus rhythm; heart rate 90bpm
- Abdominal X-ray (Fig. 41.1).

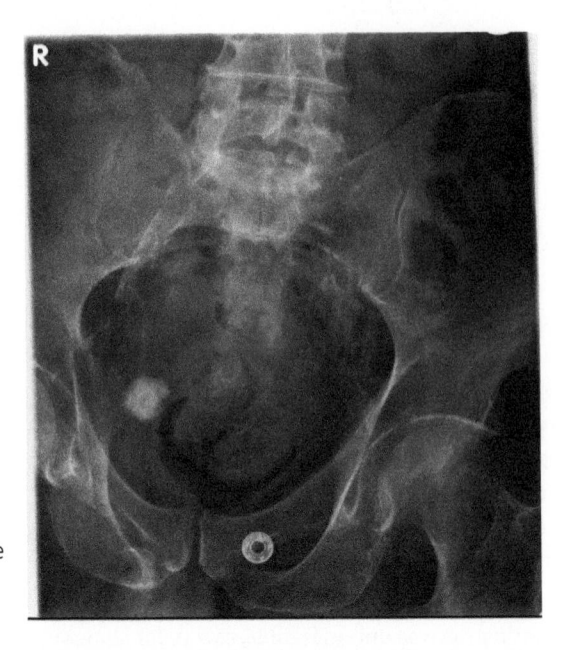

Fig. 41.1 Plain X-ray of the abdomen/pelvis from the patient.

Questions

1 What is the major abnormality on the abdominal X-ray in Figure 41.1?
2 Considering the history and investigation findings, what is the most likely cause of his present distress?
3 How should this patient be managed?
4 What general principles in the management of symptoms in palliative care could be applied in this case?
5 How would you control pain?
6 List adjuvant analgesics and the indications for their prescription for pain control in elderly patients.
7 How would you estimate life expectancy of a patient receiving palliative care and why is this important?
8 What clinical features would suggest that death is imminent?
9 What are the most common differences in the palliative care of older compared with younger adults?

Answers

1 What is the major abnormality on the abdominal X-ray in Figure 41.1?

The abdominal X-ray shows a bladder stone (Fig. 41.2) (arrow), which was confirmed on pelvic ultrasound (Fig. 41.3).

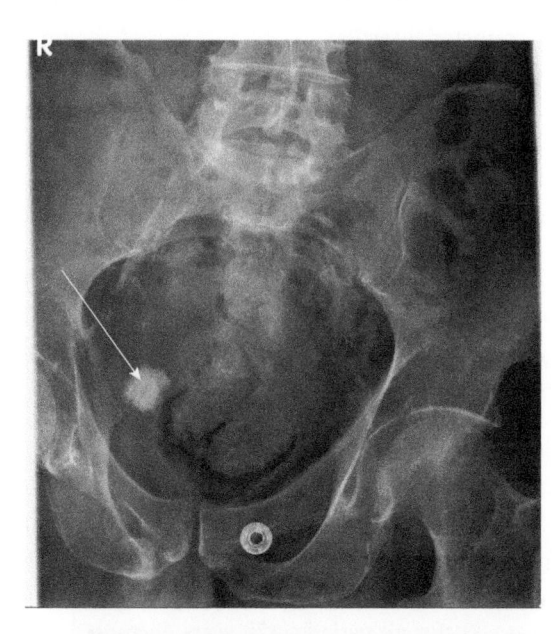

Fig. 41.2 The plain abdominal X-ray shows a bladder stone (white arrow), also heavy calcification of the iliac arteries, degenerative changes in the lumbosacral spine and faecal loading.

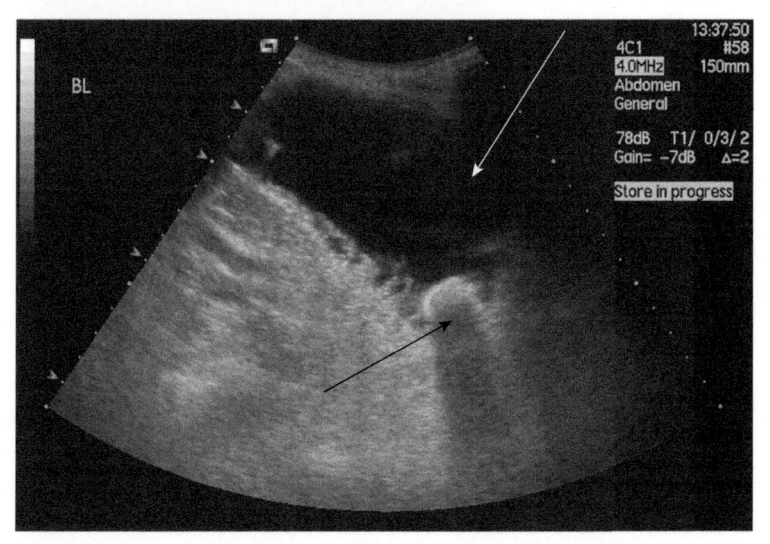

Fig. 41.3 Pelvic ultrasound: full bladder (big white arrow) with a stone shadow (small black arrow).

2 Considering the history and investigation findings, what is the most likely cause of his present distress?

The most likely underlying and remediable cause of the distress in this patient was a bladder calculus causing lower abdominal discomfort/pain. This was thought to have been repeatedly tearing the catheter balloon, causing the catheter to fall out. A bladder calculus should always be considered in patients needing multiple urinary catheter insertions over short periods of time. Other symptoms include suprapubic pain and pain radiating to the tip of the penis, scrotum, perineum, back, or hip and aggravated by sudden movements, dysuria, intermittency, frequency, hesitancy, nocturia, urinary retention, haematuria, and sudden termination of voiding.

This patient had a long-term urinary catheter and prostatic enlargement, known risks for urinary bladder stone formation. Other risk factors include congenital anomalies (e.g. ureterocele), acquired anomalies (e.g. vesical diverticula), history of urethral implantation, urethral stricture, neurogenic bladder, and vaginal reconstruction in women. The diagnosis is usually made on abdominal X-ray or ultrasound.

3 How should this patient be managed?

The assessment and management of older patients with metastatic cancer requiring palliative care is often complicated by cognitive impairment and communication difficulties, as in the current case. The International Society for Geriatric Oncology recommends performing a Comprehensive Geriatric Assessment (CGA) (see case 33) for all patients >70 years diagnosed with cancer. Symptom evaluation and control is of paramount importance. In this patient, pain was probably from multiple causes—bladder calculus, cervical fracture, and bone metastases—and it was difficult to establish how much each was contributing to his distress. Studies suggest that systematic assessment detects many more symptoms compared to spontaneous complaints voiced by patients receiving palliative care, although the precise cause of each symptom may be difficult to pin down.

Discussion with the son and daughter was undertaken regarding the patient's previously expressed wishes, since he was confused and deemed to lack capacity regarding treatment decisions (see case 13). There was no advanced directive or lasting power of attorney. As his distress became much worse when the urinary catheter fell out and his pain seemed most prominent in the abdomen, it was decided that it would be in his best interests to remove the bladder stone under local/regional anaesthesia. It was important to ensure that the family understood that the aim of this treatment was symptom control and not prolongation of life. After discussion, the son and daughter agreed with the plan, so avoiding any need to ask the Court of Protection to arbitrate in defining the patient's best interest in case of disagreement (see case 13).

The bladder stone was removed without complications and a new urinary catheter inserted. The patient became much more settled and was able to take adequate food and fluids. Pain was well controlled on oral medications. It transpired that the daughter's main concern was that her father should be sedated to avoid any distress. However, once pain was controlled, he was no longer distressed and sedation was not required or appropriate.

4 What general principles in the management of symptoms in palliative care could be applied in this case?

The following general principles for palliative care could be applied (ascribed the acronym EEMMA, adapted from Twycross):

Evaluation: the pathogenesis of a symptom should be established if possible before any treatment (e.g. the Assessment of Pain, Twycross R; Box 41.1).

Box 41.1 (Adapted from Twycross R), OPQRST questions—the Assessment of Pain

Onset

Palliative or provocative factors: 'What makes it better or worse?'

Quality: 'What exactly is it like?'

Radiation: 'Does it spread anywhere?'

Severity: 'How bad it is?, e.g. scale 0–10'

Temporal factors: 'Is it there all the time, or does it come and go?'—'Is it worse at any particular time of the day or night?'

In practice, it may be best to start with **T** and **P**.

Clinicians should be always alert to the possibility of a new cause for a new problem in any patient, regardless of any previously recognized condition. Evaluation can be difficult, as with this patient, owing to poor cognition, and difficulties in communication; diagnosis often has to be made on a basis of pattern recognition and probability. In such cases, direct observation for tachycardia, restlessness, moaning, guarding, grimacing, whether when the patient is at rest or being moved, together with information about pain control from carers, nursing staff, or family members, may be useful. In some cases where assessment of pain is not possible, careful observation before and after an empirical trial of an analgesic may be helpful.

For patients with adequate communication who are in pain, it is important to accept their estimation of its severity and to establish its cause, location, radiation, and response to treatment and its significance for daily living. The impact of non-physical factors, the patient's mood and morale, and the meaning of pain for the patient should also be considered.

Research has shown that the biggest difference between patients and professionals is in the assessment of severe pain, with health care professionals underestimating it in around 70% of cases. However, studies have shown that family members also underestimate patients' pain.

- *Explanation:* should be given to patients or family members/carers, about the probable underlying mechanisms of pain (or other symptoms) and options for management. For a patient who can understand and retain information, this should be done before starting treatment in order to improve compliance, demystify the condition, and ensure the patient's sense of participation.
- *Management:* is individual in identifying and treating causes of symptoms and in selecting between drug and non-drug treatment options.
- *Monitoring:* of the impact of intervention and to identify any new problems, especially adverse effects of intervention, such as confusion or drowsiness caused by analgesics.
- *Attention to detail.* The question 'why?' should be asked of everything that is happening with a patient at all times.

In some cases problems may be:

- Mechanical, requiring mechanical solutions, such as pain caused by fracture that will improve with immobilization.
- Anticipated in advance (e.g. while starting opioid analgesia, starting laxative at the same time will prevent constipation and its consequences, including further pain, discomfort, nausea, overflow diarrhoea, confusion, etc.).

5 How would you control pain?

Pain in palliative care patients is managed according to the analgesic ladder (Box 41.2) and should be started after the following assessment:

- Where possible, treatment should be directed at the cause of pain, not just the pain itself. This may not be possible for various reasons, for example the patient may be too unwell or may refuse further investigation or treatment.

- Verbal and written information about analgesics to the patient, family, and carers, may lead to better outcomes. Frequent review of analgesic therapy is important, with dose reduction in the context of developing hepatic or renal failure. The review should include the route of drug delivery and management of adverse effects. These are more common with older patients owing to changes in body fat distribution, liver mass, and renal function, with consequent elevation of blood drug levels. In some difficult cases, a second medical opinion may be helpful. There is no firm evidence on how to start pain control for older patients. Most clinicians start with a low dose of analgesic (some authors recommend 30–50% of the recommended starting dose for younger adults) and titrate it according to response. In addition to oral medication, sublingual, transdermal, rectal, injection, and subcutaneous infusions may need to be considered (e.g. lack of IV access, intolerance of certain medications, etc.).

Box 41.2 The WHO analgesic ladder for cancer pain

Step 1 Non-opioid (antipyretic) ± adjuvants
Step 2 Weak opioid + non-opioid ± adjuvants
Step 3 Strong opioid + non-opioid ± adjuvants.

6 List adjuvant analgesics and the indications for their prescription for pain control in elderly patients.

Adjuvant agents for pain control and indications for their use include:

- Anticonvulsants such as gabapentin; antidepressants (tricyclic, serotonin and norepinephrine reuptake inhibitors); TENS (transcutaneous electrical nerve stimulation) for neuropathic pain, as well as spinal analgesia for severe unresponsive neuropathic pain. N-methyl-D-aspartate (NMDA)-receptor-channel-blockers (e.g. methadone, amantadine, ketamine) can help if pain is poorly responsive to analgesics but should be used under specialist advice.
- Bisphosphonates for pain from bone metastases.
- Steroids are used in increased intracranial pressure, spinal cord compression, and neuropathic pain if associated with limb weakness. Usually, these are started at high dose, and then reduced to a satisfactory maintenance level.
- Muscle relaxants (for painful muscle spasm patient may benefit from local heat application and massage)

- Antispasmodics in colic
- Benzodiazepines if pain is worsened by anxiety
- Palliative radiotherapy for painful bony metastases
- Palliative systemic radionucltides for painful bony metastases
- Regional nerve blocks for severe localized pain, caused by a single nerve
- Local anaesthetics, e.g. lidocaine patches, capsaicin
- Counselling for stress and anxiety.

7 How would you estimate life expectancy of a patient receiving palliative care and why is this important?

Older patients with advanced cancer often want an accurate and honest prognosis, as do their families and carers. However, clinicians may avoid making predictions since they may be inaccurate and there may be a tendency to overestimate survival. Conversely, patients may make a surprisingly successful recovery from an acute episode of deterioration, caused by infection for example. Subjective prognostic predictions by clinicians are influenced by his or her seniority, training, experience and level of acquaintance with the patient, and are usually better with substantial experience in end-of-life care. Accurate prediction of survival might improve clinical care in advanced cancer by enabling future care planning, and helping the patient and family to prepare for death; however, inaccurate predictions may be as harmful as a mistaken diagnosis or inappropriate therapy. Although prognostic tools exist (e.g. The National Hospice and Palliative Care Organization tool, Palliative Prognostic Index), there is little evidence that they perform better than experienced clinicians' estimates.

The present recommendation from the European Association of Palliative Care is that the clinical prediction of survival is used plus, added use of other prognostic factors or a second opinion from an experienced clinician. The most important poor prognostic clinical signs and symptoms for survival in cancer patients are anorexia–cachexia syndrome, the presence of delirium, dyspnoea, poor performance status, poor swallowing, and xerostomia. Other prognostic tools shown to be significant include subjective estimates from clinicians and laboratory results, leucocytosis, lymphocytopenia, low albumin, high C-reactive protein, and high bilirubin. Rate of change in a patient's functional abilities can be one of the most important tools in helping to estimate prognosis.

8 What clinical features suggest that death is imminent?

Signs predicting death within a few days include swallowing difficulties, drowsiness, diminished oral intake, and global weakness. Signs of death within several hours are clouding of consciousness (worsening as death approaches); respiratory pattern changes; death rattle caused by sagging of the soft palate and tongue; pooling of secretions as cough and gag reflexes decline; decreased interaction; decreased oral intake; decreased urine output; cooling and cyanotic extremities; and weak or impalpable radial pulse.

In the current case, the following four questions were asked (adapted from Boyd K, Murray SA) in an attempt to determine whether death was imminent (if all four answers are positive, the patient is probably in the process of dying).

Question 1: Is it likely that this patient is in the last days of life? For example, the patient is increasingly drowsy, incapable of self-care, is confined to bed or chair, not taking oral drugs, and has difficulties with taking oral fluids.

Question 2: Was this patient's condition expected to deteriorate in this way?

Question 3: Is further prolongation of life expected to be ineffective or burdensome, is there an advanced directive refusing treatment or does the patient refuse it now?

Question 4: Have potentially reversible causes of deterioration been excluded? (e.g. dehydration; drugs; haemorrhage; anaemia; delirium; infection; depression; constipation; and biochemical disorders such as hyponatraemia).

For this patient, the answer was yes to all four questions and in agreement with the family; urgent transfer to his home was organized with the appropriate equipment and care. He died there peacefully two weeks later.

9 What are the most common differences in the palliative care of older compared with younger adults?

Palliative care is defined by WHO as 'an approach that improves the quality of life of patients and their families facing problems associated with life-threatening illness, through the prevention and relief of suffering by means of early identification, assessment and treatment of pain and other problems, physical, psychosocial, and spiritual'. The intention is to identify and relieve symptoms, facilitate access to information, to set achievable goals, plan a 'good death', to improve the quality of life of patients with advanced and incurable conditions (and their families and carers), taking into account their needs and preferences, through involving a multidisciplinary team approach.

Palliative care also aids decision making regarding therapies (benefits and burdens), and with multiple transitions between different models of care (e.g.

acute hospital ward; rehabilitation ward; home), by ensuring continuity. Palliative care for older adults, when compared with younger, has the following differences:

- Older patients more commonly have co-existing chronic conditions (e.g. dementia, as in the current case) in addition to the condition for which palliative care is needed, and so require a more complex input.
- In some studies, older people are less likely to favour dying at home. This is culturally determined and in Western societies may reflect a preference for receiving intimate or undignified bodily care from professionals rather than family members.
- More commonly have a higher prevalence of diverse symptoms. In one study, 80% of older patients reported at least one symptom as moderate or severe, while 69% had at least two such symptoms, most commonly reduced activity, fatigue, and physical discomfort.
- The assessment of older people may be more difficult as they have a higher prevalence of communication problems, agitation, acute or chronic cognitive, motor, visual or auditory impairment and disabilities. Commonly used assessment tools may need to be modified, for example by using large print questionnaires or pictures.
- The onset of new pain or the worsening of previous pain may present in different ways, such as functional decline, decreased mobility, increased confusion and agitation, delirium (see case 1) or other changes in behaviour.
- More commonly need palliative care for conditions other than cancer, for example heart failure, COPD, Parkinson's disease, dementia, and stroke.
- Have a higher prevalence of risks arising from co-morbidities, for example risk of falls or of adverse effects of drugs.
- The greater likelihood of difficulty in prognostication in non-cancer conditions, particularly in the presence of multiple co-morbidities.
- More difficulties in defining the goals of care and more frequent involvement of families and carers, as well as other individuals' granted lasting power of attorney.
- More commonly need a decision to stop an unnecessary drug with the consequent need for further communication and explanation to patients, family, and carers of the reason for doing so.
- Have a higher risk of iatrogenic and nosocomial conditions.
- 'Minor' problems may have apparently disproportionate psychological impact.

- Significant poverty and social isolation are more common in later life.
- More commonly fear addiction to opioid drugs.
- More commonly under-report pain, or suffer from unrecognized pain, leading them to require more frequent assessments.

Further reading

Barazzetti G, Borreani C, Miccinesi G, Toscani F (2010). What 'best practice' could be in Palliative Care: an analysis of statements on practice and ethics expressed by the main Health Organizations. *BMC Palliat Care*; **9**: 1.

Boyd K, Murray SA (2010). Recognising and managing key transitions in end of life care. *BMJ*; **341**: 649–652.

Coventry PA, Grande GE, Richards DA, Todd CJ (2005). Prediction of appropriate timing of palliative care for older adults with non-malignant life threatening disease: A systematic review. *Age Ageing*; **34**: 218–227.

Extermann M, Aapro M, Bernabei R, *et al.* (2005). Use of comprehensive geriatric assessment in older cancer patients: recommendations from the task force on CGA of the International Society of Geriatric Oncology (SIOG). *Critic Rev Oncol Haematol*; **55**(3): 241–252.

Gwilliam B, Keeley V, Todd C, *et al.* (2011). Development of prognosis in palliative care study (PiPS) predictor models to improve prognostication in advanced cancer: prospective cohort study. *BMJ*; **343**: d4920.

Lynn J (2001). Serving patients who may die soon and their families: the role of hospice and other services. *JAMA*; **285**: 925–932.

Ruiz M, Reske T, Cefalu C, Estrada J (2013). Management of elderly and frail elderly cancer patients: the importance of comprehensive geriatrics assessment and the need for guidelines. *Am J Med Sci*; **346**(1): 66–69.

Shaw KL, Clifford C, Thomas K, Meehan H (2010). Improving end-of-life care: a critical review of the gold standards framework in primary care. *Palliat Med*; **24**(3): 317–329.

Smith R (2000). A good death. An important aim for health services and for us all. *BMJ*; **320**: 129–130.

Twycross R. Introducing Palliative Care (2003). 4th Edition. Milton Keynes, UK: Radcliffe Medical Press.

Case 42

A 78-year-old man was noted by his GP to have an irregularly irregular pulse, which was confirmed on 12-lead ECG to be atrial fibrillation with a ventricular rate of 88bpm. Blood pressure was 150/78mmHg and there were no cardiac symptoms. Past medical history included a TIA one year previously, hypertension, type 2 diabetes (diet-controlled), and constipation. Medications included aspirin, amlodipine, and simvastatin. He was a retired civil servant who lived with his wife in a four-bedroom house. They had no carers, and were beginning to struggle with the upkeep of the house, and general daily tasks. The patient's mobility had declined over the past year owing to pain in the right hip from osteoarthritis. He had fallen four times in the past three months, but had not sustained any significant injury.

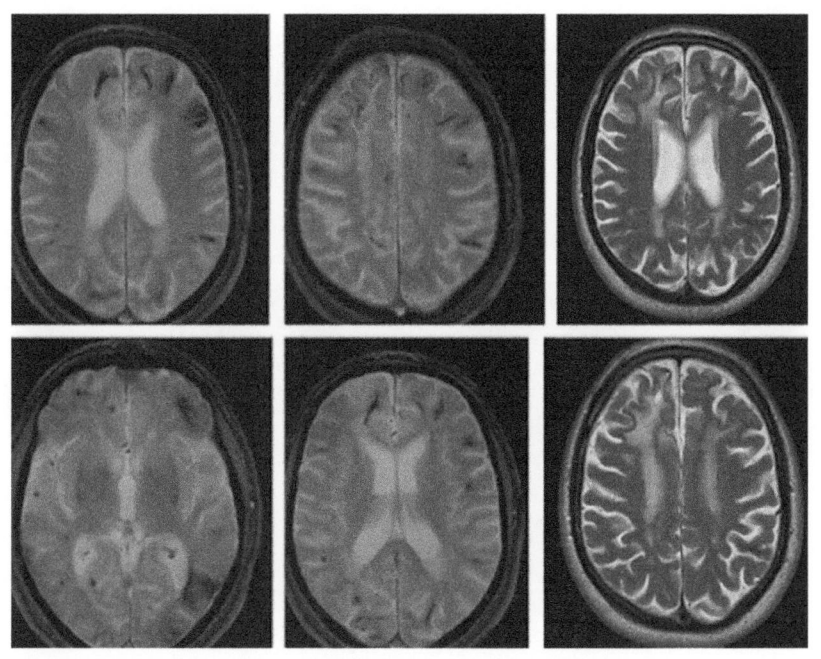

Fig. 42.1 Gradient echo (GRE) and T2-weighted axial (right images) MRI brain scan slices obtained at the time of the patient's TIA.

Questions

1 What is this man's risk of stroke in the absence of anticoagulant treatment?
2 What reduction in risk of stroke is associated with antithrombotic therapy?
3 What is the likelihood of a significant complication while taking antithrombotic therapy?
4 How would you manage this patient?
5 MRI brain scan obtained at the time of his TIA is shown in Figure 42.1. Does this change your management?

Answers

1 What is this man's risk of stroke in the absence of anticoagulant treatment?

Non-rheumatic atrial fibrillation (AF) is the most common cardioembolic cause of stroke and has the highest prevalence in the old. However, some of the association between AF and stroke must be coincidental, because AF can be caused by coronary and hypertensive heart disease, both of which may be associated with atheromatous disease, or primary intracerebral haemorrhage. This man is at high risk of a thromboembolic event associated with AF given his age, previous TIA, and other vascular risk factors. The average annual risk of stroke in patients with non-rheumatic AF (including paroxysmal AF) in the absence of anticoagulants or antiplatelet medication is overall around 4–5%, which is five to six times greater than for otherwise similar patients in sinus rhythm (risks are substantially higher in rheumatic AF). However, the risk of stroke with non-rheumatic AF in a given individual varies widely according to the presence of other risk factors. A quick tool for assessing risk is the CHADS$_2$ score (Table 42.1), which risk stratifies patients as shown in Table 42.2.

Table 42.1 The CHADS$_2$ score for stroke risk in non-rheumatic AF

Congestive heart failure	1
H—Hypertension systolic >160mmHg	1
A—Age >75 years	1
D—Diabetes	1
S—Previous cerebral ischaemia	2

Table 42.2 Risk of stroke by CHADS score

CHADS score	Adjusted annual stroke rate (95% CI)
0	1.9 (1.2–3.0)
1	2.8 (2.0–3.8)
2	4.0 (3.1–5.1)
3	5.9 (4.6–7.3)
4	8.5 (6.3–11.1)
5	12.5 (8.2–17.5)
6	18.2 (10.5–27.4)

(Data sourced from Gage et al., JAMA 2001; 285: 2864–2870.)

The patient in the current case has a CHADS score of four, and therefore an annual stroke risk of 8.5% in the absence of antithrombotic therapy. A newer, extended score, CHA$_2$DS$_2$-VASc (Table 42.3), includes three other variables (vascular disease, age 65–74, and female sex), and gives two points instead of one to age 75 and older (Table 42.4). The CHA$_2$DS$_2$-VASc is superior for identifying patients at truly low risk and at very high risk.

Table 42.3 CHA$_2$DS$_2$-VASc score

CHA$_2$DS$_2$-VASc score[3] risk factor	Points
C—Congestive heart failure or left ventricular dysfunction	1
H—Hypertension	1
A$_2$—Age ≥75	2
D—Diabetes mellitus	1
S$_2$—Stroke, transient ischaemic attack, or thromboembolism	2
V—Vascular disease (prior myocardial infarction, peripheral arterial disease, aortic plaque)	1

Table 42.4 Risk of stroke by CHA$_2$DS$_2$-VASc score

CHA$_2$DS$_2$-VASc Score	Participants, n	Event rate of hospital admission and death due to thromboembolism per 100 person-years (95% CI)	Recommended antithrombotic therapy (European Society of Cardiology, 2010)
0	6,369	0.78 (0.58–1.04)	No antithrombotic therapy (preferred) or aspirin 75–325mg/d
1	8,203	2.01 (1.70–2.36)	Oral anticoagulant (preferred) or aspirin 75–325mg/d
2	12,771	3.71 (3.36–4.09)	Oral anticoagulant
3	17,371	5.92 (5.53–6.34)	Oral anticoagulant
4	13,887	9.27 (8.71–9.86)	Oral anticoagulant
5	8,942	15.26 (14.35–16.24)	Oral anticoagulant
6	4,244	19.74 (18.21–21.41)	Oral anticoagulant
7	1,420	21.50 (18.75–24.64)	Oral anticoagulant
8	285	22.38 (16.29–30.76)	Oral anticoagulant
9	46	23.64 (10.62–52.61)	Oral anticoagulant

Paroxysmal atrial fibrillation (PAF) carries the same stroke risk as persistent AF and should be treated similarly. There is no evidence that conversion to sinus rhythm followed by pharmacotherapy to try and maintain such rhythm is superior to rate control in terms of mortality and stroke risk.

2 What reduction in risk of stroke is associated with antithrombotic therapy?

Warfarin therapy is more beneficial than aspirin and will decrease the risk of stroke in patients with AF by approximately two-thirds versus a placebo, compared with reduction of around one-fifth for aspirin, and is also superior to aspirin plus clopidogrel. Warfarin produces greater relative and absolute risk reductions for patients at high versus lower risk (Table 42.5). The Birmingham Atrial Fibrillation Treatment of the Aged (BAFTA) has corroborated these findings in individuals with AF aged 75 and older.

Table 42.5 Reductions in stroke risk with warfarin versus aspirin

Risk group	Untreated	Aspirin	Warfarin	NNT*
Very high—previous ischaemic stroke or TIA	12%	10%	5%	13
High age over 65 and one other risk factor: • hypertension • diabetes mellitus • heart failure • LV dysfunction	5–8%	4–6%	2–3%	22–47
Moderate • Age over 65, no other risk factors • Age under 65, other risk factors	3–5%	2–4%	1–2%	47–83
Low age under 65, no other risk factors	1.2%	1%	c. 0.5%	200

* Number needed to treat with warfarin instead of aspirin for one year to prevent one stroke. Adapted from Consensus Statement of the Royal College of Physicians of Edinburgh.

Recently, new anticoagulants have been developed that do not require monitoring using the INR. In 2009, the Randomized Evaluation of Long-term Anticoagulant TherapY (RE-LY) trial was published. This compared the efficacy and safety of dabigatran, a direct thrombin inhibitor, with warfarin in patients with non-valvular AF. In this trial two doses of dabigatran were used, 110mg bd, and 150mg bd. Over 18,000 patients were included in the trial and randomly assigned to either dose of the dabigatran or warfarin therapy. The patients were followed up for a median of two years. The rate of stroke or systemic embolism was 1.54%, 1.11% and 1.71% in patients receiving 110mg bd dabigatran, 150mg dabigatran bd, and warfarin therapy respectively. Dabigatran at 150mg bd appeared superior, and dabigatran at 110mg bd non-inferior, to warfarin. In patients over the age of 75 years, there were higher rates of extracranial bleeding with 150mg versus 110mg dabigatran, but the 150mg dose appeared equally safe as warfarin. Dabigatran and similar drugs have advantages over warfarin in not requiring monitoring of INR to ensure therapeutic levels and are less affected by dietary changes. However, dabigatran has a twice daily regimen and there is no available reversible agent for use in case of bleeding.

Subsequently other novel anticoagulants (NOACs) have been developed, including rivaroxaban and apixaban, which are both direct Xa inhibitors. The ROCKET AF trial published in 2010 compared rivaroxaban with warfarin and demonstrated non-inferiority with no significant difference between major and non-major clinically relevant bleeding rates. The ARISTOTLE trial originally published in 2011 demonstrates that apixaban is superior in preventing thromboembolic stroke in patients with AF, when compared to warfarin (HR 0.79; 95%CI 0.66–0.95). However, there was no difference in the rate of systemic embolism (HR 0.89; 95%CI 0.44–1.75), but there was a significant reduction in all-cause mortality in patients in the apixaban group, compared to the warfarin group (HR 0.89; 95%CI 0.80–0.998). The ARISTOTLE trial also demonstrated that apixaban treatment significantly reduced the risk of major bleeds compared to warfarin treatment (HR 0.69; 95%CI 0.6–0.8), with a significantly lower rate of intracranial bleeding, but with no difference between rates of GI bleeding.

A comparison of the new oral anticoagulants and warfarin is summarized in Table 42.6. Head-to-head comparisons have not been performed. Safety information remains limited, as these drugs have not been in widespread use for long. Warfarin is still significantly cheaper than any of the new anticoagulants.

Anticoagulation is not effective in secondary prevention of stroke for patients in sinus rhythm. Warfarin treatment to a target INR of 3–4.5 was associated with significant harm because of a large increase in major bleeding complications, especially intracerebral haemorrhage, in patients with previous TIA or ischaemic stroke in the SPIRIT trial. The subsequent Warfarin-Aspirin Recurrent Stroke Study (WARSS) trial of aspirin versus warfarin for patients in sinus rhythm and without a cardioembolic source, or >50% carotid stenosis showed no additional benefit for warfarin at a target INR of 1.4–2.8.

Anticoagulant therapy is underused in elderly adults with AF. Various studies have suggested that warfarin is prescribed to only two-thirds of individuals with AF who are eligible for anticoagulation in part because of the inherent difficulties and inconvenience associated with warfarin use.

Table 42.6 Comparison of warfarin with three new oral anticoagulants in non-valvular atrial fibrillation (AF)

Comparison parameter	Warfarin (Coumadin; FDA approved)	Dabigatran (Pradaxa; FDA approved)	Rivaroxaban (Xarelto; FDA approved)	Apixaban (Eliquis; under FDA review)
1. Cost of 30-day supply in the United States, $	4	264	246	–
Mechanism of action	Vitamin K antagonist (inhibits vitamin K-dependent hepatic synthesis of factors II, VII, IX, and X, and proteins C and S)	Direct thrombin inhibitor	Factor Xa inhibitor	Factor Xa inhibitor
Dose	Once daily, dose adjusted to INR	150mg twice daily (FDA approved); 110mg twice daily (not FDA approved)	20 mg/d	5mg twice daily
Use in renal impairment	Not contraindicated	75mg twice daily if CrCl 15–30mL/min	15mg/d if CrCl 15–50mL/min	Lower dose (e.g. 2.5mg twice daily)
Use in hepatic impairment	Extreme caution	Not contraindicated	Avoid in moderate or severe hepatic impairment	Avoid in severe hepatic impairment
Bioavailability, %	~100	3–7	80–100	50
Time to peak plasma concentration, hours	72–96	0.5–2	2–4	3–4
Half-life, hours	20–60	12 to 17 if CrCl 50–80mL/min; 18 to 24 if CrCl 30–49mL/min; >24 if CrCl <30mL/min	5–9; 11–13 (elderly)	9–14
Metabolism by cytochrome P450	CYP2C9, 2C19, 2C8, 2C18, 1A2, 3A4	No	CYP3A4, 3A5, 2J2	CYP3A4, 3A5, 1A2, 2C8, 2C9, 2C19, 2J2
Elimination	Hepatic	Renal (80%)	Renal and hepatic	Renal and hepatic
Laboratory monitoring of anticoagulant effect	INR	Ecarin clotting time, activated partial thromboplastin time, or thrombin time might be helpful; HEMOCLOT direct thrombin inhibitor assay can accurately estimate plasma concentrations of dabigatran[40]	Factor Xa activity and PT might be helpful	Factor Xa activity and PT might be helpful

(continued)

Table 42.6 (continued)

Comparison parameter	Warfarin (Coumadin; FDA approved)	Dabigatran (Pradaxa; FDA approved)	Rivaroxaban (Xarelto; FDA approved)	Apixaban (Eliquis; under FDA review)
Reversal agent	Vitamin K, PCCs, FFP	FFP?, PCCs?, rVIIa?	PCCs?, rVIIa?	
Drug interactions	Multiple	P-glycoprotein inducers and inhibitors	P-glycoprotein and CYP3A4 inducers and inhibitors	P-glycoprotein and CYP3A4 inducers and inhibitors
Food interactions	Multiple	None reported	None reported	None reported
Randomized trial that tested drug efficacy in AF		RE-LY trial (vs. warfarin; n = 18,113 for entire trial)	ROCKET AF (vs. warfarin; n = 14,264 for entire trial)	ARISTOTLE trial (vs. warfarin; n = 18,201 for entire trial)
Event rates compared with warfarin				
Stroke and systemic embolism		⇓ (D150) ⇔ (D110)	⇔	⇔
Haemorrhagic stroke		⇓ (D150) ⇓ (D110)	⇓	⇓
Ischaemic stroke		⇓ (D150) ⇔ (D110)	⇔	⇔
Major haemorrhage		⇔ (D150) ⇓ (D110)	⇔	⇓
Intracranial haemorrhage		⇓ (D150) ⇓ (D110)	⇓	⇓
All-cause mortality		⇔ (D150) ⇔ (D110)	⇔	⇓

ARISTOTLE = Apixaban for Reduction in Stroke and Other Thromboembolic Events in Atrial Fibrillation; CrCl = creatinine clearance; FDA = Food and Drug Administration; FFP = fresh frozen plasma; INR = international normalized ratio; PCCs = prothrombin complex concentrates; PT = prothrombin time; rVIIa = human recombinant activated factor VII; RE-LY = Randomized Evaluation of Long-term Anticoagulant TherapY; ROCKET AF = Rivaroxaban Once Daily Oral Direct Factor Xa Inhibition Compared with Vitamin K Antagonism for Prevention of Stroke and Embolism Trial in Atrial Fibrillation; ⇓ = significant reduction; ⇔ = no significant difference.

Another important barrier relates to physician perceptions of benefits and risks—specifically, physicians tend to fear causing warfarin-related bleeding and to under-appreciate the risk of stroke in the absence of therapy.

3 What is the likelihood of a significant complication while taking antithrombotic therapy?

The Birmingham Atrial Fibrillation Treatment of the Aged Study (BAFTA), and Warfarin versus Aspirin for Stroke Prevention in Octogenarians with AF (WASPO) have shown that warfarin is as safe as aspirin in elderly patients with AF. If warfarin is taken correctly and anticoagulation kept in the therapeutic range, then the risk of a major haemorrhage is around 1% when used for primary prevention. However, in the case of secondary prevention, the risk of a major haemorrhage increases to 2.5%.

Several scoring systems have been developed to predict bleeding risk with anticoagulation therapy, including the HAS-BLED score (Table 42.7).

Table 42.7 HAS-BLED score for bleeding risk

HAS-BLED Score	
Risk factor	Points
H—Hypertension (uncontrolled, systolic blood pressure >160mmHg)	1
A—Abnormal renal function or abnormal liver function—1 point each	1 or 2
S—Stroke	1
B—Bleeding history or predisposition to bleeding (e.g. bleeding diathesis, anaemia)	1
L—Labile INRs (unstable or high INRs or poor time in therapeutic range, e.g. <60%)	1
E—Elderly (age >65)	1
D—Drugs (antiplatelet agents, non-steroidal anti-inflammatory drugs) or alcohol abuse—1 point each	1 or 2

However, as will be seen from the scores for stroke risk and for bleeding, many of the factors that increase the risk of ischaemic stroke also increase the risk of bleeding on anticoagulation. Older patients also often experience intercurrent illness that increases the response to warfarin or results in changes to medications and dietary sources of vitamin K, explaining the frequently observed derangement in INR in older people on warfarin admitted to hospital as an emergency.

The risk of major bleeding on combined antiplatelet and warfarin therapy is 1.8–3.7 times as high as on warfarin monotherapy, and should therefore be carefully justified. Warfarin and antiplatelet agent may be considered in AF and recent acute coronary syndrome, recent coronary or peripheral arterial stenting, and recent coronary artery bypass surgery. Drug-eluting stents, which require prolonged dual antiplatelet therapy, should be avoided unless the benefit over bare-metal stents is significant.

4 How would you manage this patient?

This patient is at high risk of stroke and anticoagulation would normally be warranted, but he has also had recent falls. The risk of intracranial haemorrhage in older people prone to falls is a major deterrent to the use of anticoagulation. A detailed account of the falls and a thorough examination including full neurological and cognitive assessment are needed to establish the cause, and referral to a falls clinic considered if necessary. If a treatable cause is found, warfarin may be started without hesitation assuming the patient is in agreement. Where the risk of falls is likely to persist, a careful discussion with the patient of the risks and benefits of warfarin is necessary, bearing in mind that the evidence suggests that doctors overestimate the risks and underestimate the benefits of warfarin. The advent of NOAC drugs is useful in this situation. As although at present there is no drug to reverse their anticoagulation effects, they have lower rates of intracranial bleeding when compared to warfarin therapy, so they may be safer to use in these situations.

Analytical models evaluating different antithrombotic strategies for individuals with AF aged 65 and older who were at risk for falls showed that warfarin provided higher quality-adjusted life years than aspirin or no antithrombotic therapy. In another study of elderly adults with AF, a decision to withhold warfarin was more likely to be detrimental because the rates of ischaemic stroke (13.7 and 6.9 per 100 patient-years in those at high risk for falls and other individuals, respectively) easily exceeded the rates of intracerebral haemorrhage (ICH). In individuals who were at high risk for falls, but were also at moderate-to-high risk for a stroke based on a $CHADS_2$ score of 2 or greater, warfarin was associated with a 25% relative risk reduction in the composite outcome of stroke, ICH, myocardial infarction, and death.

5 MRI brain scan obtained at the time of his TIA is shown in Figure 42.2. Does this change your management?

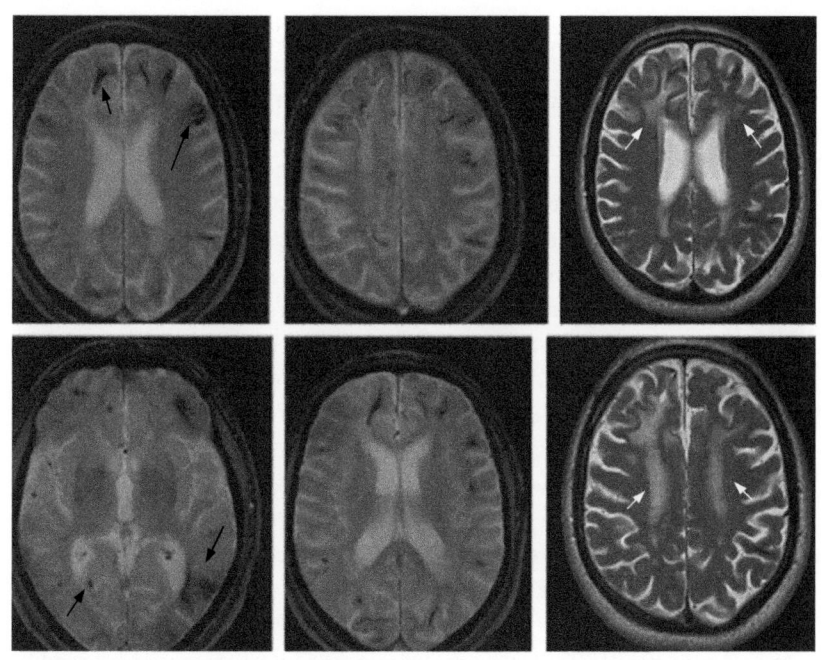

Fig. 42.2 Gradient echo (GRE) and T2-weighted axial (right images) MRI brain scan slices obtained at the time of the patient's TIA. There are multiple areas of old haemorrhage including subcortical haemorrhages and microbleeds (black arrows) and widespread white matter changes (white arrows).

The MRI brain scan has been performed using gradient echo imaging (GRE) and shows changes consistent with cerebral amyloid angiopathy (CAA) with multiple microbleeds (BMBs), subcortical haemorrhage and widespread white matter changes and this was felt to increase the risk of intracranial haemorrhage on warfarin and thus to influence the risk-benefit evaluation for this patient.

CAA is defined by the deposition of amyloid in the walls of leptomeningeal and cortical arteries, arterioles, capillaries, and veins. This central nervous system vasculopathy is associated with a number of clinical syndromes, including recurrent lobar haemorrhage, subcortical ischaemia, migraine, BMBs, and dementia. CAA may be hereditary or sporadic. Hereditary forms, mostly associated with amyloid precursor protein mutations, are rare, but the sporadic form increases exponentially with age. It is rare before the age of 50 years and common in those aged ≥90 years.

BMBs are small homogeneous round foci of low signal intensity on haem-sensitive gradient echo (GRE-T2*) sequences on MRI, which represent perivascular collections of haemosiderin deposits. Using conventional MR sequences, the prevalence of BMBs is about 5% in healthy people, but increases with age. Microbleeds are associated with stroke: overall around 34% of patients with ischaemic strokes and 60% with haemorrhagic strokes have microbleeds. The prevalence is less in first-ever compared with recurrent strokes, suggesting that BMBs are a marker for severity of the underlying cerebrovascular disease. Microbleeds are particularly common in CAA and are also seen in hypertension and Alzheimer's disease, affecting around a fifth of patients with this condition. The diagnostic and prognostic characteristics of BMBs are uncertain and thus their presence can give rise to clinical dilemmas, as illustrated in the current case.

In a population-based cross-sectional sample of 1,062 people aged 60 years and older without dementia, BMBs were more prevalent among users of antiplatelet drugs (adjusted odds ratio 1.71; 95% CI 1.2–2.4). However, these findings do not necessarily indicate that patients with BMBs are at increased risk of bleeding when treated with antiplatelet drugs, since BMBs may be related to the underlying vascular disease.

Recently, Lovelock *et al.* (2010) undertook a pooled analysis of 3,817 patients with ischaemic stroke or TIA, and 1,460 patients with ICH, and found an excess of BMBs in warfarin-associated ICH that was not found in patients who had an ischaemic stroke or TIA while on warfarin. These preliminary data indicate that warfarin may be hazardous in patients with BMBs. Similar but weaker associations between BMB frequency and antiplatelet-associated ICH were also seen, but significant heterogeneity between cohorts means that these results should be interpreted with caution. Available prospective data are few, but support the hypothesis that the presence of BMBs increases the risk of future ICH with antithrombotic drug use. More prospective data on the safety of antithrombotic drugs in patients with BMBs are required, and anticoagulation should not be withheld in situations where there is established overall benefit.

Antithrombotic treatment decisions are particularly difficult in CAA where there are high risks of both ischaemic and haemorrhagic strokes, and there are few data to guide decisions. Antithrombotic agents appear to increase the risk of recurrent haemorrhage in CAA. Warfarin appears to increase both the frequency and severity of cerebral haemorrhage, and should be avoided, if possible, in patients with CAA. Aspirin at commonly prescribed doses increases the risk of haemorrhage to a lesser extent. In one prospective cohort of patients with primary lobar ICH, aspirin was associated with an increased risk of ICH recurrence (HR = 3.95; 95% CI 1.6–8.3) when controlling for other haemorrhage risk factors. Nonetheless, aspirin use can be considered in selected patients with CAA, if they have clear indications for antiplatelet therapy.

Although the vascular pathology in CAA does not appear to be linked to hypertension, control of blood pressure is nonetheless advisable. Support for lowering of blood pressure in patients diagnosed with CAA came from a secondary analysis of data from the PROGRESS trial. Randomization to active treatment (perindopril plus indapamide) when there was either no indication, or a contraindication to diuretics in this study resulted in a 77% reduction in the risk of probable CAA-related ICH.

The current patient decided to continue aspirin rather than starting warfarin after discussion with the TIA and stroke clinic team owing to the large number of BMBs and evidence of previous haemorrhage on the MRI scan. Simvastatin was stopped due to presence of multiple BMBs and increased risk of intracranial haemorrhage. The falls were felt to be secondary to mechanical difficulties from the hip, in combination with loose carpets and poor lighting, which were rectified. A once a day care package and help with meals and cleaning were instituted.

Further reading

Gage BF, Birman-Deych E, Kerzner R, Radford MJ, Nilasena DS, Rich MW (2005). Incidence of intracranial hemorrhage in patients with atrial fibrillation who are prone to fall. *Am J Med*; **118**: 612–617.

Gage B, Waterman A, Shannon W, Boechler M, Rich M, Radford M (2001). Validation of clinical classification schemes for predicting stroke. *JAMA*; **285**: 2864–2870.

Hansen ML, Sørensen R, Clausen MT, *et al.* (2010). Risk of bleeding with single, dual, or triple therapy with warfarin, aspirin, and clopidogrel in patients with atrial fibrillation. *Arch Intern Med*; **170**: 1433–1441.

Hart RG, Pearce LA, Aguilar MI (2007). Meta-analysis: antithrombotic therapy to prevent stroke in patients who have nonvalvular atrial fibrillation. *Ann Intern Med*; **146**: 857–867.

Knudsen KA, Rosand J, Karluk D, Greenberg SM (2001). Clinical diagnosis of cerebral amyloid angiopathy: validation of the Boston criteria. *Neurology*; **56**: 537–539.

Lovelock CE, Cordonnier C, Naka H, *et al.* (2010). Antithrombotic drug use, cerebral microbleeds, and intracerebral hemorrhage: a systematic review of published and unpublished studies. *Stroke*; **41**: 1222–1228.

Man-Son-Hing M, Laupacis A (2003). Anticoagulant-related bleeding in older persons with atrial fibrillation: Physicians' fears often unfounded. *Arch Intern Med*; **163**: 1580–1586.

Man-Son-Hing M, Nichol G, Lau A, Laupacis A (1999). Choosing antithrombotic therapy for elderly patients with atrial fibrillation who are at risk for falls. *Arch Intern Med*; **159**: 677–685.

Mant J, Hobbs FD, Fletcher K, *et al.* (2007). Warfarin versus aspirin for stroke prevention in an elderly community population with atrial fibrillation (the Birmingham Atrial Fibrillation Treatment of the Aged Study, BAFTA): a randomised controlled trial. *Lancet*; **370**: 493–503.

Morrison C, Gainsborough N, Rajkumar C (2007). Warfarin versus aspirin in the elderly in primary prophylaxis in atrial fibrillation. *Age Ageing*; **36**(2): 117–119.

NICE guideline 36, section 3 (2006). Atrial Fibrillation: The management of atrial fibrillation. Antithrombotic therapy. Atrial fibrillation prophylaxis of systemic embolism.

Pisters R, Lane DA, Nieuwlaat R, de Vos CB, Crijns HJ, Lip GY (2010). A novel user-friendly score (HAS-BLED) to assess 1-year risk of major bleeding in patients with atrial fibrillation: The Euro Heart Survey. *Chest*; **138**: 1093–1100.

Thijs V, Lemmens R, Schoofs C, *et al.* (2010). Microbleeds and the risk of recurrent stroke. *Stroke*; **41**: 2005–2009.

Vernooij MW, Haag MD, van der Lugt A, *et al.* (2009). Use of antithrombotic drugs and the presence of cerebral microbleeds: the Rotterdam Scan Study. *Arch Neurol*; **66**: 714–720.

Case 43

Case 43.A

A 64-year-old history teacher was reviewed in the out-patient clinic. He had not been able to work for a year, as there had been increasing concern about his behaviour although not about his teaching ability. His wife accompanied him to the out-patient appointment, and while she stated that he had always been eccentric, she too was worried. He had become aggressive towards his pupils, and had been found on several occasions wandering naked in the street outside, early in the morning. He had also developed occasional urinary incontinence, and had become withdrawn, and low in mood. His wife reported that he had trouble in remembering the names of everyday objects. He had no significant past medical history and was not on any regular medication. There was no family history of note.

On examination, observations were unremarkable. It was noted that he repeated the commands given by the examining doctor before performing the required action. There were no cranial nerve abnormalities and tone, power, coordination, and sensation were normal. Reflexes were slightly brisk, but equal throughout, and a palmar grasp and snout reflex were elicited. MMSE score was 28.

Case 43.B

A 67-year-old woman was referred to the geratology clinic with odd behaviour on a background of previous depression. She worked in a hotel kitchen and had started behaving strangely at work. On a couple of occasions, she had been seen eating food waste out of the food disposal unit. Her daughters reported that she had been singing the same 'little ditties' repeatedly, and was repeating phrases she heard on the television. The patient was unaware of any problem. There was a history of severe postpartum depression many decades earlier and her daughters had been concerned that her mood had been low more recently. On examination, she was pleasant, co-operative, and unconcerned about being at the clinic. There was nil to find on examination and MoCA was 25/30.

Questions

1 What investigation would you perform urgently in both cases?

Answers

1 What investigation would you perform urgently in both cases?

CT or MRI brain imaging is required.

Behavioural change accompanied by urinary incontinence should always prompt assessment for a space-occupying lesion in the frontal lobe. Focal neurological signs are frequently absent even in the presence of large tumours.

Both patients had a CT brain scan (see Fig. 43.1 from case B, in which MRI was also performed), which showed no evidence of a focal lesion.

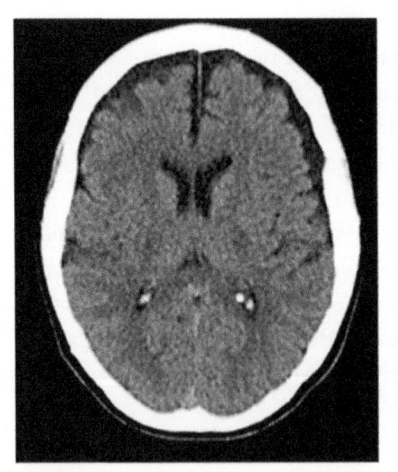

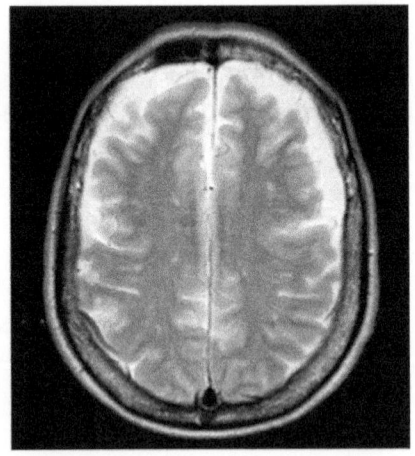

Fig. 43.1 CT axial brain scan slice from case B (left image), for which MRI was also performed, (right image, T2-weighted axial slice), showing no evidence of a focal lesion but significant frontal atrophy.

Questions continued

2 Given that the brain scans showed no evidence of a frontal lobe tumour, what is the most likely diagnosis in both cases? List other possible diagnoses.
3 What further investigations might you consider?
4 What management strategy would you undertake?
5 What is the prognosis in this condition?

Answers continued

2 Given that the brain scans show no evidence of a frontal lobe tumour, what is the most likely diagnosis in both cases? List other possible diagnoses.

The most likely diagnosis in both cases is frontotemporal dementia (FTD).

Patient A developed prominent behavioural changes accompanied by difficulty naming everyday objects, but with preservation of his teaching abilities and functional status. Patient B developed odd behaviour, but her ability to perform her job was unaffected. In both patients, cognitive function appeared relatively well preserved as evidenced by the MMSE and MoCA scores. Given that a space-occupying lesion had been excluded, the most likely diagnosis is frontotemporal dementia.

Frontotemporal lobe dementia comprises a heterogeneous group of dementias (including what used to be termed Pick's disease), which accounts for 20% of cases of dementia diagnosed before the age of 65 years. This form of dementia can occur in later years, but symptoms are most likely to occur between 45–65 years of age. There are three major sub-types of this condition, although there is often a degree of overlap:

- Primary progressive aphasia
- Semantic dementia
- Fronto-behavioural variant.

Primary progressive aphasia is characterized by progressive difficulty producing speech with preserved comprehension and in advanced stages, patients become almost mute. In semantic dementia, there is loss of the understanding of the meaning of words, so for example a patient does not know what the word 'bicycle' means, although retains understanding of visual information, i.e. can recognize a bicycle or image of one. Speech is fluent, but increasingly devoid of content. Patients with the frontal variant have prominent behavioural difficulties with lack of insight, repetitive mannerisms, and blunting of the normal emotional response.

Depression may be an early feature of frontal temporal dementia and can occur prior to cognitive or behavioural changes, as in case B. General intellectual function is often relatively well preserved in the early stages; hence the MMSE or other short cognitive tests may be misleading in diagnosis or assessment of severity of impairment as seen in the current cases. Compared with Alzheimer's disease, urinary incontinence occurs early. Primitive frontal reflexes such as the snout reflex, palmar grasp and glabella tap all reflect non-specific damage to the frontal lobes, and are often seen in cases of frontotemporal lobe dementias, as in case A.

The differential diagnosis for dementia at a relatively young age with normal CT is broad and includes:

- *Alzheimer's disease,* although prominent early behavioural changes would not be expected.
- *Vascular dementia* may be associated with behavioural abnormalities including apathy, depression, disinhibition and/or emotional lability. However, patients A and B had no vascular risk factors, or history of cerebrovascular disease, and brain imaging did not suggest this as the underlying cause.
- *Creutzfeldt-Jakob disease.* This may cause early mood changes, but patients often have sensory symptoms or myoclonus (see case 33, Oxford University Press's *Neurological Case Histories*).
- *Normal pressure hydrocephalus* (see case 6). Early incontinence is a feature of this condition, but pronounced behavioural abnormalities would not be expected.
- *AIDS-related dementia* (see case 30).
- *Neurosyphilis* (see case 30).
- *Voltage-gated channelopathies.*
- *Intracerebral pathology,* e.g. lymphoma (see case 26).
- *Primary psychiatric disorder.* Although patient B had a history of depression, there were no specific features, such as hallucinations or delusions, to suggest psychosis. Urinary incontinence or abnormalities on neurological examination would not be expected.

3 What further investigations might you consider?

Investigations to be considered include:

- Blood tests to exclude a metabolic disorder, infection, or inflammation, e.g. serum vitamin B_{12}, folate, caeruloplasmin, and thyroid function tests.
- Formal neuropsychological testing.
- EEG—this is characteristically abnormal in sporadic CJD, but otherwise shows non-specific changes in dementia.
- Further brain imaging with MRI.

Initial investigations should aim to exclude any reversible or contributing causes of cognitive impairment, although the behavioural features of these cases make such causes relatively less likely. Brain and cerebral vessel imaging with MRI/MRA may be considered to look for lymphoma, tumour, small vessel disease, and vasculitis. EEG is usually non-specific, but is useful where sporadic CJD is suspected as diagnostic abnormalities may be seen (characteristic spike and wave pattern).

MRI in FTD often demonstrates bilateral frontal and temporal lobe atrophy. Such changes may be subtle although in more advanced cases, are obvious (Figs. 43.1 and 43.2). Functional imaging with SPECT (single-photon emission computer tomography) and PET (positron emission tomography) demonstrate focal lobar areas of hypometabolism or hypoperfusion, and may be used in cases of diagnostic uncertainty, but these investigations are not routinely available or necessary. Figure 43.3 shows characteristic images from a patient with FTD.

Formal neuropsychological testing is helpful where there is diagnostic uncertainty or to provide a more detailed picture of specific cognitive deficits and a baseline level of function. This is particularly important in FTD, given the relative insensitivity of short cognitive tests owing to a lack of frontal specific tests.

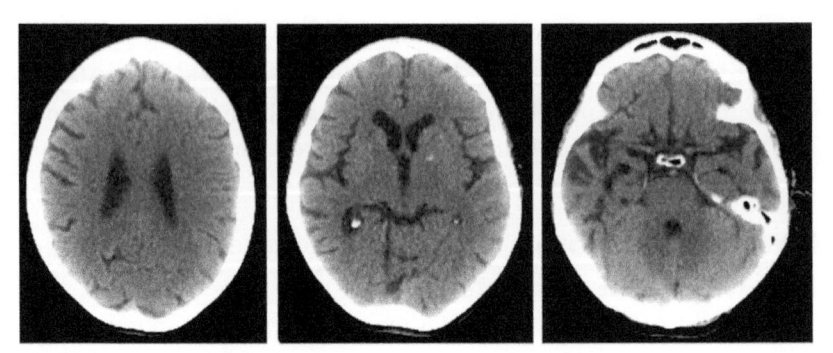

Fig. 43.2 CT brain scan from another patient with FTD showing pronounced frontal and temporal lobe atrophy.

CASE 43 | 449

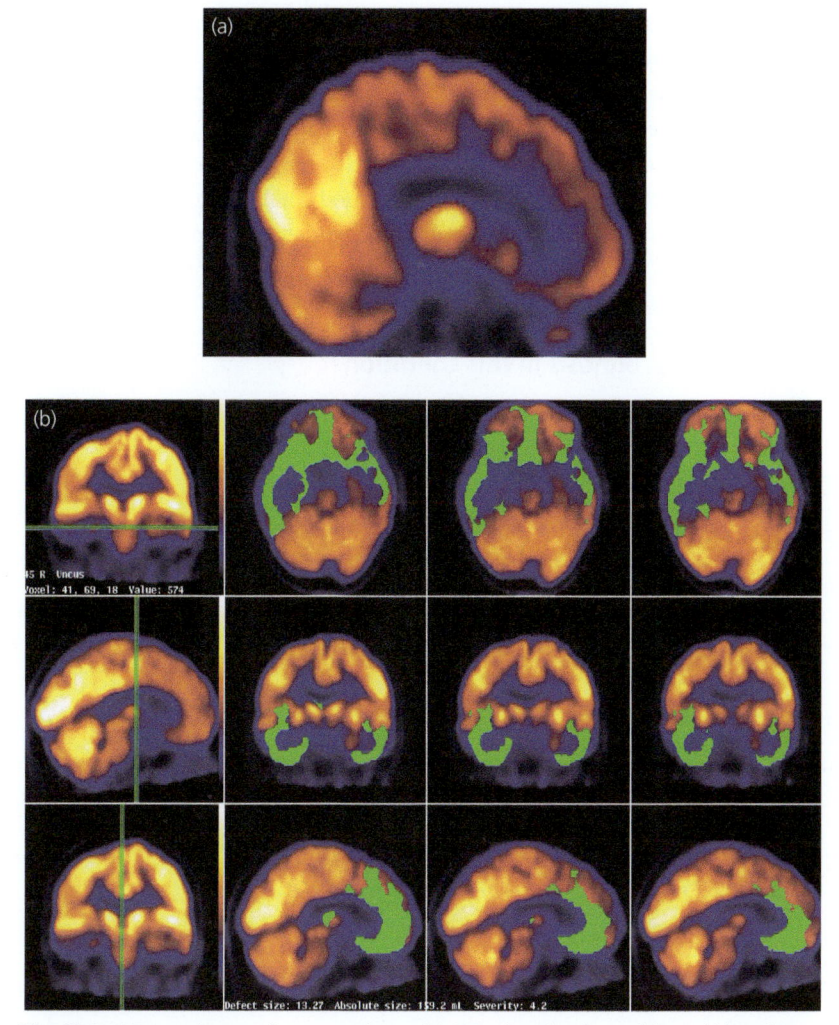

Fig. 43.3 PET scan images from a patient with FTD showing frontal (a and b) and temporal (b) hypometabolism.

4 What management strategy would you undertake?

There is no specific treatment for frontotemporal dementia. Care should be focused on providing support for the patient and the family, and this is best provided by a specialist clinic with a dementia specialist (old age psychiatry, geriatrics, or neurology), with access to dementia advisors and groups, including Young Dementia UK. Carer support is extremely important and may sometimes include cognitive behavioural therapy. Management of challenging behaviour including aggression and wandering is very difficult, and employment issues may also arise.

Although there are no disease-modifying treatments for frontotemporal dementia, there is some evidence for pharmacological agents in the treatment of mood disorders and behaviour, which may help relieve distress in patients and carers. SSRIs have been shown to be helpful in depression and may also improve behaviour. Trazodone may help aggression and sleep. There is no evidence for acetylcholinesterase inhibitors, which may in fact, make things worse.

5 What is the prognosis in this condition?

The prognosis for patients with frontotemporal dementias is poor, with a median survival of 6–11 years from onset of symptoms and three to four years from time of diagnosis.

Further reading

NICE guideline 42: Dementia: Supporting people with dementia and their carers in health and social care (2006). http://www.nice.org.uk/guidance/cg42

Rabinovici G, Miller B (2010). Frontotemporal lobar degeneration: epidemiology, pathophysiology, diagnosis and management. *CNS Drugs*; 1; **24**(5): 375–398.

SIGN guideline 86: Management of people with dementia (2006). http://www.sign.ac.uk/pdf/sign86.pdf

Weder N, Aziz R, Wilkins K, Tampi R (2007). Frontotemporal dementias: a review. *Ann Gen Psychiatry*; **6**: 15.

Case 44

An 80-year-old retired university lecturer was referred to the geratology rapid access clinic for further assessment following an admission to the emergency department two days earlier. While sitting with his family, he had suddenly lost consciousness and slumped to one side, and had begun shaking with jerking of all limbs and eyes rolling backwards for about five minutes, accompanied by incontinence of urine. In the emergency department, he was confused, and blood tests (glucose, normal full blood count, biochemistry), urine dipstick, chest X-ray, blood pressure, ECG, and CT brain scan, were unremarkable. The confusion resolved over the following hours and he was discharged home.

Past medical history included a myocardial infarction and a left hip total replacement two years before. Medications were aspirin, statin, ramipril, and paracetamol.

Further history revealed that he had had a similar episode the previous year while he was on holiday: his wife had witnessed sudden unprovoked loss of consciousness with tongue biting and urinary incontinence followed by confusion, which lasted for several hours. Extensive investigations including a week of cardiac monitoring were reportedly normal. Unfortunately, his wife had died suddenly shortly after their return from holiday and he had not attended further follow-up. He admitted worrying that his driving licence might be taken away.

Physical examination was unremarkable. Blood pressure was 130/70mmHg, without postural drop, and AMTS was 10/10.

Investigations in clinic revealed the following:

- CXR: normal
- ECG—sinus rhythm, heart rate 72bpm regular; Q waves in leads II, II, and aVF (long-standing).

Questions

1 What is the most likely diagnosis in this case and why? List differences in this condition in younger and older adults.
2 Give a differential diagnosis for this condition in older people.
3 List the assessments necessary to confirm the diagnosis.
4 List the most common causes of this condition in older people.
5 What is the most appropriate treatment and management strategy for this condition in this patient and generally in older people?

Answers

1 What is the most likely diagnosis in this case and why? List differences in this condition in younger and older adults.

Clinical presentation and available investigation results suggest that the most likely diagnosis is epilepsy. After stroke, epilepsy is globally the most common neurological disorder, and occurs in many forms. Epilepsy presents potentially life-shortening brain disorder of multifactorial origins with the main symptom being seizures.

The prevalence of epilepsy in developed countries is estimated at around 700 per 100,000, rising to around 1,200 for people over 60 years old. Annual incidence rises to 90 per 100,000 for people aged 65–69, and 150 per 100,000 at ages above 80 years. Around 500,000 people are estimated to have epilepsy in England. Although the condition carries a good prognosis in general, older people with epilepsy report a poorer quality of life in comparison with the general population. Possible reasons include isolation, vulnerability to falls, adverse effects of antiepileptic drugs, anxiety, and depression (see case 18), with prevalence twice as high as in the general population.

New epilepsy in older people usually presents as focal seizures with or without secondary generalization, although a quarter present with tonic-clonic seizures. Common presenting features include episodes of confusion, unresponsiveness, incontinence, syncope, or Todd's paresis. In comparison with younger patients with epilepsy, older patients are much less likely to experience auras, but usually have more prolonged postictal periods (sometimes lasting up to two weeks) occasionally presenting with changed behaviour including wandering. Epilepsy in older people is associated with past or future cerebrovascular events owing to the age-related rise in incidence of vascular risk factors.

There is some evidence to suggest that epilepsy is associated with cognitive decline possibly related to seizure activity, drug treatment, and more rapid accumulation of amyloid plaques, especially in those with the apolipoprotein epsilon 4 allele.

2 Give a differential diagnosis of this condition in older people.

The differential diagnosis of seizures in older people is wide and includes:
- cardiac syncope (see case 11), e.g. cardiac arrhythmias, critical aortic stenosis, orthostatic hypotension, vasovagal syncope, carotid sinus syndrome, migraine, transient global amnesia
- biochemical abnormalities, e.g. hypoglycaemia, hypocalcaemia, hyponatraemia, hypomagnesaemia

- certain sleep disorders (see case 37), e.g. periodic limb movement disorder, rapid eye movement disorder, narcolepsy
- factitious disorders, including psychogenic non-epileptic attack disorder (pseudo-seizures), especially if accompanied by tremor.

Diagnosis in older people may be difficult owing to the presence of co-morbidities, cognitive impairment, lack of a witness account in those living alone, and the reluctance of some older patients to admit symptoms or ask for help. In addition, some older people do not act on symptoms because of the stigma attached to the diagnosis and for fear of losing their driving licence.

3 List the assessments necessary to confirm the diagnosis.

In this patient, initial investigations were normal. As the history was suggestive of epilepsy, electroencephalography (EEG) was organized on the day of his clinic appointment, which confirmed epileptiform activity in the temporal region.

The further assessment of epilepsy usually includes:

- Taking a careful history from the patient and a carer/witness. Epilepsy is suggested by recurrent episodes of twitching, sensory disturbance of face or limbs, involuntary movements, amnesia, and confusion enduring for more than one hour after the event, behavioural change, and prolonged loss or disturbance of consciousness. Epilepsy should also be considered where events occur during sleep (although periodic leg movement disorder or REM sleep disorder may be differential diagnoses), or are associated with a particular posture (including lying down). Epilepsy should also be considered in patients with unexplained recurrent falls.
- Full drug history. A history of alcohol abuse or alcohol withdrawal increases the risk of seizure, as do certain antidepressants or antibiotics (e.g. ciprofloxacin) and some illicit, or over the counter substances (e.g. gingko biloba).
- Blood and urine tests, chest X-ray, and ECG are required to look for abnormal serum glucose, calcium, magnesium, sodium, infection, or arrhythmia. Echocardiogram, carotid sinus massage, or tilt-table testing may be required.
- Brain imaging. All patients with suspected epilepsy should have brain imaging with magnetic resonance imaging or CT, particularly after the onset of focal seizures. Around 5–8% of strokes provoke seizures within two weeks. Brain imaging may need to be repeated when seizures continue, despite appropriate treatment.

- Electroencephalography (EEG) should be considered, although negative results do not exclude the diagnosis. EEG in older people often shows non-specific abnormalities. The use of video-EEG monitoring may also be helpful in selected cases.

The diagnosis of epilepsy is mainly clinical, and where a definite diagnosis cannot be achieved, referral to an epilepsy specialist should be considered.

4 List the most common causes of this condition in older people.

The most common causes of epilepsy in older people are:

1 Cerebrovascular disease (30–40%)
2 Brain space-occupying lesions (~15% of those aged over 60 years presenting with a first seizure)
3 Head injury (1–3%), e.g. brain contusion, subdural haematoma
4 Neurodegenerative changes (~15%)
5 Hypertensive encephalopathy
6 Cerebral vasculitis
7 Central nervous system infection
8 Limbic encephalitis causing temporal lobe seizures, anterograde memory impairment, and behavioural change.

No cause is identified in up to 30–50% of cases of epilepsy in older people owing to the diagnostic difficulties noted earlier and the often less exhaustive approach to investigation in the older population. It has been proposed that 'micro-infarcts' are the most likely underlying cause of epilepsy in patients with vascular risk factors, even in the absence of visible pathology on brain imaging.

5 What is the most appropriate treatment and management strategy for this condition in this patient and generally in older people?

The management strategy includes explaining the condition to the patient and starting pharmacotherapy. This patient was started on low dose lamotrigine with a plan for slow up-titration. He remained seizure-free six months later. He was given lifestyle advice, including regarding the need to cease driving and to be seizure-free for one year before driving could be reconsidered, and was referred to the epilepsy nurse specialist for follow-up in the community, and annual follow-up with his GP.

When starting epilepsy treatment in older people, the presence of co-morbidities, polypharmacy, risk of drug interactions, the patient's wishes (e.g. for a simple drug regime) and possible side-effect (e.g. confusion, falls) should be considered. The aim is to control seizures with monotherapy if possible, and the rule for introducing new drugs to older people ('start low (usually with half of the recommended dose for adults) and go slow') applies.

The SANAD trial revealed that around half of patients, regardless of the drug used (newer drugs such as gabapentin or lamotrigine, or older drugs including valproate or carbamazepine) reported one or more adverse effects. However, there is some evidence that first line and well-tolerated medications (causing less side-effects) are lamotrigine, levetiracetam, gabapentin, and low dose topiramate.

Treatment choice in new onset and refractory epilepsy in adults will also depend on the type of epilepsy. Lamotrigine, levetiracetam, gabapentin, and carbamazepine are recommended for new onset partial seizures, clobazam and pregabalin for refractory partial seizures, lamotrigine and valproate for new onset idiopathic generalized epilepsies, and levetiracetam and clobazam for refractory idiopathic generalized epilepsy. Some antiepileptic drugs impair attention and memory, effects that seem to be less prominent with some newer drugs.

It is not clear whether first seizures should be treated, but the chance of recurrence is high at around 80%. The single seizure trial and the Multicentre Study of Early Epilepsy showed reduced risk of a second seizure in patients started on drug therapy after a first seizure, reduced time to achieve a two-year seizure-free period, and increased interval to first occurrence of tonic-clonic seizure or a second seizure. Monotherapy achieves seizure-free outcome in 65–80% of older patients, compared with only 30% in younger people, and with generally lower serum concentrations of antiepileptic drugs.

Many antiepileptic drugs accelerate bone loss. In The Women's Health Initiative, the use of these drugs was associated with increased incidence of falls and fractures among postmenopausal women aged 50–79 years although it was not clear whether the epilepsy itself was the cause, or unsteady gait, ataxia, and dizziness caused by the drugs. The evidence for an association with bone loss is stronger for older antiepileptic drugs (carbamazepine, phenytoin, and valproate), but emerging evidence suggests that levetiracetam, gabapentin, and oxcarbazepine are also implicated, so prophylactic treatment with calcium and vitamin D is recommended for all patients. Evidence for a ketogenic diet is unavailable for older patients.

Therapeutic failure of one drug may lead either to changing to an alternative in order to avoid polytherapy, or to the introduction of an add-on drug, but treatment is often guided by 'trial and error'. Around 20–30% of newly diagnosed patients have drug resistant epilepsy and are at increased risk of somatic and psychiatric co-morbidities, as well as death. Referral to a specialist is required for those with difficult epilepsy, diagnostic uncertainty, significant adverse effects from drugs, and the presence of psychiatric co-morbidities. A small number of patients may benefit from surgical intervention, but this is usually appropriate in younger rather than older patients.

Further reading

Bagshaw J, Crawford P, Chappell B (2009). Care in people 60 years of age and over with chronic or recently diagnosed epilepsy: a note review in United Kingdom general practice. *Seizure*; **18**: 57–60.

Clearly P, Tallis RC, Shorvon SD (2004). Late onset seizures as a predictor of future stroke. *Lancet*; **363**: 1184–1186.

Gosney M, Harper A, Conroy S (2012). Oxford Desk Reference: Geriatric Medicine. Oxford, UK: Oxford University Press.

Kim LG, Johnson TL, Marson AG, Chadwick DW, MRC MESS Study group (2006). Prediction of risk of seizure recurrence after a single seizure and early epilepsy: further results from the MESS trial. *Lancet Neurol*; **5**: 317–322.

Murray CJ, Vos T, Lozano R, *et al.* (2012). Disability-adjusted life years (DALYs) for 291 diseases and injuries in 21 regions, 1990–1992-1-: a systematic analysis for Global Burden of Disease Study 2010. *Lancet Neurol*; **380**: 2197–2223.

Nunes VD, Sawyer L, Neilson J, Sarri G, Cross JH (2012). Diagnosis and management of the epilepsies in adults and children: summary of updates NICE guidance. *BMJ*; **344**: e281.

Ramsay RE, Rowan AJ, Pryor FM (2004). Special considerations in treating the elderly patient with epilepsy. *Neurology*; 9: **62**(5 Suppl 2): S24–S29.

Schmidt D, Schachter S (2014). Drug treatment of epilepsy in adults. *BMJ*; **348**: g254.

Tebartz van Elst, Baker G, Kerr M (2009). The psychosocial impact of epilepsy in older people. *Epilepsy Behav*; **15**: S17–S19.

Case 45

A 75-year-old retired chemist was referred by her GP to the emergency multi-disciplinary team unit with a sudden onset of shortness of breath (SOB). She denied chest pain or fever, but had a chronic history of cough productive of sputum.

Past medical history comprised hypertension, asthma since childhood, hay fever, breast cancer (treated surgically several years before), two episodes of deep vein thrombosis, atrial fibrillation, osteoporosis with wedge fractures of L4 and L5, and varicose eczema of the lower legs. She previously smoked at least 20 cigarettes a day for more than 50 years, but had reduced it to five cigarettes a day in the last two years. Alcohol intake was an occasional glass of sherry. She lived with her husband in a ground floor flat. Her father had died of asthma at age 60.

Medications were alendronic acid, vitamin D and calcium supplements, amlodipine, omeprazole, warfarin, paracetamol, lactulose, senna, tamoxifen and 'some inhalers', which she did not bring to the hospital. INR was 3.2 from the previous day.

On examination, she was short of breath at rest with a respiratory rate of 26 breaths per minute and oxygen saturation on room air of 75%. She walked with the help of her husband into the emergency unit and was using accessory muscles on inspiration. Blood pressure was 100/70mmHg, jugular venous pressure was not elevated, and heart rate was 120bpm irregularly irregular with normal heart sounds. The trachea was not examined but chest expansion was reduced on the right with hyper-resonance, and reduced breath sounds.

Initial investigations showed the following:

- Blood gas: pH 7.32; pCO_2 6.9 pO_2 8; HCO_3 28.3; BE + 4
- Initial blood tests: awaited
- ECG: atrial fibrillation; heart rate 120bpm; normal axis and conduction
- CXR: awaited.

Questions

1 What do you think is the most likely diagnosis?
2 What are the main differences in this condition in older versus younger patients?
3 How would you treat this patient?

Answers

1 What do you think is the most likely diagnosis?

The most likely diagnosis is pneumothorax secondary to underlying lung disease of which asthma, chronic obstructive pulmonary disease (COPD), pulmonary fibrosis, tuberculosis, malignancy, and connective tissue disorders are most commonly implicated. Primary spontaneous pneumothorax occurs mainly in younger, tall, and previously well males.

Shortness of breath together with the blood gas results in this patient could indicate an acute exacerbation of underlying airways disease, but the onset of shortness of breath was sudden and there was no wheeze on examination although in severe airways disease, wheeze may be absent. Pulmonary embolism should always be considered in cases of sudden onset of shortness of breath, but the lack of chest pain, and therapeutic INR made this diagnosis less likely. Chest infection was also unlikely in view of the sudden onset of symptoms and absence of other features, and there was nil to suggest pulmonary oedema, secondary to arrhythmia, or myocardial infarction.

Spontaneous pneumothorax was felt to be the most likely diagnosis in view of the sudden onset of symptoms on a background of underlying airways disease and history of heavy smoking, accompanied by the clinical signs. The diagnosis was confirmed by chest X-ray (Fig. 45.1).

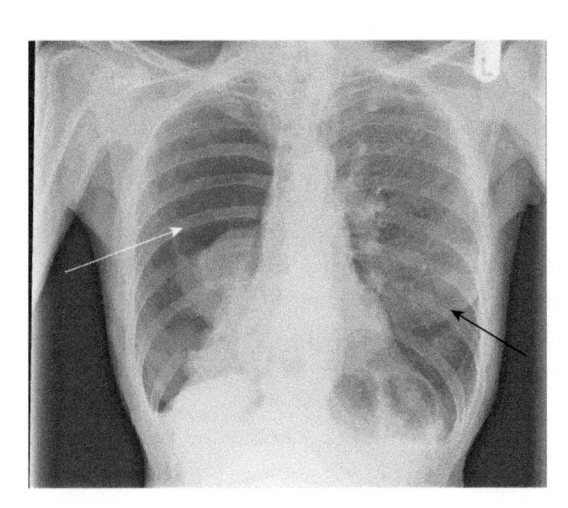

Fig. 45.1 Chest X-ray, showing a right side pneumothorax (white arrow). The heart size is normal. Asymmetrical breast shadows were noted (black arrow).

In cases of suspected pneumothorax where upright plain chest X-ray is inconclusive, lateral or lateral decubitus chest X-rays may be performed, but CT of the chest is the investigation of choice as it discriminates pneumothorax from bullae and provides an accurate assessment of the size of pneumothorax.

2 What are the main differences in this condition in older versus younger patients?

The most frequent differences between older and younger patients with pneumothorax are that older patients more often:

- present without pleuritic chest pain
- present with only SOB
- have severe SOB
- have underlying COPD, but may also have pulmonary fibrosis, neoplasm, or pneumonia
- are misdiagnosed clinically before chest X-ray is available
- require prolonged hospitalization
- have poor respiratory function
- also have heart failure.

The majority of older patients with pneumothorax are male (as is the case for younger patients) as historically more male patients smoked and therefore had COPD. However, unlike younger men, older individuals are often malnourished (see case 5) and are already on oxygen therapy for chronic respiratory failure. If surgical treatment is required, such patients have high post-surgery mortality rate of around 15%. Pneumothorax has a bimodal incidence that peaks in young adults and in those over 60 years, the later being attributable to underlying lung disease. Guidelines issued by the British Thoracic Society classify pneumothorax according to size as: 1. complete (airless lung, separate from diaphragm); 2. large ≥ 2cm; 3. small <2cm; and, according to the presence or absence of underlying lung condition, as primary or secondary. Treatments vary according to the category of pneumothorax.

In a minority of older patients, a tension pneumothorax (a progressive rise in intrapleural pressure) can develop, which requires emergency treatment—high flow oxygen, insertion of a cannula in the second mid clavicular anterior intercostal space, followed by an intercostal tube insertion. Tension pneumothorax should be suspected if the patient presents with the rapid development of:

- laboured breathing
- tachycardia
- progressive cyanosis
- pleuritic chest pain
- signs of mediastinal shift
- unilateral lack of movement on the affected side
- haemodynamic instability.

3 How would you treat this patient?

This patient was given oxygen supplementation while waiting for chest X-ray, after which a chest drain was inserted with immediate effect (Fig. 45.2). Recovery was complicated by chest infection, fast atrial fibrillation, and acute heart failure, but pre-morbid function was gained after four weeks, and the chest X-ray had normalized (Fig. 45.3).

Complications of chest drain insertion include: drain-related empyema; injury to major organs; interpleural bleed due to intercostal artery laceration; surgical emphysema; re-expansion pulmonary oedema; prolonged air leak; and failure of the lung to expand.

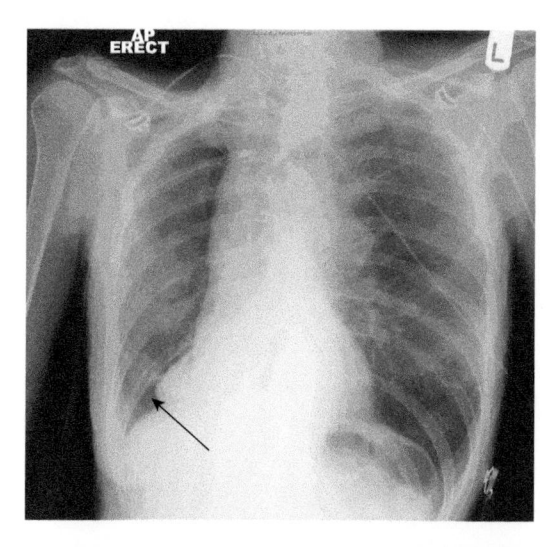

Fig. 45.2 Chest X-ray of the same patient after chest drain insertion, showing the tip of the right chest tube medially. There is a small area of subcutaneous emphysema in the right axilla/subclavian area, collapse of the right lower lobe, and the right upper lobe has expanded. There is right residual pneumothorax (black arrow). The left lung and pleural space are clear.

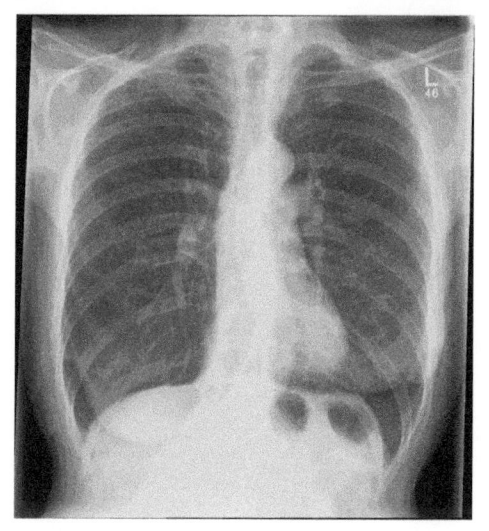

Fig. 45.3 Chest X-ray of the same patient three weeks later showing resolution of the pneumothorax and lung changes consistent with COPD.

Treatment for small, asymptomatic, primary spontaneous pneumothoraces consists of observation and follow-up X-ray (after six and 48 hours) looking for enlargement, while large and symptomatic primary spontaneous pneumothorax require catheter aspiration or chest drain insertion.

Case development

The patient was seen six months later in the geratology out-patient clinic with her daughter, who worked as a physiotherapist in another hospital.

Questions continued

1 The daughter wished to know the role of age in her mother's lung condition. List the most common age-related changes in the respiratory system and why these are important.

2 The daughter and the patient asked about the diagnosis of chronic obstructive pulmonary disease versus the diagnosis of asthma. List the main reasons why it may be difficult to distinguish asthma from chronic obstructive pulmonary disease in this and other older patients.

3 Which initial questions in the history may help in distinguishing asthma from chronic obstructive pulmonary disease in this and other older patients?

4 How might investigations help discriminate between asthma and chronic obstructive pulmonary disease in older patients and why is this distinction important?

5 Describe the further management of this patient.

Answers continued

1 The daughter wished to know the role of age in her mother's lung condition. List the most common age-related changes in the respiratory system and why these are important.

Age-related changes in the respiratory system contribute to increased susceptibility to infection, reduced exercise capacity and respiratory reserve, and these include:

- Increased chest wall stiffness and reduction in forced vital capacity (FVC) owing to osteoporosis and degenerative changes (e.g. ossification of the costal cartilages, loss of intervertebral disc spaces), rib fractures, kyphosis, and impaired mobility of the thoracic cage.
- A reduction in type IIa fibres and a reduction in production of muscle myosin, impairing the endurance and strength of respiratory muscles.
- Impaired chemoreceptors and microbial defence because of reduced number of glandular cells and production of mucus, reduced mucociliary clearance, impaired phagocytosis, and impaired macrophage function.
- Decreased elastic recoil (rate of decline is 0.2% per year of the ratio of FEV_1 to FVC) and loss of alveolar area. This reduces gas exchange and increases ventilation-perfusion mismatch.
- Altered response of the respiratory centre to hypercapnia and hypoxia.
- Increased airway hyper-responsiveness.
- Increased pro-inflammatory cytokines (hyper-inflammatory state).

In addition, older patients have generally decreased fitness, some may have previous lung disease including tuberculosis, and, like this patient, are more likely to have been smokers. Asthmatics who smoke have accelerated decline in lung function. As a consequence of age-related physiological changes in lung function, over 50% of >80 year-olds and 25% of >70 year-olds have FEV_1/FVC <70%, resulting in the over-diagnosis of COPD.

It is important to explain to the patient and daughter that the main reason for respiratory functional impairment in this case is disease and smoking, rather than ageing.

2 The daughter and the patient asked about the diagnosis of chronic obstructive pulmonary disease versus the diagnosis of asthma. List the main reasons why it may be difficult to distinguish asthma from chronic obstructive pulmonary disease in this and other older patients.

Chronic obstructive pulmonary disease is defined by the Global Initiative for Chronic Lung Disease (GOLD) as 'a preventable and treatable disease, characterized by airflow limitation that is not fully reversible'. It is a progressive systemic disease that results in debility over time and is usually related to smoking, developing in later life. It is one of the leading causes of hospital admission in older people in the UK. A comparison of the clinical features seen in COPD and asthma is shown in Table 45.1.

Table 45.1 Clinical features of asthma versus COPD

	Asthma	COPD
Age of onset	Usually at early age, but may occasionally affect older people	Rarely before the age of 50
Shortness of breath	Intermittent; but persistent in untreated chronic asthma	Persistent (usually)
Nocturnal symptoms	Common	Rare
Gender	Females (more common)	Males (more common)
History of allergic conditions e.g. hay fever	More common	
Winter exacerbations	Rare	Common
Spirometry	Variable, during remission usually normal	Usually abnormal and with no variability
Cough and sputum production	Dry cough, small volume sputum	Often high volume sputum and frequent cough
Interference with normal activity	None, if well controlled	Common, owing to symptoms
Chest X-ray	Usually normal	Usually abnormal

Asthma presents an allergic disease with airway inflammation, airway hyper-responsiveness, variable airflow obstruction, and episodic course. It is diagnosed on the basis of clinical presence of two or more of the following symptoms: cough; wheeze; chest tightness; and SOB. Asthma in older patients is under-diagnosed, being regarded by many as a condition of younger adults and under-treated. It has high morbidity, mortality, and risk of hospitalization: mortality rate during acute asthma attacks for older patients is higher than in younger patients, partly because the clinical signs (tachypnoea and tachycardia) are less marked for the same level of bronchoconstriction and older asthmatics are also more likely to underplay their symptoms. Older patients with asthma have often had asthma since childhood, although late-onset asthma starting at or after middle age is recognized. Churg–Strauss syndrome should always be considered in those with late-onset asthma. Older asthmatics are more likely to be female and less likely to have been smokers, and may develop irreversible airways obstruction at some point. The prevalence of asthma in the older population is similar to that for younger adults at between 5% and 10%. Deaths in such patients occur most frequently from December to February, coinciding with the highest incidence of respiratory infection.

Distinguishing asthma and COPD can be difficult, as symptoms in both conditions are similar: SOB; chest tightness; cough (with and without sputum production); wheeze (intermittent or chronic); and nocturnal exacerbations or exercise-induced symptoms. Some older patients with asthma may present with persistent, irreversible airflow obstruction as a consequence of chronic airways inflammation, bronchial thickening, and subepithelial fibrosis, simulating COPD, while conversely some patients with COPD may have a degree of reversibility simulating asthma.

The diagnostic difficulty, particularly in older patients, may be compounded by the absence of abnormalities on examination in less advanced disease and the presence of other conditions, such as heart failure, pulmonary embolism, or cancer, which may also cause similar symptoms. So for example, a night-time intermittent wheeze may easily be confused with paroxysmal nocturnal dyspnoea.

3 Which initial questions in the history may help in distinguishing asthma from chronic obstructive pulmonary disease in this and other older patients?

The initial assessment of an older patient with possible asthma or COPD requires a detailed history including:

- Smoking (>90% COPD, but also some patients with asthma)
- Presence of wheezing
- History of night-time intermittent deterioration with SOB and/or wheezing -more common in asthma
- Chronic, slowly progressive, SOB, and wheezing symptoms present during minimal or moderate physical efforts suggest COPD

- Age of onset (asthma usually begins in childhood or in early adulthood, but may begin later)
- During exacerbations, are the symptoms of SOB variable and occasional? (more common in asthma)
- Is coughing or SOB provoked by allergens or drugs (e.g. beta-blockers—oral or topical—ocular, NSAIDs), exercise, irritants, or cold air? (more common with asthma)
- History of exposure to chemicals, industrial dust, or tobacco smoke? (more common with COPD)
- Is there a diurnal variation of symptoms? (more common with asthma)
- Quality of life (progressively poorer in COPD, and more likely to be variable in asthma)
- Is coughing a constant feature? (more common in COPD)
- Is there a history of hay fever or other allergic conditions, or personal/family history of asthma (more common in asthma)?

The comprehensive guidelines published by the Global Initiative for Chronic Obstructive Lung Disease (GOLD) (2001, updated 2011), state that the presence of any of the following increases the probability of COPD:

- History of chronic cough (may be unproductive or be intermittent)
- SOB—persistent or getting worse over time or with exercise
- Chronic sputum production
- Family history of COPD
- History of exposure to risk factors such as domestic smoke, tobacco smoke, or chemicals.

4 How might investigations help discriminate between asthma and chronic obstructive pulmonary disease in older patients and why is this distinction important?

All patients should have CXR, ECG, FBC, oximetry, and if oxygen saturation is below 92%, arterial blood gas levels. Peak expiratory flow rate should be measured two to four times a day over two weeks to assess variability in flow rate. A >20% diurnal variation on > three days in a week for two weeks suggests asthma. Spirometry is more sensitive, although some older patients may find it difficult to perform. It should be performed before and after inhalation of a short-acting bronchodilator, and the following spirometry findings support diagnosis of asthma:

- reduced FEV_1
- reduced FEV_1/FVC ratio

- decreased FVC (if gas trapping)
- improvement in FEV_1 of >12% or an increase ≥10% of predicted FEV_1 in response to bronchodilator treatment.

Also, patients should have flow-volume loops reviewed in order to exclude a common mimic of asthma—vocal cord dysfunction.

Diagnosis of asthma is straightforward in many cases, but in many older patients it is difficult to be certain of the cause of the underlying lung disease. Eosinophilia and raised serum total IgE level often accompany asthma, but may not be present in late-onset cases.

Diagnosis of COPD is suspected in patients with characteristic history, chest X-ray, and is confirmed with spirometry findings of:

- FEV_1 is <80% predicted (e.g. when below 1L, patients experience SOB with activities of daily living)
- FVC reduced
- Reduced ratio of FEV_1/FVC.

Some studies have suggested that reduced diffusing capacity for carbon monoxide (DLco), higher respiratory volume, higher functional residual capacity, and airflow obstruction in older COPD patients, and absence of hypercapnia among older asthmatic patients may aid in distinguishing the two conditions. DLco may be particularly useful, usually reduced in COPD, and normal or elevated in asthma patients.

Discriminating asthma from COPD in older patients is important, since COPD carries a worse prognosis being a progressive condition with 60% fatality at 10 years; the treatment of the two conditions is also different.

This patient's spirometry showed: FEV_1 39%; FVC 62%; PEF 47%; FEV_1/FVC 0.56. Following bronchodilators, the results were FEV_1 45%; FVC 64%; PEF 53%; FEV1/FVC 0.59—the changes not being sufficient to distinguish COPD from asthma. Furthermore, she showed no significant improvement after a four-week course of steroids. She therefore had findings consistent with the combined syndrome of asthma and COPD.

5 Describe the further management of this patient.

Combined asthma and COPD findings are common in older patients, but since such patients are generally excluded from clinical trials, there is a lack of evidence for efficacy of treatments. Steroid therapy risks and benefits should always be evaluated, since such therapy is associated with harmful side effects including osteoporosis (this patient had a high risk of osteoporosis owing to her age, sex, heavy smoking habit, and immobility). Older patients also have an increased risk of pneumonia on long-term inhaled steroids.

Asthma treatment has a stepped approach, with inhaled beta agonists, inhaled steroids, oral steroids, beta agonists, leukotriene-receptor antagonists, and theophyllines. The likelihood of side effects, interactions with other drugs, and toxicity of theophyllines for a given drug level is greater in older versus younger patients.

In COPD, only oxygen supplementation and smoking cessation have any impact on disease progression. In mild disease, short-acting beta2 agonist or short-acting muscarinic antagonist as required are given, and as the disease progresses either of these medications in long-acting form may be added, followed by inhaled corticosteroid in cases of severe disease and recurrent exacerbations. In acute exacerbations, non-invasive ventilation may be necessary, and is generally equally beneficial and tolerable in older as for younger patients, although not in the presence of certain co-morbidities, including severe dementia.

In the clinic, she reported feeling better in herself and less short of breath. Oxygen saturation on room air was 92%. Treatment included:

- Smoking cessation advice and the offer of nicotine replacement therapy.
- Regular inhalers (inhaled beta agonists, inhaled steroids, and muscarinic antagonist), together with a leukotriene-receptor antagonist and theophylline.
- Checking inhaler technique. This may be affected in older patients by impairment of grip strength, vision, coordination, cognition, and poor timing. Spacer or powder devices increase intrapulmonary drug delivery and may be considered in such cases, although some studies have shown that older patients often do not use the spacer provided or have difficulties with using them.
- Pulmonary rehabilitation while in hospital and after discharge home. Pulmonary rehabilitation should be offered to patients with functional disability with COPD. It improves functional outcome, reduces hospital admissions, and mortality after exacerbations. Rehabilitation may include inspiratory muscle training and Nordic walking.
- Influenza and pneumococcal vaccination (although recent evidence has cast doubt on the ability of pneumococcal vaccination to reduce the risk of pneumonia, exacerbations of the disease, or mortality).

Further reading

Beauchamp MK, Janaudis-Ferreira T, Goldstein RS, Brooks D (2011). Optimal duration of pulmonary rehabilitation for individuals with chronic obstructive pulmonary disease—a systematic review. *Chronic Respir Dis*; **8**: 129–140.

British Thoracic Society/SIGN British Guideline on the Management of Asthma (May 2008). SIGN 101: www.sign.ac.uk

Gibson PG, Simpson JL (2009). The overlap syndrome of asthma and COPD: what are its features and how important is it? *Thorax*; **64**: 728–735.

Gosselink R, De Vos J, van den Heuvel SP, Segers J, Decramer M, Kwakkel G (2011). Impact of inspiratory muscle training in patients with chronic obstructive pulmonary disease: what is the evidence? *Eur Respir J*; **37**: 416–425.

Hardie JA, Vollmer WM, Buist AS, Bakke P, Mørkve O (2005). Respiratory symptoms and obstructive pulmonary disease in a population aged over 70 years. *Respir Med*; **99**(2): 186–195.

Liston R, McLoughlin, Clinch D (1994). Acute pneumothorax: a comparison of older with younger patients. *Age Ageing*; **23**: 393–395.

Rice KL, Dewan N, Bloomfield HE, *et al.* (2010). Disease management program for chronic obstructive pulmonary disease: a randomized controlled trial. *Am J Respir Crit Care Med*; **182**: 890–896.

Sin BA, Akkoca Ö, Saryal s, Öner f, Misirligil Z (2006). Differences between asthma and chronic obstructive pulmonary disease in the older. *J Investig Allergol Clin Immunol*; **16**; 44–50.

Thomas MJ, Simpson J, Riley R, Grant E (2010). The impact of home-based physiotherapy interventions on breathlessness during activities of daily living in severe chronic obstructive pulmonary disease: a systematic review. *Physiotherapy*; **96**: 108–119.

Waterhouse JC, Walters SJ, Oluboyede Y, Lawson RA (2010). A randomized 2 x 2 trial of community versus hospital pulmonary rehabilitation for chronic obstructive pulmonary disease followed by telephone or conventional follow-up. *Health Technol Assess*; **14**: (6): i–v, vii–xi, 1–140.

Case 46

A 75-year-old man was admitted to the general medical team via his GP. He had taken to his bed three days previously having become non-specifically unwell. His mobility and ability to transfer had significantly declined over the preceding six months, and just prior to admission, he was only able to mobilize short distances around the house with a stick. There was no formal diagnosis of dementia, but his wife said that he had become much more forgetful over the previous 18 months, and at times was unable to recognize his grandchildren. The past medical history included atrial fibrillation, myocardial infarction, and TIA. He was a retired painter and decorator who lived with his wife and continued to smoke.

On admission, the AMTS was 3/10, and he appeared cachectic and drowsy. Heart rate was 110bpm irregularly irregular, oxygen saturation was 94% on air, respiratory rate was 28 breaths per minute, and temperature was 37.9°C. General systems examination revealed crackles at the base and midzone on the right. There was a sacral pressure sore, which his wife said had been present for the last six months.

On the ward, he was given antibiotics and intravenous fluids for lower respiratory tract infection and accompanying delirium. His condition improved such that after 10 days he was more alert; MMSE was 11/30 and IQCODE was 4.2. The clinical picture, and in particular the history from the wife suggesting progression over months, was felt to be consistent with established dementia. A CT brain scan showed global atrophy and moderate small vessel disease.

Despite resolution of his respiratory symptoms, his appetite remained poor, and he required considerable prompting and assistance with meals. Ten days after his admission, he had a prolonged coughing episode at lunch and the following day he was diagnosed with a recurrence of right lower pneumonia. His swallow was deemed unsafe and intravenous fluids were started, pending consideration of alternative feeding methods.

Questions

1. Discuss the physiology of swallowing and how this changes in dementia.
2. What is the IQCODE?
3. Give some other common causes of swallowing difficulties in older patients with dementia.
4. Discuss the role of enteral feeding in dementia.
5. What are the next steps in the management of this case?

Answers

1 Discuss the physiology of swallowing and how this changes in dementia.

Normal swallowing involves 30 different muscles and has three phases: oral; pharyngeal; and oesophageal. The oral phase can be further sub-divided into two stages. Food is chewed and formed into a bolus, which is then held against the roof of the hard palate with the tongue in the first oral (preparatory) phase. In the second part of the oral (transit) phase, the tongue propels the food bolus backwards towards the pharynx. This is a voluntary action, which is controlled by centres in the cerebral cortex.

The pharyngeal phase of swallowing occurs in less than one second, during which the food bolus is pushed towards the back of the pharynx by the pharyngeal constrictor muscle. The larynx closes at the level of the vocal cords, preventing the food bolus from entering the trachea. The larynx is then elevated and the cricopharyngeal muscle is relaxed allowing passage of the food bolus into the oesophagus.

In the oesophageal (third) phase of swallowing, peristalsis begins in the oesophagus and pushes the food bolus down the oesophagus, through the oesophageal gastric sphincter, and down into the stomach. This phase is controlled by the brainstem and the myenteric plexus.

Dementia impacts on the neural control of swallowing, including the coordination of the swallow reflex and deterioration in swallow integrity with risk of aspiration. All stages of swallowing may be affected. In the first (oral) phase, poor coordination and weakness of the muscles of mastication result in food pooling and leakage, increasing the risk of aspiration during inhalation, especially in patients who have impaired consciousness. In the second phase, pharyngeal constrictor muscle weakness can result in build up of food residue, which in turn can be aspirated. The third phase of swallowing may be affected by upper GI tract changes common in older people, including achalasia, or a lax oesophageal gastric sphincter muscle, which also increase the risk of aspiration.

Swallowing problems in dementia often worsen, or may appear *de novo* with acute intracurrent illness, but may also improve as recovery occurs, so the swallow should be reassessed at intervals.

2 What is the IQCODE?

The IQCODE is the informant questionnaire for cognitive decline in the elderly. This is a questionnaire for relatives or friends, which asks the informant to compare how the patient is now with how they were 10 years earlier for

16 different areas of cognitive function. The informant circles a choice of answers scoring from 1 for 'much improved' and 5 for 'much worse'. An average item score of ≥ 3.6 is consistent with progressive dementia. The IQCODE is useful in establishing prior cognitive decline in the memory clinic, but is also helpful in the hospitalized population to provide information on premorbid cognitive function, particularly when the patients may be too unwell or unwilling to undertake cognitive testing or where the effects of acute illness and delirium may impact on cognitive scores.

3 Give some other common causes of swallowing difficulties in older patients with dementia.

Patients with dementia may develop swallowing problems unrelated to dementia and diagnostic difficulties are magnified where the patient is unable to give a clear account of symptoms. Establishing the time course of onset can be helpful. Common problems include:

- Acute onset
  - oral candida/oral or dental infection
  - reduced consciousness owing to acute illness (sleepy delirium)
  - stroke/TIA
  - medication (antipsychotics, sedatives, anticholinergics)
  - oesophageal foreign body, e.g. false teeth
- Chronic course
  - persisting dysphagia post stroke
  - oesophageal stricture or tumour
  - Parkinson's disease
  - other progressive neurological conditions, e.g. MND, MS
  - depression (loss appetite, food refusal, or abnormal perception of food).

4 Discuss the role of enteral feeding in dementia.

There is no evidence to support long-term enteral feeding in dementia. Difficulty eating and dysphagia are signs of advanced dementia and are often accompanied by a reduced desire to eat. This makes maintenance of adequate nutrition problematic (see also case 5 for discussion of malnutrition in older people). Referral to a speech and language therapist and a dietitian can be helpful, but there is no benefit to acute hospital admission for dysphagia caused by dementia in the absence of new acute pathology. However, since decreased oral intake may also occur with depression or concurrent acute illness, potentially reversible conditions should be looked for and treated if necessary. In such situations, temporary placement of a feeding tube may be appropriate to provide short-term nutritional support. Where depression is a contributing factor, mirtazapine is felt by some clinicians to be helpful in stimulating appetite.

In the absence of reversible pathology, persisting poor nutritional intake, or ongoing aspiration risk, the question of longer-term enteral feeding is often raised by relatives who are concerned that failure to provide adequate nutrition is wrong, and that the patient will be distressed by hunger and thirst. Relatives may feel that enteral feeding will improve the patient's quality of life. However, available evidence suggests no benefit from tube feeding in advanced dementia on survival, quality of life, nutritional status, or reduced pressure sore risk. Risk of pneumonia from feed aspiration and death may even be increased. Tubes may also become blocked, cause perforation, or the insertion site may become infected. Careful hand feeding is therefore the recommended method of feeding in advanced dementia, even in those deemed to have an 'unsafe' swallow and this ensures continuation of human contact, social interaction, stimulation and comfort, and helps provide/maintain some quality of life.

Feeding patients with advanced dementia is time consuming and impacts on staffing requirements in the general hospital. The quality of relationship between feeder and patient is an important predictor of food intake; people with dementia respond best when the person helping is interested, involved, flexible, calm, co-operative, and supportive. Patients should be sat upright, with small and regular portions of food being offered. A speech and language review may also be helpful to guide food consistency to optimize swallowing and hence safety. Dietitian input can help with maximizing nutritional input in the event of swallowing difficulty and reduced appetite.

5 What are the next steps in the management of this case?

An open and honest discussion with the patient and family is needed regarding the diagnosis, future management, and ceilings of treatment. The feeding strategy should be discussed. Reversible or exacerbating causes of cognitive decline and low mood should be excluded. Supportive management for any future infection including antibiotics would appear to be reasonable in the first instance, but in the case of recurrent infection this may need review. Resuscitation decisions should be discussed, and in the event of clinical deterioration, discussions regarding appropriateness for escalation of care to ICU should be undertaken. Careful assessment of needs will be required for effective discharge planning. Cholinesterase inhibitor therapy is not usually started in the hospital environment, because recovery from acute illness may make assessment of treatment benefit difficult and it is usually left until the patient's condition has stabilized in the community.

Further reading

Royal College of Physicians and British Society of Gastroenterology (2010). Oral feeding difficulties and dilemmas: A guide to practical care, particularly towards the end of life. London: *Royal College of Physicians.*

Sampson EL, Candy B, Jones L (2009). Enteral tube feeding for older people with advanced dementia. *Cochrane Database Syst Rev*; **15**(2):CD007209.

Smith HA, Kindell J, Baldwin RC, Waterman D, Makin AJ (2009). Swallowing problems and dementia in acute hospital settings: practical guidance for the management of dysphagia. *Clin Med*; **9**: 544–548.

Case 47

A 72-year-old woman was out shopping at the local market, when she began to feel light-headed, and noticed that her heart was racing. She turned around quickly to sit on a bench behind her, but lost her footing, and fell to the ground. An ambulance was called by a passer-by, as she was unable to get up owing to severe left leg pain. She was taken to the local accident and emergency department, and subsequently admitted to the trauma and orthopaedic ward with a left fractured neck of femur.

She lived alone in a second floor flat and was independent in walking, occasionally using a stick when the osteoarthritis in her knees was painful. She had no formal carers, but more recently her daughters had been helping out with shopping, and chores around the house.

There was a 20-year history of type 2 diabetes. Initially blood sugar was well controlled on metformin 1g bd and gliclazide 160mg bd, but three months earlier, the GP had added in glargine (a long-acting insulin), prescribing 12 units at night. Other medications included oxybutynin 5mg od, bendroflumethiazide 2.5mg od, citalopram 20mg od, salbutamol inhaler PRN, and ipratropium bromide inhaler tds, with lactulose and senna taken as needed.

On examination, she was uncomfortable. The left leg was shortened and externally rotated. Respiratory rate was 22 breaths per minute, heart rate was 148bpm, and blood pressure was 152/88mmHg. Heart sounds were normal and lung fields clear on auscultation.

The admission investigations were as follows:

- Hb: 8.2g/dL, WCC: 12.9×10^9/L, MCV: 79×10^{-15}/L, Neut: 6.8×10^9/L, Na: 134mmol/L, K: 4.2mmol/L, Urea: 7.3mmol/L, Creat: 125μmol/L
- Calcium: 2.1mmol/L
- ALT: 47IU/L, Bili: 16μmol/L, Alk phosp: 188U/L, Albumin: 34g/L
- CRP: 26mg/L
- BM: 11.8
- ECG showed fast atrial fibrillation (AF).

480 | CASE HISTORIES IN GERIATRIC MEDICINE

X-rays of the left hip are shown in Figures 47.1 and 47.2. She had been reviewed by the trauma and orthopaedic registrar, and was listed for a total hip replacement the following day.

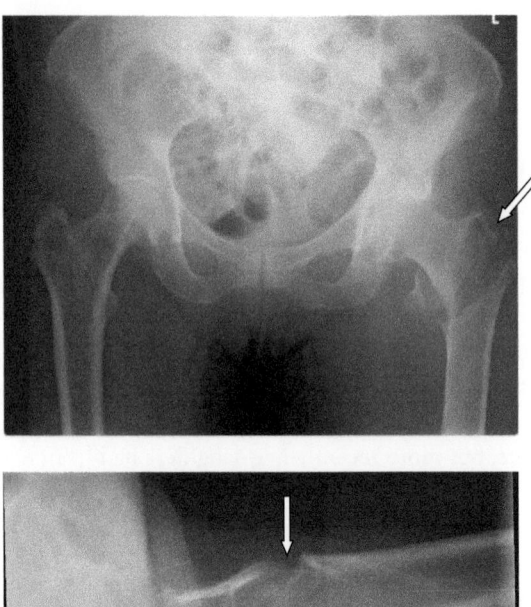

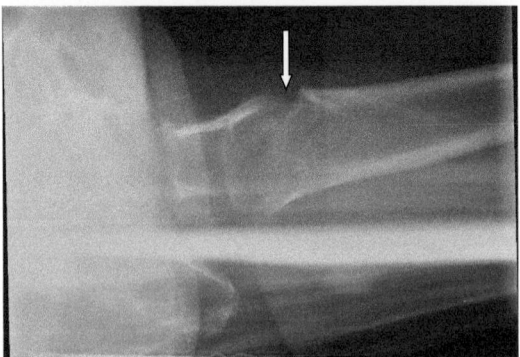

Figs 47.1 and 47.2 X-rays of the patient's pelvis and left hip showing neck of femur fracture (arrows).

Questions

1 What factors need to be addressed prior to surgery for the hip fracture?
2 What further investigations would you request to help elucidate the cause of the fall?

Answers

1 What factors need to be addressed prior to surgery for the hip fracture?

This patient has sustained a hip fracture as a result of a low impact fall from standing height indicating that she has osteoporosis. Hip fracture is very common with around 70,000–75,000 hip fractures occurring each year in the UK, and is associated with considerable morbidity and mortality. Some 95% of fractures occur in patients aged over 60 years and 75% of patients are female. Mortality is around 10% at one month and around 30% at one year.

Prompt surgical management is key (ideally within 36–48 hours) as meta-analyses demonstrate that delay in surgery is associated with increased length of stay, postoperative complications such as pressure sores, thromboembolic events and pneumonia, and increased mortality. Surgery is also the best treatment for relieving pain. Hip fracture patients are often frail and around one third have at least one co-morbidity, one fifth have two, and nearly a tenth have three or more. One quarter of patients have some degree of cognitive impairment. Intensive rehabilitation is required postoperatively to enable patients to regain their previous level of function and independence. Hip fracture patients are therefore best managed by a multidisciplinary team composed of surgeons, orthogeriatricians, nurses, physiotherapists, occupational therapists, and social workers.

This patient has a microcytic anaemia with haemoglobin of 8.2g/dl. Preoperative anaemia is not uncommon in patients with fractured neck of femur being seen in approximately 40%. Haemorrhage and haemodilution may cause the haemoglobin to decrease by 2.5g/dl such that those with preoperative anaemia are at risk of severe postoperative anaemia, which may lead to increased risk of myocardial ischaemia and stroke. Older patients should be considered for transfusion if Hb <9g/dl or <10g/dl in patients with a background of ischaemic heart disease and this patient was given two units of blood prior to theatre. Possible causes for iron deficiency anaemia should be explored after surgery. In this case, a more detailed history revealed unintentional weight loss of 1.5 stones and blood in the stools, and subsequent colonoscopy revealed a sigmoid malignancy.

The patient was in fast atrial fibrillation with a rate of 148bpm, which should be slowed to <100bpm prior to the operation. In this patient, the heart rate settled after transfusion of two units of blood, and there was no need for rate limiting medication such as beta-blockers or digoxin. Other factors including pain, sepsis, hypovolaemia, hypoxaemia, and electrolyte disturbance may cause atrial fibrillation in the perioperative period and should be addressed accordingly.

The patient is diabetic and blood glucose (BM) on admission was 11.8. Just under 10% of patients with hip fracture are diabetic. Hyperglycaemia in itself should not be a reason to delay surgery, unless the patient has diabetic ketoacidosis or hyperosmolar hyperglycaemic state (see case 2) in which case stabilization is required before theatre. Many hospitals have their own local guidelines and practices for diabetic patients having elective and emergency surgery. In general, if a patient is likely to be nil by mouth for > six hours or has a blood glucose >10mmols/L, then an insulin sliding scale should be used in the perioperative period. This patient's procedure was carried out the morning after admission, and since the blood sugars had remained erratic and she was required to be nil by mouth from midnight, a sliding scale was used. The evening after the operation, she was able to eat and drink normally, the sliding scale was taken down, and her long-acting insulin was restarted. The metformin was withheld for a further two days before being reinstated alongside with the gliclazide. Metformin should only be restarted if renal function is normal, or at baseline for the patient, since it may cause lactic acidosis.

The pre-admission medication included inhalers, suggesting a diagnosis of airways disease. This increases vulnerability to basal atelectasis and chest infections in the postoperative period, and careful supplemental oxygen with regular nebulizers 24–48 hours after the operation would be advisable.

Routine blood tests should be reviewed: patients with hip fracture may have lain on the floor for a long period, resulting in rhabdomyolysis and renal impairment. Creatinine kinase should always be checked in such cases.

It is important to ask about alcohol intake as it is a risk factor for falls, and untreated alcohol withdrawal may cause significant perioperative morbidity and mortality (see case 27).

Five per cent of patients with hip fracture take anticoagulants. Generally INR should be <2 for surgery and the effects of warfarin should be reversed with vitamin K if necessary. Depending on the indication for anticoagulation, low molecular weight heparin, or even a continuous heparin infusion may be used in the perioperative period, although this is not usually required, and anticoagulants can be recommenced 24 hours after surgery.

Heart murmurs often raise concerns regarding possible aortic stenosis. However, surgery should not generally be delayed while waiting for a routine echocardiogram to evaluate a murmur and should proceed with careful general anaesthesia and invasive blood pressure monitoring. A preoperative echocardiogram may rarely be indicated in patients who are breathless at rest or on minimal exertion, or if symptomatic aortic stenosis is suggested by the history (e.g. angina on exertion, unexplained syncope which might be the cause of the hip fracture, see case 11).

All patients with fractured neck of femur should have a baseline cognitive assessment given the high prevalence of cognitive impairment, both pre-existing and resulting from delirium (see case 1); and in the UK, on admission and in the postoperative period, AMTS is mandatory. Identification of cognitive impairment is particularly important in surgical patients, since consent is required to undergo surgery. Impaired patients may lack the capacity to weigh up the risks and benefits of the procedure (see case 13). In such cases, patients should be treated in their best interests and decisions should be discussed with the next-of-kin.

The Nottingham Hip Fracture Score is a validated tool, which uses readily available patient characteristics such as age, sex, pre-fracture cognitive function, haemoglobin level, place of residence, number of co-morbidities, and malignancy to predict postoperative mortality, return to home and length of stay, and may be helpful in discharge planning.

2 What further investigations would you request to help elucidate the cause of the fall?

This case illustrates the potentially serious consequences of falls, the risks of which increase with age. Around one third of people aged >65 years and a half of those aged >80 years fall at least once a year. The patient described in this case reported that her heart was racing and that she felt light-headed prior to the fall. ECG on admission showed fast atrial fibrillation in keeping with her symptoms and it is likely that this caused the fall. Medications on admission did not include any rate control therapy, aspirin or warfarin, suggesting that the atrial fibrillation was probably new, but this should be checked with the patient, and hospital and GP records. Thought should be given to the cause of the atrial fibrillation. In this case, the anaemia could be a contributing factor and thyroid function should be checked with a routine electrolyte screen, and infection should be excluded. The patient is a diabetic and a silent myocardial infarction precipitating atrial fibrillation cannot be excluded, so troponin level and repeat ECG after rate control should be considered. A postoperative non-urgent echocardiogram should be done to examine left atrium size, valvular function, and ventricular/septal contractility. Direct current (DC) cardioversion could be considered for persistent AF, although this is unlikely to be successful in the medium to longer term if there is left atrial dilatation or other structural heart disease.

Falls affecting frail older people with multiple co-morbidities tend to be multifactorial in origin and a comprehensive geriatric assessment is required, including a thorough history to establish the circumstances of the fall. Management should focus on identifying and treating reversible causes in order to prevent further falls. Assessment should include postural blood pressure measurements, medication review, review of footwear, balance assessment, need for walking aids, and a visual assessment (see case 27).

Case progression

Two days after the operation, the nursing staff became increasingly concerned about the patient and asked for a medical review. She had not slept well the previous night and had become agitated, pulling out her cannula when the physiotherapist arrived.

Repeat blood tests were as follows:

- Hb: 9.8g/dL, WCC: 10.6 × 10^9/L, MCV: 82 × 10^{-15}/L, Neut: 4.7 × 10^9/L, Na: 124mmol/L, K: 3.6mmol/L, Urea: 7.3mmol/L, Creat: 136μmol/L
- CRP: 28mg/L
- BM: 14.1.

Questions continued

3 What is the cause of the deterioration?
4 Once the patient has recovered from surgery, what medical issues should be addressed prior to discharge?

Answers continued

3 What is the cause of the deterioration?

This patient has developed delirium (see case 1). It is likely that it is in part, secondary to hyponatraemia. Hyponatraemia is a common electrolyte disturbance with one quarter of hospital cases occurring during the postoperative period owing to loss of solute in excess of water, or from water retention, or excess water administration. Surgery causes release of pituitary antidiuretic hormone (ADH) that continues for several days after the operation, leading to water retention. This may be exacerbated by certain medications including citalopram, bendroflumethiazide, and oxybutynin, as seen in the current case. A retrospective study by Rudge and Kim in 2012 looked at 254 patients who were admitted to their orthopaedic unit for hip surgery following trauma. They identified patients who developed hyponatraemia within 10 days of surgery and compared them with those who remained normonatraemic pre- and postoperatively. They found a mean postoperative drop of serum sodium of 1.8mmol/L (95% CI: 1.3–2.3mmol/L $p < 0.001$) compared with preoperative levels. The incidence of moderate (<135–130mmol/L) and severe (<130mmol/L) hyponatraemia was 27% (95% CI: 21.7–32.5%) and 9% (95% CI: 5.7–12.8%) respectively. They found that length of hospital stay was significantly increased among those with moderate postoperative hyponatraemia compared to normonatraemic patients (30 versus 21 days, $p<0.001$). Ethnicity, gender, fracture type, operative procedure, or functional status did not statistically increase new postoperative hyponatraemia. However, statistical analysis did reveal significant associations between the use of proton pump inhibitors, selective serotonin re-uptake inhibitors, and number of medications.

Other factors important to consider in relation to the delirium include:

- *Constipation.* The patient was using laxatives prior to admission and postoperatively has probably required opiate analgesic medication.
- *Postoperative infection.* Although the blood results do not suggest infection, this should always be considered and the hip wound should be examined as part of the septic screen.
- *Pain* is an important contributor to delirium. This should usually be obvious, but may be less so in cognitively impaired patients.
- *Analgesic agents,* especially opiates.
- *Alcohol dependency* should always be considered (see case 27). There are no indicators in the history in this patient, but the symptoms have developed within the right time period postoperatively and a collateral history from friends or relatives should be sought.

4 Once the patient has recovered from surgery, what medical issues should be addressed prior to discharge?

The two factors that need to be addressed prior to discharge are secondary prevention of osteoporosis, and prevention of thromboembolic events secondary to atrial fibrillation.

Osteoporosis is a condition of reduced bone density (see case 24) prevalent in the older population, especially in post-menopausal women. In youth, bone formation exceeds bone resorption, but this balance switches by the third decade and there is a gradual loss of bone mass thereafter. The World Health Organization defines osteoporosis as a T score of ≥2.5 standard deviations below the mean bone mineral density of young adults at their peak bone mass on dual-energy X-ray absorptiometry (DXA) scanning. In patients aged <75 years with a fragility fracture (vertebrae, hip, and distal radius in order of frequency). DXA scanning should be performed but this is not required in those aged ≥75 years in whom osteoporosis is assumed. Osteoporosis is commonly asymptomatic, presenting only after a low impact fall and fracture. Secondary prevention includes advice on lifestyle measures (smoking cessation, reduction in alcohol intake, and regular exercise) as well as medication.

Given that this patient is 72 years old, she should have a DXA scan prior to commencing any secondary preventative medication. If DXA scanning confirms osteoporosis, daily calcium and vitamin D supplements should be prescribed together with a bisphosphonate, which alters osteoclast activation and function. In the UK, alendronate is recommended first line. It is a weekly preparation that should be taken first thing in the morning on an empty stomach with at least 200ml of water. Common side effects include gastrointestinal (GI) upset and resultant poor compliance. Alendronate is contraindicated in patients with oesophageal abnormalities or other factors delaying gut transit and risedronate should be used with caution. Bisphosphonates need to be taken for around 12–18 months before beneficial effects are seen. There is little evidence regarding the use of bisphosphonates in patients with normal bone density or osteopaenia.

Strontium ranelate may be considered for those unable to take bisphosphonates. It has a dual effect on bone metabolism, increasing bone formation, and decreasing bone resorption. It should not be used in severe renal impairment or where there is increased risk of venous thromboembolism.

Other medications used in secondary prevention of osteoporosis are selective oestrogen receptor modulators such as raloxifene. They aim to optimize the beneficial effects of oestrogen on the bone with minimal adverse effects on the breast and endometrium. They have been shown to increase the risk of venous thromboembolism, especially within the first four months of treatment and are contraindicated in patients with hepatic or severe renal impairment, unexplained uterine bleeding, or endometrial cancer. Teriparatide, a recombinant fragment of human parathyroid hormone, stimulates new bone formation. It is not widely used as it is expensive and is administered by daily subcutaneous injections in the thigh or abdomen, requiring patients to be able to self-administer via this route. It is contraindicated in severe renal impairment, hypercalcaemia, Paget's disease of the bone, and previous radiation treatment to the skeleton.

This patient's CHA_2DS_2VASc score was 4, making her high risk for a thromboembolic event (9.3%/year) (see case 42) and she should ideally be anticoagulated to reduce the stroke risk. However, she was anaemic, and further investigation revealed a sigmoid tumour, which was resected four months after the hip surgery. Warfarin was started after recovery from this procedure.

Further reading

Association of Anaesthetists of Great Britain and Ireland (2011). Management of proximal femoral fractures.

NICE clinical guideline 124 (2011). Hip fracture: The management of hip fracture in adults (amended March 2014).

NICE clinical guideline 161 (June 2013). Falls: Assessment and prevention of falls in older people.

NICE technology appraisal guidance 161 (2011). Alendronate, etidronate, risedronate, raloxifene, strontium ranelate and teriparatide for the secondary prevention of osteoporotic fragility fractures in postmenopausal women (amended).

Rudge J, Kim D (2014). New-onset hyponatraemia after surgery for traumatic hip fracture. *Age Ageing*; **43**: 821–826.

Case 48

A GP was called to see an 81-year-old care home resident, who had become increasingly muddled, and was apparently talking to her husband who had died some years previously. The staff reported a rapid deterioration in her condition: the previous day, she had been her normal self and had been enjoying the hot summer weather in the garden with other residents.

The patient had moved into the care home following a fall and fractured neck of femur two years earlier. There was a past history of diabetes, hypertension, and osteoporosis. Medication included bendroflumethiazide, alendronate, aspirin, metformin, gliclazide, simvastatin, and paracetamol.

On examination, the patient was confused with an AMTS of 5/10 and temperature of 40°C. The heart rate was elevated at 140bpm and respiratory rate at 32 breaths per minute, with a blood pressure of 118/68mmHg. Neurological examination showed horizontal nystagmus, normal power in the upper limbs and mildly reduced power globally in the lower limbs. She was unsteady on standing, and unable to walk unassisted.

She was admitted to hospital, where investigations showed:

- Hb: 11g/dL, WCC: 9×10^9/L, Neut: 6×10^9/L, HCt: 0.45/L, Na: 148mmol/L, K: 2.9mmol/L, Urea: 26mmol/L, Creat: 378μmol/L, ALT: 104IU/L, Bili: 88μmol/L, Alk phos: 459U/L
- CK: 494μmol/L
- CRP: 45mg/L
- ABG: on air.

pH: 7.51, PO_2: 9.2KPa, pCO_2: 2.9KPa, HCO_3: 20.1mmol/L, ECG: sinus tachycarda, CXR: unremarkable, Urine dipstick: no nitrites.

Questions

1. What is the most likely diagnosis and why?
2. What are the features of this condition?
3. Describe the pathophysiology underlying the diagnosis.
4. Why are older people particularly vulnerable to this condition?
5. What is the cause of this patient's renal failure?
6. How would you manage this condition?
7. What is the prognosis?
8. List the prognostic indicators.

Answers
1 What is the most likely diagnosis and why?
The most likely diagnosis is heat stroke. The differential diagnosis includes:
- heat-related conditions
- dehydration secondary to hot weather
- heat exhaustion
- heat stroke
- CNS infection
- encephalitis
- meningitis
- systemic infection
- thyroid storm.

The most likely answer in this case is heat stroke, the patient having been exposed to hot weather in the garden the afternoon prior to her deterioration. Heat stroke is the most extreme form of heat-related illness and occurs when mild heat exhaustion is allowed to progress unchecked. The severity of symptoms and signs seen in the current case, including central nervous system involvement, would not be seen in heat exhaustion or dehydration.

Although the CRP is raised suggesting the possibility of infection, both the white cell count and neutrophil level are within normal range, CXR was unremarkable, and urinary dipstick was nitrite negative making an infective cause less likely. Also the arterial blood gas demonstrates a respiratory alkalosis secondary to hyperventilation caused by CNS stimulation. In cases of sepsis, the arterial blood gas is more likely to show a metabolic acidosis.

Neuroleptic malignant syndrome is again unlikely, although this might cause similar symptoms, as there is no suggestion that this patient is taking, or has taken, a neuroleptic agent in the recent past. Also in neuroleptic malignant syndrome (see case 36), the arterial blood gas would demonstrate a metabolic acidosis.

Thyrotoxic storm (see case 20, Oxford University Press' *Neurological Case Histories*) could account for the fever, agitation, CNS signs, and tachycardia, however, no obvious precipitating factor such as infection, trauma, or recent surgery is suggested in the case history. Although thyroid storm can occur at any age, it is most likely to occur between the third and sixth decade.

Similar signs and symptoms may be seen with anticholinergic or aspirin overdose. However, in the present case, there was no suggestion of previous low mood or depression, and the patient was not on anticholinergic medication.

2 What are the features of this condition?

Heat stroke is clinically defined when the core body temperature is greater than 40°C. There is associated neurological impairment and multiorgan dysfunction. In severe cases death may occur.

There are two types of heat stroke. The first, exertional heatstroke (EHS) often affects the young and is seen after prolonged strenuous activity in hot weather. The second type, non-exertional heat stroke (NEHS) is commonly seen in the elderly or those with chronic disease who are unable to regulate their own body temperature correctly. The elderly patients are particularly susceptible to the effects of heat because of co-morbidity and the use of medications, such as diuretics (as seen in the current case) and anticholinergics, which interfere with the normal physiological cooling response. Heat stroke affects many organ systems in the body and causes multiple blood abnormalities, as shown in Box 48.1 and 48.2.

Box 48.1 Impact of heat stroke on organ systems

Central nervous system

- Cerebellar signs are common
- Delirium, confusion, hallucinations
- Decreased GCS, and ultimately coma secondary to cerebral oedema and herniation

Cardiovascular system

- Hyperdynamic state with sinus tachycardia 130–140bpm
- Hypodynamic state in patients unable to mount a tachycardia secondary to medication, or underlying cardiac pathology, or seen before cardiovascular collapse

Pulmonary system

- Respiratory alkalosis caused by direct CNS stimulation, or as a compensatory mechanism for lactic acidosis
- Pulmonary oedema
- Acute Respiratory Distress Syndrome (ARDS)

> **Box 48.1 Impact of heat stroke on organ systems** *(continued)*
>
> **Renal system**
>
> - Acute renal failure secondary to dehydration and rhabdomyolysis
>
> **Gastrointestinal system**
>
> - GI haemorrhage may occur
> - Increased permeability of gut leading to systemic release of endotoxin
> - Hepatic ischaemic injury is common: this is often limited to raised transaminases and hyperbilirubinaemia (as seen in the current case). However, severe cases can result in fulminant liver failure with encephalopathy, hypoglycaemia, and DIC

> **Box 48.2 Blood abnormalities associated with heat stroke**
>
> **ABG**
>
> Respiratory alkalosis—CNS stimulation
> Hypoxia—pulmonary oedema/lung injury
> Metabolic acidosis—lactic acidosis
>
> **FBC**
>
> Increased WCC
> Low platelets
>
> **Electrolytes**
>
> Hypernatraemia—dehydration
> Hyponatraemia—diuretics, excessive sweating resulting in salt losses
> Hypokalaemia—initial stages, especially if concomitant diuretic medication
> Hyperkalaemia—later stages due to renal failure
> Hypercalcaemia—initially due to dehydration
> Hypocalcaemia—later stages due to increased calcium binding in injured muscle

> **Box 48.2 Blood abnormalities associated with heat stroke** *(continued)*
>
> Hypomagnesaemia
> Hypophosphataemia
>
> **Liver function tests**
>
> Raised liver enzymes, peaking at around 48 hours
> Increased bilirubin
> Hypoglycaemia
>
> **Renal function tests**
>
> Increased urea
> Increased creatinine
> Increased CK

3 Describe the pathophysiology underlying the diagnosis.

Normal thermoregulation allows the body temperature to be kept at 37°C. The heat of the body is the total of the sum gained from the environment and that produced by the body during metabolism and/or during exercise. If the blood temperature is allowed to rise by less than 1°C, activation of peripheral and hypothalamic receptors takes place. This diverts blood away from the internal organs to the skin surface, allowing cooling to occur via convection and radiation. Heat is also dissipated by sweating and evaporation, resulting in loss of salt and water which must be adequately replaced in order to maintain the thermoregulatory process. However, this method of heat loss becomes less efficient in humid environments when heat loss is aided by increasing respiratory and heart rates, raising cardiac output up to 20L per minute, shunting blood to the periphery. This decreases blood flow to the internal organs, particularly the kidneys and intestines.

When the body temperature rises to above 41°C, cellular enzyme processes become unregulated, and apoptotic and inflammatory cascades are initiated. Increased gut permeability allows endotoxins into the systemic circulation. Pro-inflammatory cytokines including IL-6 released from damaged muscle may cross the blood brain barrier and directly affect the hypothalamus' ability to set body temperature.

4 Why are older people particularly vulnerable to this condition?

Older people are particularly vulnerable to heat stroke owing to lower physiological reserve and chronic illness, such as cardiovascular disease, and are often taking medications that limit the body's thermoregulatory ability. Staff in care homes especially need to be aware of the risk of heat stroke, as many of their patients are unable to change their surrounding environment because of limited mobility and are reliant on staff to provide them with adequate hydration.

5 What is the cause of this patient's renal failure?

The patient's renal failure is likely to be due to a combination of dehydration during the hot weather, diuretic use, and rhabdomyolysis. Although rhabdomyolysis is more commonly seen as a complication of EHS, it is becoming more commonly recognized as contributing to renal failure seen in NEHS. As the core body temperature increases, there is disruption of the muscle membrane integrity, leading to muscle protein breakdown and myoglobinuria.

6 How would you manage this condition?

The primary aim in the management of heat stroke is to rapidly reduce the core body temperature, since this will reduce the likelihood of complications.

Cooling is best done by removing clothing, applying ice packs or cool water to the body, and using a fan. However, care must be taken to ensure that the patient does not start to shiver, as this will increase the metabolic heat produced. In practice, the patient is either cooled using the application of ice packs and cool compresses, while a fan is used to blow warmer air over them, or ice and cold water are used for short periods of time, and the patient is allowed to warm slightly in between.

Appropriate support of failing organ systems and close monitoring for electrolyte disturbance is also required.

Antipyretics should not routinely be used as they maybe harmful in patients with hepatic injury and may increase the risk of gastrointestinal (GI) bleed in patients with disseminated intravascular coagulation (DIC).

7 What is the prognosis?

It is difficult to give exact mortality figures for heat-related deaths in the elderly patients, as cases are often under reported or poorly recognized as a major contributing factor to death. However, data from the 2003 heat wave in England and Wales show that there were more than 2000 deaths during this period attributable to heat-related illnesses.

The prognosis of elderly patients with heat stroke is poor, with residual brain damage occurring in approximately 20%. Brain damage is thought to occur as a result of raised intracranial pressure secondary to oedema, coupled with a decrease in mean arterial pressure from vasodilatation of the peripheral vasculature, brain hypoperfusion, and ischaemia. Brain imaging in older patients with heat stroke shows changes consistent with cerebral oedema, white matter changes in the corpus striatum and cerebral hemispheres, and ischaemic microinfarcts. In severe cases, particularly where there is associated DIC, imaging may reveal microhaemorrhages and central pontine myelinolysis. Follow-up imaging at four to six weeks in those with persistent neurological deficits (incoordination, clumsiness, personality change and in severe cases cortical blindness) may show cerebral atrophy.

8 List the prognostic indicators.

Poor prognostic indicators include:

1 Temperature >41°C

2 Pulmonary oedema

3 Deranged liver tests with AST >1,000 within the first 24 hours

4 Decreased GCS and coma >2 hours duration

5 Cardiovascular compromise.

Further reading

Axelrod BN, Woodard JL (1993). Neuropsychological sequelae of heatstroke. *Int J Neurosci*; **70**(3–4): 223-325.
Bouchama A, Knochel J (2002). Heat stroke. *N Engl J Med*; **346**: 1978–1988.
Dematte JE, O'Mara K, Buescher J, et al. (1998). Near-fatal heat stroke during the 1995 heat wave in Chicago. *Ann Intern Med*; 1; **129**(3): 173–181.
Glazer JL (2005). Management of heatstroke and heat exhaustion (2005). *Am Fam Physician*; **71**(11): 2133–2140.
Hajat S, Kovats RS, Lachowycz K (2007). Heat-related and cold-related deaths in England and Wales: Who is at risk? *Occup Environ Med*; **64**: 93–100.
Tan W, Herzlich BC, Funaro R, et al. (1995). Rhabdomyolsis and myoglobinuric acute renal failure associated with classic heat stroke. *South Med J*; **88**(10): 1065–1068.
Trujillo MH, Bellorin-Font E, Fragachan CF, Perett-Gentill R (2009). Multiple organ failure following near fatal exertional heat stroke. *J Intensive Care Med*; **24**: 72–78.

List of cases by diagnosis

Case 1:   Delirium
Case 2:   Hyperosmolar Hyperglycaemic State (HHS)
Case 3:   Abuse
Case 4:   Digoxin toxicity
Case 5:   Nutrition, Sarcopenia, Cachexia
Case 6:   Normal pressure hydrocephalus
Case 7:   Urinary incontinence
Case 8:   Hypercalcaemia
Case 9:   Drug induced SLE
Case 10: Infective endocarditis
Case 11: Syncope, postprandial
Case 12: Paget's disease
Case 13: Mental capacity and its assessment, Cardiopulmonary resuscitation decisions
Case 14: Pressure ulcers
Case 15: Heart failure
Case 16: Fever of unknown origin
Case 17: Systemic sclerosis
Case 18: Depression
Case 19: Cerebellar infarct
Case 20: Charles Bonnet syndrome
Case 21: Diabetes mellitus and hypoglycaemia
Case 22: Coeliac disease
Case 23: B_{12} deficiency, hypocalcaemia
Case 24: Pubic rami and sacral fractures
Case 25: Dementia with Lewy bodies
Case 26: Intravascular B-cell lymphoma
Case 27: Fall and alcohol excess
Case 28: Polymyalgia rheumatica
Case 29: Chronic renal failure
Case 30: Acquired Immuno Deficiency Syndrome (AIDS), Syphilis
Case 31: Leptomeningeal carcinomatosis, Seizures
Case 32: Faecal incontinence
Case 33: Motor neuron disease

Case 34: Pruritus
Case 35: Aortic stenosis/TAVI
Case 36: Serotonin syndrome
Case 37: Sleep disorders
Case 38: Pyoderma gangrenosum
Case 39: Giant cell arteritis
Case 40: Multiple System Atrophy
Case 41: Palliative care
Case 42: Atrial fibrillation and Cerebral amyloid angiopathy, Stroke, Anticoagulation
Case 43: Frontotemporal dementia
Case 44: Epilepsy
Case 45: Pneumothorax/COPD/Asthma
Case 46: Dementia and PEG feeding
Case 47: Falls, Osteoporosis, Hyponatraemia
Case 48: Heat stroke

List of cases by presentation/aetiology

Falls/Syncope: *1, 11, 24, 27, 47*
Cognitive impairment: *1, 5, 6, 13, 25, 26, 27, 43, 46*
Cerebrovascular disease: *19, 26, 42*
Metabolic/Endocrine disorder: *2, 8, 12, 21, 23, 47, 48*
Drugs/Toxin effects: *4, 9, 21, 27, 36*
Skin disorders: *9, 14, 22, 30, 34, 38*
Autoimmune/Inflammatory/Infectious disorders: *8, 10, 16, 17, 24, 34, 28, 30, 38, 39*
Neurodegeneration: *25, 37, 40, 43*
Frailty syndromes: *5, 7, 13, 14, 20, 24, 25, 32, 35, 41, 46, 48*
Ethical issues, abuse: *2, 3, 13, 41, 46*
System ageing: *5, 7, 15, 20, 29, 30, 32, 34, 35, 42, 45, 47, 48*
Palliative care: *13, 16, 41*
Cancer: *16, 26, 31, 41*
Rehabilitation: *24, 33*

Index

A
Abbreviated Mental Test Score (AMTS) 1, 6–8, 483
Abuse 27–36
  forms 32–4
  management 35–6
  prevalence and risk factors 29–30
Acute Respiratory Distress Syndrome (ARDS) 492
Serotonin syndrome 375–80
Addisonian crisis 78
Advance Directive 137–41
AIDS 317–22
Alcohol excess/intoxicaton, hallucinations 219, 288, 289, 293
Alcohol withdrawal 296, 328, 454
Alkaline phosphatase levels 291
Alzheimer's disease
  amyloid PET imaging 273–4
  delirium in 14
  depression in 201
  differential diagnosis 60, 266
  hippocampal atrophy 268
  short-term memory 266
  visual hallucinations 219, 266
  with/without delirium 14–15
  see also dementia
Amyloid deposition 263–4
Amyotrophic lateral sclerosis 349
Anaemia
  of chronic disease 193
  iron deficiency anaemia 481
  microcytic anaemia 481
  normocytic anaemia 193
  pernicious anaemia 241, 244–5
  postoperative anaemia 481
Analgesics 12
  adjuvant 423–4
  analgesic ladder for cancer pain 423
  back pain 292–4
Anocutaneous reflex 338
Anti-neutrophil cytoplasmic antibodies (ANCAs) 87, 192
Anti-SCL-70 184, 185
Anti-tissue transglutaminase autoantibodies 236
Anti-topoisomerase I antibody 185
Antibody-mediated immune disorders 192
Anticentromere antibody (ACA) 184, 185
Antihypertensive therapy, clinical trials 310
Antinuclear antibodies (ANA) 87, 184, 185, 192
Antithrombotic therapy 433–7
  comparisons 433–6
  complications 437–8
  HAS-BLED score for bleeding risk 437
Aortic stenosis 367–70
  management algorithm 370
  TAVI 369
Arthropathies 300
  assessment 393
  Cognitive impairment 10, 13
  Comprehensive Geriatric Assessment (CGA) 257–8, 420
  mental capacity assessment 130–41
  pain 422–4
  polyarthropathy 88
Asthma 459–71
  treatment 470–1
  vs COPD 467–70
Atherosclerotic risk factors 368
Atrial fibrillation 209, 214, 429–41
  antithrombotic therapy 433–7
  falls 483
  paroxysmal 433
  prevention of thromboembolic events 487
  risk of stroke 433–7
  treatment 438–41
Autoimmune disorders 239
  and ageing 191–3
  see also coeliac disease; systemic lupus erythematosus (SLE); systemic sclerosis; vasculitis
Autonomy, vs beneficence 126–7

B
B-cell lymphoma, intravascular (IVBCL) 277, 283–4
Back pain 289–90
Beneficence, vs autonomy 126–7
Bladder capacity 70
  incomplete bladder emptying 72
  overactive bladder syndrome (OAB) 71
  retraining 73
Bladder injury 252
Bladder stone 419–21
Blood glucose (BM) 20–1, 225, 229, 472
Body mass index (BMI) 167
Borrelia burgdorferi 169, 315

Brain imaging 62, 444–50
  Epilepsy 453
  Frontotemporal dementias 446–9
  Heat stroke 496
  Hippocampal atrophy 268
  MRI 280
  Progressive bulbar palsy 349
  Progressive supranuclear palsy (PSP) 411–12
  Space-occupying lesions 209, 444
  Ventriculomegaly 62
Brain microbleeds (BMBs) 439–41
Brainstem encephalitis 209
Breast cancer, leptomeningeal carcinomatosis 328–9
Breathlessness
  aortic stenosis 367
  shortness of breath (SoB) 459–71

C

C-reactive protein 83, 153, 171, 300, 397, 424
Cachexia 47–8
Calcium
  vitamin D intoxication 79
  see also hypercalcaemia; hypocalcaemia
Cancer
  Comprehensive Geriatric Assessment (CGA) 420
  Fever of unknown origin 177–8
  Intravascular B-cell lymphoma 277, 283–6
  Leptomeningeal carcinomatosis 328–32
  see also malignancy; palliative care
Cardiopulmonary resuscitation (CPR) 138–41
Carotid sinus syndrome 104
Catatonia 376
Cell-mediated immune disorders 192
Cerebellar infarct/stroke 209–13
  complications 210–12
  differential diagnosis 209–10
  management 212
Cerebellar stroke 209–12
Cerebral amyloid angiopathy 278, 439–41
Cerebral autosomal dominant arteriopathy 277
Cerebrospinal fluid, defective resorption in NPH 64
Cerebrovascular disease
  cause of epilepsy 327
  differential diagnosis 60
  intravascular B-cell lymphoma 277, 283–6
  see also cerebellar infarct/stroke; cerebral amyloid angiopathy
Cervical spine disease 348–9
CHADS score, risk of stroke 431–2
Charles Bonnet syndrome 217–22
  diagnostic criteria 221
  pathophysiology 221–2
  treatment 222

CHARM trial, heart failure 165
Chest infection, hypercalcaemia and 77
Chronic kidney disease (CKD) 303–12
  NICE classification 307, 308
  uraemic pruritus 358
Chronic obstructive pulmonary disease (COPD) 167, 459–71
  defined 467
  treatment 470–1
  vs asthma 466, 468–70
Churg–Strauss syndrome 468
Cockcroft and Gault equation 305
Coeliac disease 233–9
  criteria for diagnosis 236–7
  defined 236
  differential diagnosis 238–9
  refractory disease 239
  skin disorders 238
  T-cell lymphoma 238
  thyroid disorders 239
Cognitive impairment 10
  confusion associated with acute stroke 275
  differential diagnosis 60
  DLB 263, 266–7
  falls 60
  in heart failure 167
  Large B-cell lymphoma 283, 286
  Malnutrition 50–2
  Normal pressure hydrocephalus (NPH) 60–6
  see also hyper/hypothyroidism; hypercalcaemia; hypoglycaemia; hyponatraemia; mental capacity assessment; renal failure
Confusion, associated with acute stroke 273–86
Confusion Assessment Method (CAM) screen 6–7
Consent issues 130–1, 132–6, 140
Conversion disorder 278
Corona mortis artery (obturator) 253
Corticobasal degeneration 412
Cramp fasciculation syndrome 349
Cranial arteritis 397–405
CREST syndrome 183, 185
Creutzfeldt-Jakob disease 277, 283, 359, 447

D

Death, imminence 424–5
Dehydration see heat stroke; hyperglycaemic hyperosmolar state
Delirium 1–14, 219
  AMTS vs MoCA 8
  associated factors 9–11
  CAM screen 6
  cognitive screen for admission 7
  DSM IV criteria 3–4

intervention programme (reduction of incidence) 12
prognostic implications 13–14
risk/precipitating factors 9, 294
secondary to hyponatraemia 486
Dementia
  Alzheimer's disease 14–15, 60
  cause of epilepsy 327
  differential diagnosis 60, 447
  differentiation from delirium 6, 8–9
  Frontotemporal 349, 446–8
  hallucinations 219
  IQCODE 473, 475–6
  role of enteral feeding 476–7
  swallowing difficulties 476–7
  types 263, 266–7
  Vascular 61
  see also Alzheimer's disease
Dementia with Lewy bodies (DLB) 219, 261–71
  consensus criteria 264–5
  differential diagnosis 6, 266
  falls 270
  investigations 267–70
  management 270
  prognosis 270–1
Demyelinating disorders 209, 277
Depression 6, 195–204
  assessment 197–8
  mimics of 198–9
  older vs younger patients 201–2
  rating scales 197–8
  risk factors 200–1
  treatment 202–4
Dermatitis herpetiformis 238
Diabetes mellitus
  CKD 225–34, 309
  hip fracture 479–88
  hyperglycaemic hyperosmolar state (HHS) 17–24
  hypoglycaemia 227–32
  treatment 227–30
    algorithm 228
    beta-blockers 230
Digoxin toxicity 39–43
  ECG 40
  treatment 43
Diphyllobothrium latum 244
Disc herniation 348
  see also spinal
Discitis, infective 293
Domestic abuse *see* abuse
Driving, advice 106, 450
Drug-induced disorders
  delirium 12, 13
  digoxin toxicity 39–43
  gastric lavage 43
  myopathies 300, 349
  nephritis 87

pruritus 359
Serotonin syndrome 373–80
SLE 85–8
Duodenal biopsy 235

E

Echocardiography 93, 94, 483
Elder abuse and neglect 27–36
Encephalopathies
  cause of epilepsy 327–8
  metabolic, toxic, and endocrine 277
Endocarditis *see* infective endocarditis
Endocrine and metabolic encephalopathies 277
  see also hypoglycaemia, renal
Epilepsy 219, 325–33, 451–7
  causes 327–9, 455
  differential diagnosis 327–9, 453–5
  investigations 331, 453–5
  new-onset 327–8
  partial seizures 330
Escherichia coli, multi-drug resistant extended-spectrum alpha-lactamase-producing 254, 256
Ethical issues
  abuse 27–36
  advanced directive 134, 138, 420, 425
  CPR 138–9
  dementia and PEG 475–6
  Deprivation of Liberty Safeguards (DOLS) 136
  mental capacity assessment 127–41
  neglect 32
Exercise, normal response 367

F

Faecal incontinence 335–44
Falls 477–88
  abuse 29
  alcohol excess 289–96
  atrial fibrillation 479
  cognitive impairment 60
  epilepsy 453, 454
  motor neurone disease 348–52
  postural hypotension 104–5, 168
  postural instability in NPH 61, 66
  pubic rami fractures 247–58
  serotonin syndrome 203
FDG-PET/CT 174, 266
Fever of unknown origin 169–78
  aetiology 173–4
  differential diagnosis 172–3
  malignancy-related 175–8
  types 171–2
Frailty syndromes
  defined 368
  Fried clinical phenotype 368–9
  see also delirium

Frontotemporal dementia (FTD) 349, 433–50
  depression in 443, 446
  investigations 444–7
  sub-types 446

G

Gait abnormality
  in DLB 266
  in NPH 59
Gastric lavage 43
Geriatric Depression Scale (GDS) 197
Giant cell arteritis 299, 397–405
  complications 401–2
  diagnostic criteria 400–1
  treatment 402–5
Glomerular filtration rate 305
Granulomatous lesions, hypercalcaemia 79, 112

H

Haemodialysis 83
Hakim-Adams triad, NPH 60–1
Hallucinations
  deafferentiation theory 221–2
  differential diagnosis 219–20
  in DLB 263
  migraine 220
  visual 219–20
Heart failure 153–68
  associated conditions 166–8
  classification by ejection fraction 155, 160–3, 164–6
  classification by NYHA 157
  co-morbidities 164
  defined 155
  investigations 157–9
  mimics 166
  with preserved ejection fraction 166
Heat stroke 489–96
  defined 492
  pathophysiology 494
  prognosis 495–6
  types 492
Helicobacter pylori infection 245
Hip fracture 8–9, 479–88
  rhabdomyolysis 482
HIV infection 315–22
HLA typing 237
'Hot cross bun sign' 413
  see also Multiple System Atrophy
'Hummingbird sign' 412
  see also Progressive Supranuclear Palsy
Hydralazine-induced nephritis 87
Hydrocephalus
  obstructive 210–12
  secondary 60, 331–2
  see also normal pressure hydrocephalus (NPH)

Hyperalbuminaemia 78
Hypercalcaemia 75–84
  complications 84
  investigations 79–80
  management 82–3
  presenting features 79
  rare causes 78
Hypercoagulable state 24
Hyperglycaemic hyperosmolar state (HHS) 17–24
  aetiology 20
  characteristic features 19
  osmotic diuresis 20
Hypernatraemia 24
Hyperparathyroidism 77–80, 120
Hyperproteinaemia 78
Hyperthyroidism 78
Hypocalcaemia 83, 237, 327, 453
Hypoglycaemia 225–32
  complications 231
  drug treatment 227–30
Hypokalaemia 241–5
  causes 244–5
  digitalis toxicity 41
Hypomagnesaemia, digitalis toxicity 41
Hyponatraemia 12
  secondary 486

I

Immobilization, hypercalcaemia 78–84
Immune disorders, cell-mediated 192
Immune function and ageing 191
Independent Mental Capacity Advocacy Service (IMCAS) 132–5
Infectious disorders, chest infection 77–9
Infective endocarditis 89–102
  aetiology 91–5
  clinical features 95–6
  Duke criteria 93–4
  older vs younger patients 95–6
  risk factors 95
Inflammatory disorders, non-infectious (NIID) 172
Insomnia 384
Intracranial pressure monitoring 63, 220, 330, 423, 496
Intravascular B-cell lymphoma (IVBCL) 277, 283–6
Intrinsic factor antibodies 192, 241, 245
Ischaemic stroke see stroke

K

Korsakoff's syndrome 296

L

Labyrinthitis 209, 210
Left ventricular diastolic function 162
Left ventricular failure 367

Leg ulcers 389–95
Leptomeningeal carcinomatosis 325–33
  investigations 331–2
  pathophysiology 329–30
  secondary hydrocephalus 31
  signs and symptoms 329–30
  treatment 333
Lower limb
  spasticity, NPH 61
  ulcers 389–95
Lumbar puncture, tap test in NPH 63
Lumbar spine wedge fractures 289–96, 346
Lung fibrosis 186, 187
Lymphoma, intravascular (IVBCL) 277, 283–6

M

Magnetic resonance imaging 62
Malignancy
  Fever of unknown origin 177–8
  Hypercalcaemia 77–8
  Leptomeningeal carcinomatosis 325–33
  Middle cerebral artery (MCA) infarction 214
  multiple malignant deposits 111–12
  neuroleptic malignant syndrome 375–6, 491
Malignant hyperthermia 376
Malnutrition 45–56
  defined 47
  nutritional risk screening tool 52
  prevalence 48, 49
  protein-energy malnutrition 47, 51, 56
Malnutrition Universal Screening Tool (MUST) 52–3
Mania 6
Mental Capacity Act 2005 126, 135
Mental capacity assessment 123–41
  Advance Directives 135, 138–41
  IMCAS 132–5
Metabolic encephalopathies 277
Middle cerebral artery (MCA) infarction 214
Migraine, hallucinations 220
Mini Nutritional Assessment (MNA) 54
Montreal Cognitive Assessment (MoCA) 8, 62, 263, 267, 337, 350, 407
Motor neurone disease 345–52
  investigations 350–1
  main subgroups 349
  mimics 349
  rehabilitation 351–2
Multiple system atrophy (MSA) 407–16
  differential diagnosis 409–10
  EMSA study 409
  forms 409–10
  treatment 415–16
Myasthenia gravis 349
Myopathies

drug-induced 300
MND 348

N

Natriuretic peptide (BNP, NT-proBNP, MR-proANP) 158–9
Neglect 27–36
Neurodegenerative syndromes 210
Neuroleptic malignant syndrome 376–7, 491
New York Heart Association (NYHA) classification 157
Non-infectious inflammatory disorders (NIID) 172
Normal pressure hydrocephalus (NPH) 59–66
  complications of treatment 65
  differential diagnosis 60–1, 62–3
  evidence for effectiveness of shunting 66
  pathogenesis 63–4
  results of intervention 66
  symptoms and physical findings 61
Normocytic anaemia 193
  systemic sclerosis 193
Nutritional risk screening tool (NRS) 52
Nutritional state 45–56
  assessment 52–4

O

Obstructive hydrocephalus 210–12
Obstructive sleep apnoea (OSA) 383, 384
Osteoarthritis 300
Osteoporosis 256–7, 481
  defined, WHO 487
  secondary prevention 487
Overactive bladder syndrome (OAB) 71
Overlap syndromes 183, 184

P

Paget's disease 78, 109–21
  alkaline phosphatase 112, 118
  bone deformities 119
  differential diagnosis 111–12, 116
  hypercalcaemia 119–20
  indications for treatment 118–21
  osteosarcoma 119
  prevalence and severity 117
Pain control 418–20
  adjuvant analgesics 423–4
  assessment 421–3
  back pain 291–2
  WHO analgesic ladder for cancer pain 423
Palliative care 417–27
  life expectancy 424–5
  mental capacity assessment 123–41
  older vs younger patients 425–7
  principles of management 421–2
Papilloedema 220

Parathyroid hormone
  contraindications 488
  levels 77–8, 80
Parkinsonian disorders
  Corticobasal degeneration 412
  Dementia 263, 266
  Dementia with Lewy bodies (DLB) 219, 261–71
  differential diagnosis 60
  MSA-C 410, 411, 413
  MSA-P 410–11
  Progressive supranuclear palsy (PSP) 411–12
  vascular 412
  Wilson's disease 413
Parkinson's disease 411, 414
PEP-CHF study 165
Peripheral neuropathy, differential diagnosis 60
Peritoneal dialysis 83
Pernicious anaemia 241, 243–4
Pick's disease 446
Plant toxins 43
Pneumonia, community-acquired 82–3
Pneumothorax
  older vs younger patients 462
  secondary to COPD, asthma 461
Poisoning, gastric lavage 43
Polyarthropathy 88
Polymyalgia rheumatica 299–301
Posterior fossa space-occupying lesions 209, 214
Postural hypotension 104–6, 168
Postural instability
  NPH 61
  test for 66
Pressure ulcers 143–51
  grading 145–7
  mechanical factors 149–50
Primary lateral sclerosis 349
Progressive bulbar palsy 349
Progressive supranuclear palsy (PSP) 411–12
Protein-energy malnutrition 47, 49–51
Pruritus 185, 355–63
  differential diagnosis 357–9
  drug-induced 357
  investigations and treatment 360–1, 362–3
  mechanisms 357
  uraemic 358
Pubic rami fractures 247–58
  prognostic indicators 250
'pull test' 66
Pulmonary embolism 461
Pulmonary fibrosis 183, 184, 187, 190
Pyoderma gangrenosum 392–3

R

Raynaud's phenomenon 183–7
  secondary 189

Rehabilitation 351–2
  Motor neurone disease 348–9
  Older vs younger patients 351–2
  Pubic rami fractures 258
Renal failure
  heat stroke induced 493
  immobilization and 83
  see also chronic kidney disease (CKD)
Renal impairment, chronic 166–7
Renal replacement therapy 311–12
Restless legs syndrome 384
Rhabdomyolysis 495
  acute renal failure 79, 472, 495
  calcium release 79
  patients with hip fracture 482
  serotonin syndrome 378

S

Sacral fractures 251
Sarcoidosis (calcitriol release) 79
Sarcopenia 47
Scabies 357–8
Scleroderma 183–5
Seizures see epilepsy
Self-neglect 50
Serotonin syndrome 373–80
  causes 377–8
  complications 378–9
  differential diagnosis 374–5
  falls 203
  Hunter Toxicity Criteria Decision Rules 379
  rhabdomyolysis 378
Shortness of breath (SoB) 459–71
Shunting, evidence for effectiveness in NPH 66
Skin disorders
  dermatitis herpetiformis 238
  differential diagnosis 317
  pressure ulcers 143–51
  pruritus 185, 355–63
  pyoderma gangrenosum 392–3
  rash in syphilis 317–19
  see also coeliac disease; systemic lupus erythematosus; systemic sclerosis
Sleep disorders 381–7
  associated disorders 383
  drug treatment 270
  hallucinations 217, 219
  investigations 385–6
  MSA 409–10, 414
  obstructive sleep apnoea (OSA) 384
  sleep apnoea syndromes 167
  treatment 386–7
Small bowel biopsy 236
Spinal cord compression, differential diagnosis 60
Spinal stenosis 348
Spine

disc herniation 348
infective discitis 293
vertebroplasty 293
wedge fractures 289–96, 346
Stroke
  acute 275
  cardioembolic 277
  cerebellar stroke 209–12
  cerebral MRI 93
  cognitive change vs time 5
  confusion associated with 273–86
  depression and 202
  differential diagnosis 273, 277
  with dysphagia 124
  faecal incontinence 335–44
  hypoglycaemia 231
  ischaemic stroke 214
  lacunar stroke 214
  misdiagnosis 283–4
  post-stroke dementia 14
  post-stroke epilepsy 327
  posterior fossa stroke 214
  postoperative anaemia 481
  risk
    atrial fibrillation 429–41
    CHADS score 431–2
  seizures in 327, 453
  visual hallucinations 219
  see also cerebellar infarct/stroke; heat stroke
Subdural haematoma 277
  in shunting 65
Suicide rates 199
Swallowing difficulties 124, 128, 473–8
Syncope
  aortic stenosis 367, 483
  causes 104–6
  differential diagnosis 104–5, 227, 327–8
  driving restrictions 106
  postprandial 103–6
  postural hypotension 105–6
  vs epilepsy 453
Synucleinopathies 410
Syphilis 315–22
Systemic lupus erythematosus (SLE) 172, 183, 309, 317
  drug-induced 85–8
Systemic sclerosis 181–93
  classification 183–4
  clinical features of subsets 186
  defined 185
  normocytic anaemia 193
  pathogenesis 185
  prognosis 190

T

TAVI 369–70
T-cell lymphoma 238, 239
Temporal arteritis 397–405
Thyroid disorders 210, 292, 300, 325, 483
  coeliac disease 239
Thyroid storm 491
Toxic encephalopathies, metabolic and endocrine 277
Toxins
  gastric lavage 43
  plants 43
  see also drug-induced disorders
Transcatheter aortic valve implantation (TAVI) 369–70

U

Urinary catheter, bladder stone 420–1
Urinary incontinence 69–74
  contributory causes 72–3
  diagnostic considerations 61
  frontotemporal dementia 349, 443–50
  management strategies 73–4
Urinary retention, causes 72
Urinary tract infection 256–8

V

Vascular dementia, differential diagnosis 61
Vasculitis
  cerebral 277, 285, 455
  systemic 191
Ventriculomegaly 62, 65
Ventriculoperitoneal shunt 64
Vertebral wedge fractures 289–96, 346
Vertebroplasty 293
Vitamin B12 deficiency 241–5
  causes 351
VitaminD
  deficiency 233, 237
  intoxication 78, 79

W

Wernicke's encephalopathy 210, 296
WHO analgesic ladder for cancer pain 423
Wilson's disease 413

X

Xerosis 362